About Pearson

Pearson is the world's learning company, with presence across 70 countries worldwide. Our unique insights and world-class expertise comes from a long history of working closely with renowned teachers, authors and thought leaders, as a result of which, we have emerged as the preferred choice for millions of teachers and learners across the world.

We believe learning opens up opportunities, creates fulfilling careers and hence better lives. We hence collaborate with the best of minds to deliver you class-leading products, spread across the Higher Education and K12 spectrum.

Superior learning experience and improved outcomes are at the heart of everything we do. This product is the result of one such effort.

Your feedback plays a critical role in the evolution of our products and you can contact us – reachus@pearson.com. We look forward to it.

Genetics for Nurses
Second Edition

V. Deepa Parvathi
Associate Professor
Department of Biomedical Sciences
Sri Ramachandra
Institute of Higher Education and Research(D.U.)
Chennai, Tamil Nadu

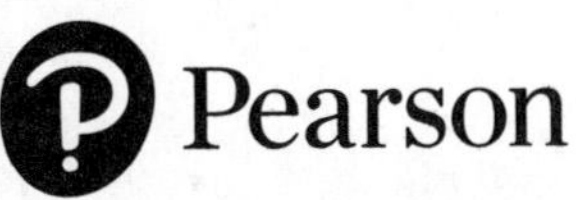

Pearson

Although the author and publisher have made every effort to ensure that the information in this book was correct at the time of editing and printing, the author and publisher do not assume and hereby disclaim any liability to any party for any loss or damage arising out of the use of this book caused by errors or omissions, whether such errors or omissions result from negligence, accident or any other cause. Further, names, pictures, images, characters, businesses, places, events and incidents are either the products of the author's imagination or used in a fictitious manner. Any resemblance to actual persons, living or dead or actual events is purely coincidental and do not intend to hurt sentiments of any individual, community, sect or religion.

In case of binding mistake, misprints or missing pages etc., the publisher's entire liability and your exclusive remedy is replacement of this book within reasonable time of purchase by similar edition/reprint of the book.

Senior Editor—Product: R. Dheepika
Senior Editor—Production: C. Purushothaman

ISBN 978-93-570-5325-9

First Impression

Published by Pearson India Education Services Pvt. Ltd, CIN: U72200TN2005PTC057128.

Head Office: 1st Floor, Berger Tower, Plot No. C-001A/2, Sector 16B, Noida - 201 301, Uttar Pradesh, India.
Registered Office: Featherlite, 'The Address' 5th Floor, Survey No 203/10B, 200 Ft MMRD Road, Zamin Pallavaram, Chennai – 600 044.
Website: in.pearson.com, Email: companysecretary.india@pearson.com

Compositor: MAP Systems, Bengaluru.
Printed in India at Sai Printo Pack Pvt Ltd

Dedicated to my beloved parents and enthusiastic students

Contents

3. Explain the Screening Methods for Genetic Defects and Diseases in Neonates and Children   124

4. Identify Genetic Disorders in Adolescents and Adults   139

Foreword

Interdisciplinary, application oriented Indian textbooks are the need of the 21st century in Indian higher education, especially in the area of medical sciences. There is also an imminent need for these textbooks to be updated by providing an international orientation of the chosen discipline for the students to whom the book is targeted.

Under this concept of textbook requirements, I am overwhelmed to record that the textbook titled **"Genetics for Nurses"** authored by **Dr. V. Deepa Parvathi** of the Department of Biomedical Sciences, Sri Ramachandra Institute of Higher Education and Research, has fully satisfied these requirements. With five units and 15 case studies, the author has oriented the book with learning objectives and learning outcomes in each chapter. Chapter objectives are clearly spelled out in the beginning and exhaustive review questions are provided at the end. Each chapter is profuse with photographic and diagrammatic illustrations. All chapters are structured as per the knowledge requirement of the student as well as the practicing nurse. Another appreciable feature of the book is the authors approach to the fundamentals of Genetics and her technique of developing it up to the requirement of a postgraduate student of the nursing profession.

Inclusion of case studies in the book is a novel approach devised to make the learner understand fully the clinical applications and relevance of genetic studies. A chapter on legal and ethical issues further adds to the academic value of the book.

I commend the quality of the book written by Dr. V. Deepa Parvathi, which has added credentials to Sri Ramachandra Institute of Higher Education and Research as well. While heartily congratulating Dr. V. Deepa Parvathi, I appeal to the nursing students and nursing professionals to be fully benefited by possessing a copy of this book for their day-to-day clinical applications.

Dr S. P. Thyagarajan

Former Chancellor, Avinashilingam Institute of Home Science and Higher Education for Women
(Former Dean(Research), Sri Ramachandra Institute of Higher Education and Research)
(Former Vice-Chancellor, University of Madras)

Preface

Genetics has emerged as a dominant force in biology, medicine, and research during the past century and its power and utility has accelerated in recent years. The dominance of genetics stems from its central importance in explaining the most basic mysteries of life and its unsurpassed methods of analysis that allow one to elucidate function and mechanisms in virtually every area of biology. Over the past few years, the field of genetics has advanced at a frenzied pace, with information and discoveries from all the genetic model systems participating together in a highly synergistic manner to explicate the mysteries of biology.

A good course in genetics has been formulated as a part of the nursing curricula. Genetics is a body of knowledge pertaining to genetic transmission, function, and mutation. The overall aim of *Genetics for Nurses*, is to provide a clear, comprehensive, rigorous, and balanced introduction to genetics at the college level. The rationale of the book is that the students must understand the basic processes of gene transmission, mutation, expression, and regulation; be able to comprehend clinical presentations and gain a sense of social context in which genetics has developed and is continuing to develop.

Each chapter has a list chapter objectives to provide the students an insight into chapter content. Also, the glossary of terms has been incorporated within each chapter to help students understand the biological terms during the course of study to enable them comprehend the content in a meaningful manner. At the end of each chapter is a complete set of review questions that help students assess themselves on the topic studied. Also, a set of ten simple case studies has been presented to help the students to identify genetic disorders, appreciate the importance of genetic counseling and understand the various genetic tests available in a clinical scenario. This would be particularly useful to students of medicine and nursing who have the opportunity to interact with patients during clinical postings and while making clinical case presentations.

The content of this book has been framed based on the curriculum designed by the Nursing Council of India. The topics have been grouped into five units in such a way that the book takes the students from classical genetics through clinical genetics and diagnosis to the latest advances in genetics adding emphasis to social and ethical issues. This helps students learn fundamental concepts in genetics, analyze and explore the different possibilities and motivate students to pursue higher education in this exciting field.

In recent decades, there has been an explosive growth in the amount of genetic knowledge acquired through systematic research. Many of the new discoveries have personal and social relevance through applications of genetics to human affairs in prenatal diagnosis, testing for carriers, and identification of genetic risk factors for complex traits, such as breast cancer and heart disease. There are also ethical controversies in gene therapy, gene manipulation, eugenics, prenatal diagnosis, artificial reproductive techniques, stem cell genetics etc. Inspired by the possibility of research and excellence, many of today's students take up the study of genetics with great enthusiasm. The challenges for the teacher are to sustain this enthusiasm by stimulating a desire to understand the principles of genetics in a comprehensive and meticulous way, and to make the students realize that genetics is not only a set of principles but also an experimental approach to solve a wide range of biological problems. He has to encourage students to think about genetic problems and about the wider social and ethical issues arising from genetics. While addressing these challenges, the author has also tried to show the magnificence, logical clarity, and integrity of the subject. Endlessly fascinating, genetics is the material basis of the continuity of life.

Many of the ideas presented in the book have been sharpened by my frequent discussions with my father, Mr. V. Venkatachalam and Ms. Dheepika R (Pearson Education). I thank them for their inputs. I also thank Prof. S. P. Thyagarajan, Former Dean(Research), Sri Ramachandra Institute of Higher Education and Research and Dr S. Rangaswami, Former Vice-Chancellor, Sri Ramachandra Institute of Higher Education and Research for their critical evaluation and comments.

ACKNOWLEDGEMENTS

I wish to express my sincere thanks and gratitude to all those who inspired me and helped me complete my work with their constant motivation and encouragement.

My sincere gratitude to Shri V. R. Venkataachalam, Chancellor, Sri Ramachandra Institute of Higher Education and Research and Mr. R.V. Sengutuvan, Pro – Chancellor, Sri Ramachandra Institute of Higher Education and Research for their constant support and motivation.

I am grateful to my beloved teachers Ms. Padmini Iyer, Dr Sankariah and Mr. R. Balabhaskar, who stirred in me my passion for biological sciences, teaching and research.

I thank my mentors, Dr M. Ravi and Dr K Rajagopal, for their dynamism and constant encouragement to my academic and research accomplishments.

I am obliged to my aunts, Mrs. Alamelu Srinivasan and Mrs. Sunanda D Rao for their constant motivation and encouragement to all my endeavors.

I am indebted to my friends R. Sumitha, Ramya Raveendran and Smitha Srinivas for all their help and support throughout my work.

My students Jennifer Sally Samson, Vaishali K, Anjani Pranitha Reddy have been very helpful with their inputs.

Dheepika R., of Pearson Education, deserves a special mention for her critical evaluation of the chapters, meticulous planning and execution towards completion of this project cheerfully. Her unbelievable patience and endurance is greatly appreciated.

I thank the publisher and Mr. C. Purushothaman and his entire production team for their valuable inputs and excellent publishing standards which were of immense help for this book to materialise.

I express my heartfelt thanks to my father-in-law, my husband and my brother for their unconditional love, undaunted support and prayers for all my accomplishments. I thank my dear son, Ishaan, for flashing his dimples.

V. Deepa Parvathi

About the Author

Dr. V. Deepa Parvathi, is a gold medallist from Sri Ramachandra Medical College and Research Institute (Deemed University) for Masters in Human Genetics and completed her doctoral studies on Nanodosimetry in the fly model. With a passion to teaching and student affairs, she has been an academician since 2006, contributing to innovative teaching methods for undergraduate and postgraduates across various disciplines of the university. She has imparted knowledge and trained students in scientific writing and encouraged undergraduate and post graduate students to publication. She is the proud recipient of Teaching Excellence Award 2020 from Sri Ramachandra Institute of Higher Education and Research (Deemed to be university).

Her areas of research interest and expertise include Cancer Biology, Human Genetics, Nutrigenomics and Nanogenotoxicology involving nanodosimetry on animal models including Drosophila and Zebra Fish. She is currently supervising 4 Ph.D. candidates and guided 1 M.Phil., 28 M.Sc. and 17 undergraduate research projects apart from consultancy based research work. She has completed extra and intra mural research grants has to her credit over 60 publications in journals of national and international repute. She has also authored three full length textbooks and three monographs published by renowned publishers. Her clinical focus to the diagnostic division of Department of Human Genetics included handling Prenatal diagnosis, Cancer cytogenetics and FISH cases. She is currently an Associate Professor at the Department of Biomedical Sciences, Sri Ramachandra Institute of Higher Education and Research (Deemed to be university), Chennai, India.

(deepakoushik305@gmail.com)

1   Nature, Principles and Perspectives of Heredity

INTRODUCTION

The need for education of nurses in genetics was ... ago. Genetic services and education have been ... health professionals including nurses. Efforts ... of nursing faculty who are well prepared in genetics substantially improve the capability of nurses to ... delivery of genetic services.

Scientific knowledge in human genetics has ... recent decades. The application of this knowledge ... viduals and families affected by or at a risk ...

Explain Nature, Principles and Perspectives of Heredity

1

INTRODUCTION

The need for education of nurses in genetics was expressed more than 25 years ago. Genetic services and education have been made available in the curricula of health professionals including nurses. Efforts have been made to develop a team of nursing faculty who are well prepared in genetics. These efforts are expected to substantially improve the capability of nurses to contribute more effectively in the delivery of genetic services.

Scientific knowledge in human genetics has expanded at a remarkable rate in recent decades. The application of this knowledge in the clinical situation to individuals and families affected by or at a risk for genetic disorders has rapidly followed. Genetic service programs are well established in all university medical centers throughout the world. As scientific and technological capabilities to identify individuals and families at risk for genetic disease continues to increase, the capacity of the health care system to inform them about the appropriate application of genetic tests will be severely inadequate unless healthcare professionals are better educated about human genetics and its clinical applications.

Previously, contributors to the Human Genetics education section have emphasized the importance of the content of genetics in medical school curricula and master's level programs in Clinical Genetics and Genetic Counselling. However, although the importance of genetic content in nursing education has been understood, the curriculum content in genetics (for nursing students) is generally inadequate today at all levels. This inadequacy is reflected when practicing nurses are queried about genetic disorders. To bridge this gap, continuing education programs have been developed to meet the needs of practicing nurses for knowledge about genetics and genetic services.

CAREER FOCUS

Opportunities for clinical experience in genetics vary widely among programs. However, all nursing students encounter patients affected by or at risk of genetic disorders during their clinical training. This is especially true in pediatrics, where at least 25% of inpatients have a disorder with a genetic component. However, in prenatal clinics rotation, students also see pregnant women at the risk of having an infant with a genetic disorder. Educating the nursing team on clinical genetics helps them identify, analyse, and understand the genetic disorder better.

In addition, there is greater flexibility for students at the graduate level to choose elective courses related to their nursing career goals but offered outside the school of nursing (in most international universities). This helps them to go on to doctoral studies in nursing, human genetics, or related fields, where they can apply the working knowledge of genetics with formal course work. Nurses specializing in maternal/child nursing can focus on genetics within their graduate nursing curriculum, which would help them take up the genetic-counselling examination given by the American Board of Medical Genetics.

INTRODUCTION TO PROKARYOTIC AND EUKARYOTIC CELL

There are two basic types of cells: prokaryotic and eukaryotic. "Karyose" comes from a Greek word, which means "kernel," as in a kernel of grain. In biology, we use this root word to refer to the nucleus of a cell. "Pro" means "before," and "eu" means "true," or "good." Therefore, "Prokaryotic" means "before a nucleus," and "eukaryotic" means "possessing a true nucleus." Prokaryotic cells have no nuclei, while eukaryotic cells do have true nuclei. Despite their apparent differences, these two cell types have a lot in common. They perform most of the same kinds of functions, and in the same ways. Both are enclosed by plasma membranes, filled with cytoplasm, and loaded with small structures called ribosomes. Both have DNA that carries the archived instructions for operating the cell. In addition, the similarities go far beyond the visible—physiologically they are very similar in many ways. For example,

Prokaryotic cell
A cell lacking a true membrane-bound nucleus, for example, Bacteria.

Eukaryotic cell
A cell with a true nucleus bound by a double membrane.

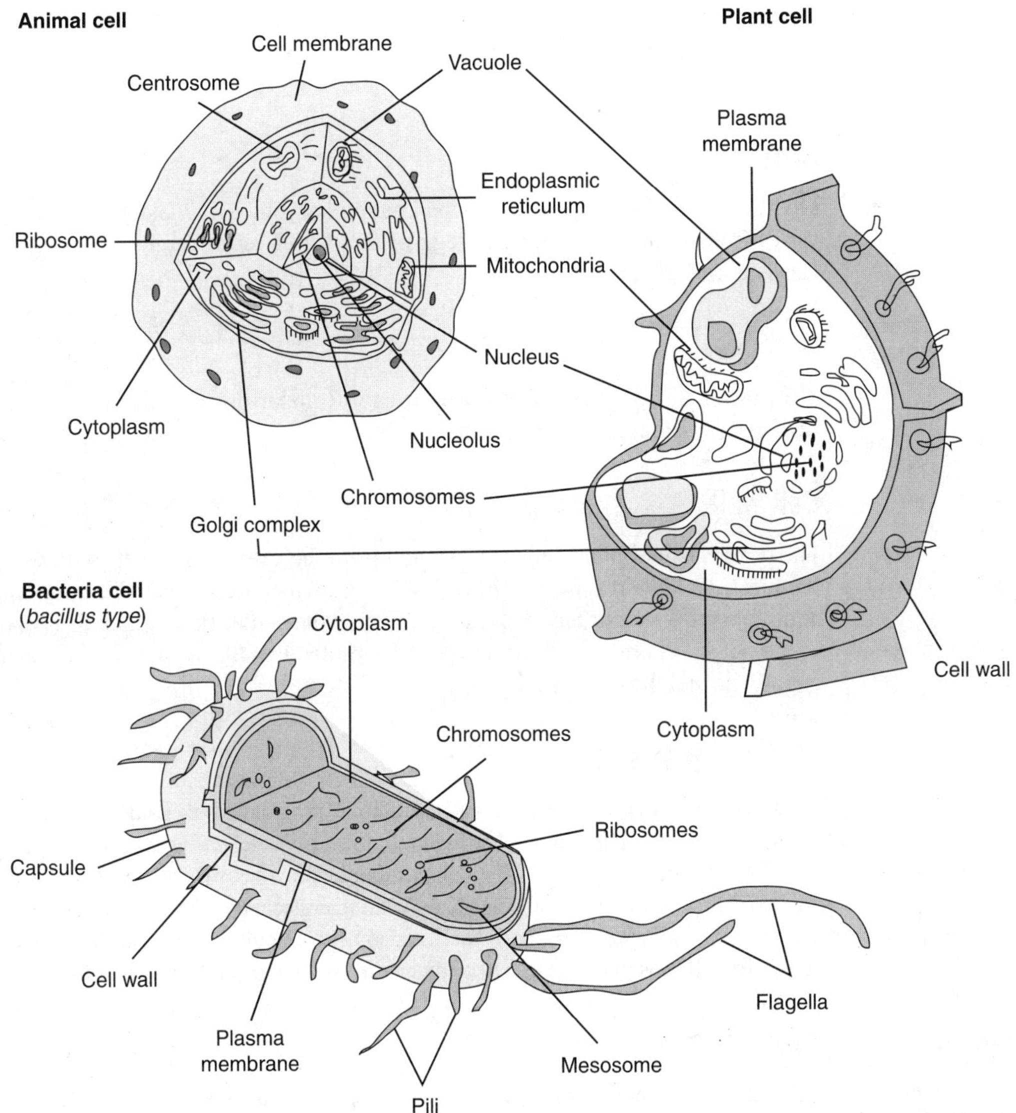

Figure 1.1 Prokaryotic and eukaryotic cells. (See page 221 for the colour image.)

the DNA in the two cell types is of precisely the same kind, and the genetic code for a prokaryotic cell is exactly the same as that used in eukaryotic cells.

Figure 1.1 illustrates the differences between a prokaryotic and a eukaryotic cell.

Shape

Eukaryotic cells are of various shapes. For example, plant cells are elongated and are almost rectangular in shape, whereas animal cells are spherical. The shape of the cell varies from organ to organ and from species to species. The shape of the cell is also correlated with its function. For example, the epithelial cells are flat and muscle cells are elongated.

Size

Mostly, eukaryotic cells are larger than the prokaryotic cells. The size of the cell varies from 1 μm to 175 mm. The egg of the ostrich is the largest cell having a diameter of 175 mm.

Number

Most of the eukaryotic cells are seen in multicellular organisms and thus many such cells exist unlike the unicellular organisms.

Cell wall

The protoplasm of plant cells is separated from the exterior by a cell wall, which is entirely lacking in animals. The cell wall is a semi-rigid, laminated, external and non-living covering of the cell. It is secreted by the cell itself and mainly consists of the polysaccharide, cellulose. It provides protection and support to the plasma membrane and the cytoplasm.

Plasma membrane

Most plant and animal cells have an external covering called plasmalemma, plasma membrane, or cell membrane. It is a living ultra-thin, elastic, porous, and semi-permeable membranous covering of the cell. It mainly provides mechanical support and form to the protoplasm. It also helps in preventing unnecessary substances from entering the cells. Since it is semi-permeable it also helps in transferring nutrients into and out of the cell. It is made up of a lipid bilayer in which many proteins are embedded.

Cytoplasm

The plasma membrane is followed by the cytoplasmic matrix. This usually fills the space between the nucleus and the plasmalemma. It is an amorphous, translucent, and homogenous colloidal liquid containing various organic and inorganic components. The cytoplasm contains many inclusions called granules that help in the storage of food and secreted substances (secretory granules and starch granules). The cytoplasm also contains many organelles that make the eukaryotic cell structurally more complex than a prokaryotic cell. Some of the organelles are as follows:

Endoplasmic reticulum (ER): The cytoplasm is traversed by a vast network of interconnecting tubules and vesicles known as the ER. It helps in the transport of various substances inside the cell and forms a link between the nucleus and the plasma membrane. Some ER have ribosomes attached to their surface and they are known as rough ER (RER).

Plasma membrane
Semi-permeable membrane enclosing the cytoplasm of a cell.

Cytoplasm
The cell substance between the cell membrane and the nucleus. It contains cytosol, organelles, cytoskeleton, and other particles.

Endoplasmic reticulum (ER)
A network of tubular membranes within the cytoplasm of a cell involved in the transport of materials. It occurs either as smooth ER (smooth surface) or rough ER (with ribosomes).

Golgi complex: This is a stack of flattened membrane-bound parallely arranged organelles also known as golgi apparatus. Each complex is composed of many lamellae, tubules, vesicles, and vacuoles. The function of the golgi complex is the storage of proteins and enzymes. It also secretes many granules and lysosomes. In plants the golgi complex is called dictyosome.

Lysosomes: These originate from the golgi complex and their function is digestion of food material by phagocytosis or pinocytosis. They are membrane-bound structures and have hydrolytic digestive enzymes.

Ribosomes: These originate in the nucleolus and consist mainly of RNA and proteins. Each ribosome has a smaller 40 s subunit and a larger 60 s subunit. Ribosomes are also found attached to the ER. The main function of ribosomes is protein synthesis.

Mitochondria: It is also called the power house of the cell. These are sausage-shaped structures bound by two membranes. The inner membrane forms folds called cristae. The main functions of mitochondria are respiration, oxidation of food, release of energy, and metabolism of energy.

Plastids: These are found in plant cells and they can be colourless (leucoplasts) or coloured (chromoplasts). Leucoplasts help in storage while chromoplasts provide colour to the various parts of the plant.

Nucleus: This is also called the heart of the cell and is a well-defined mass in the eukaryotic cell. It is surrounded by a double membrane and houses the hereditary machinery of the cell.

Nucleus

It was discovered by Robert Brown in 1831. It is here that almost the cell's entire DNA is confined, replicated, and transcribed. The nucleus thus controls different metabolic and hereditary activities of the cell.

Occurrence and position: The nucleus is found in all eukaryotic cells of plants and animals. However, some eukaryotic cells such as the lens of the eye and mammalian red blood cells (RBCs) do not contain a nucleus. Prokaryotic cells of bacteria do not have a true nucleus. Usually the nucleus remains located in the centre. However, its position can change from time to time according to the metabolism of the cell.

Example: In glandular cells, the nucleus is located in the basal portion of the cell.

Morphology: Refer Figure 1.2.

Number: Usually cells contain a single nucleus, but the number of nuclei can vary from cell to cell. According to the number of nuclei, they can be classified as mononucleate cells (most animal cells), binucleate cells, and polynucleate cells.

Shape: The shape of the nucleus is normally related to the shape of the cell. They can be spheroid, ellipsoid, or discoidal in shape.

Size: The size of the nucleus is directly proportional to that of the cytoplasm and thus varies from cell to cell.

Golgi complex
A membranous complex of vesicles, vacuoles, and flattened sacs in the cytoplasm, which is involved in intracellular secretion and transport.

Lysosome
A cell organelle containing enzymes that digest particles and also disintegrate the cell after its death.

Ribosome
An organelle that functions as the site of protein synthesis. They occur freely in small clusters or attached to the outer surface of the endoplasmic reticulum.

Mitochondria
An organelle that is responsible for energy production.

Nucleus
A specialized mass of protoplasm enclosed by a double membrane, involved in the growth, metabolism, reproduction, and transmission of genetic factors.

Euchromatin
Part of a chromosome that condenses maximally during metaphase and contains most of the genetically active material.

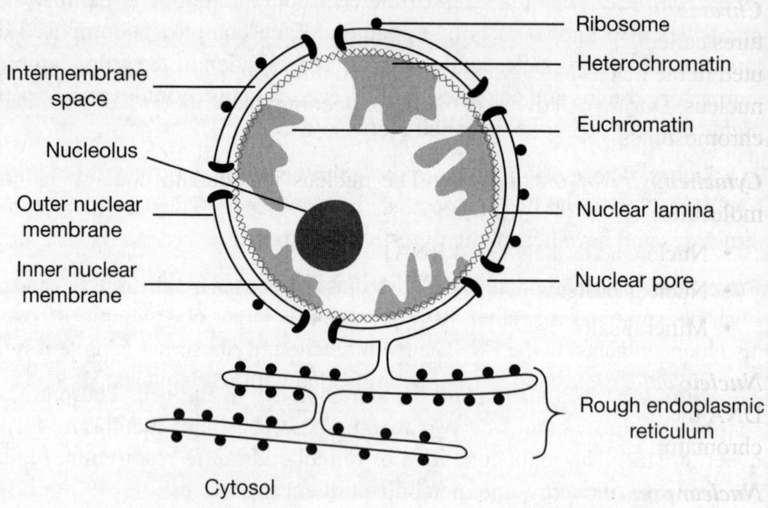

Figure 1.2 Nucleus. (See page 222 for the colour image.)

Heterochromatin
The dense highly stainable part of a chromosome.

Ultrastructure: The nucleus is composed of the following structures:

- The nuclear membrane
- The nucleolus
- The nucleoplasm
- The chromatin fibres

Nuclear membrane: It forms the nuclear envelope covering the nucleus. It is composed of two unit membranes, an outer membrane and an inner membrane, separated by a space of 100–150Å. The outer membrane is often rough because it is attached to the RER.

Nuclear pores: The nuclear membrane is broken at several places by nuclear openings or pores, but around the margin of these pores the membranes are continuous. The pores are around 600Å in diameter. The number of pores for a particular nucleus is variable and often depends on the species and type of the cell. The nuclear pores are surrounded by circular structures called annuli. The pores and the annuli are together called the pore complex.

Nucleolus
A rounded body within the nucleus of a cell.

Nucleolus: The nucleus contains a large, eccentrically situated spherical and acidophilic-dense granule called nucleolus. It was first described by Fontana in 1781. The size of the nucleolus is related to the synthetic activity of the cell; cells with higher activity have larger nucleoli. They contain 3–5% RNA and large amounts of proteins and enzymes.

Nucleoplasm: The space between the nuclear envelope and the nucleolus is filled by a transparent, semi-solid, granular, and slightly acidophilic ground substance that forms the matrix and is called the nuclear sap or nucleoplasm. Nuclear components such as chromatin fibres and the nucleolus are embedded in the nucleoplasm.

Chromatin fibres: The nucleoplasm contains many thread-like and coiled structures called chromatin. The fibres of chromatin are twisted and uniformly distributed in the nucleoplasm. These fibres can only be observed only in the interphase nucleus. During cell division the fibres become thick ribbon-like structures called chromosomes.

Cytochemistry of the nucleus: The nucleus is found to contain the following molecules:

- Nucleic acids (DNA and RNA)
- Nuclear proteins
- Mineral salts

Nucleic acids: These often remain embedded within the nuclear proteins. Besides DNA the nucleus also has RNA. The nuclear RNA is distributed in the nucleolus, chromatin, and nuclear sap.

Nuclear proteins: This part is very complex and the most commonly occurring one is the histones. They are basic in nature because of their amino acid composition. In eukaryotic nuclei there are five principal histones, namely H1, H2a, H2b, H3, and H4.

Nuclear enzymes: There are many enzymes, the most important of which are those involved in DNA replication and repair like DNA polymerase and RNA polymerase.

Mineral salts: Nuclei contain large amounts of cofactors, precursor molecules, and minerals. NAD and ATP are the most commonly found ones. Nuclei contain no lipid content.

CELL DIVISION

The ability to grow and reproduce is a fundamental property of living organisms. Cell growth is accomplished through the synthesis of new molecules of proteins,

Chromatin
Forms the chromosome during cell division. It consists of DNA, RNA, and various proteins.

Nucleic acid
A group of long, linear macromolecules that carry the genetic information directing all cellular functions. They can either be DNA or RNA.

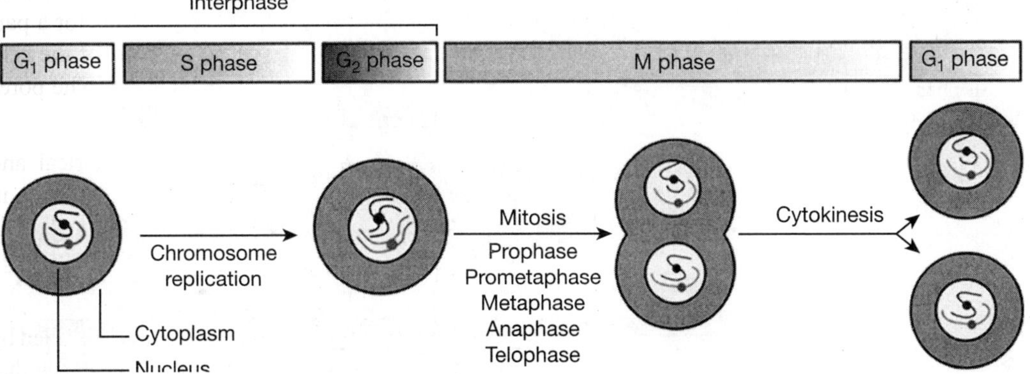

Figure 1.3 The cell division cycle. (See page 222 for the colour image.)

nucleic acids, carbohydrates, and lipids. As the accumulation of these molecules causes the volume of a cell to increase, the plasma membrane expands to prevent the cell from bursting. However, cells cannot continue to enlarge indefinitely; as a cell grows larger, there is an accompanying decrease in its surface area/volume ratio and hence in its capacity for effective exchange with the environment. For this reason, cell growth must be accompanied by **cell division** (Figure 1.3), where one cell gives rise to two new daughter cells.

When cells grow and divide, the newly formed daughter cells are usually genetic duplicates of the parent cell, containing the same DNA sequences. Therefore, all the genetic information in the nucleus of the parent cell must be duplicated and carefully distributed to the daughter cells during the division process. In accomplishing this task a cell passes through a series of discrete stages, collectively known as the **cell cycle**.

AN OVERVIEW OF THE CELL CYCLE

The **cell cycle** (Figure 1.4) begins when two new cells are formed by the division of a single parental cell and ends when one of these cells divides again into two cells. This division process, called the **M phase**, involves two overlapping events in which the nucleus divides first and the cytoplasm second. Nuclear division is called **mitosis**, and the division of the cytoplasm to produce two daughter cells is termed **cytokinesis**.

Cell cycle
The cycle of growth and reproduction of a cell. It consists of interphase M phase (5 stages), namely interphase, prophase, metaphase, anaphase, and telophase.

Mitosis
A process of cell division, which results in the production of two daughter cells from a single parent cell.

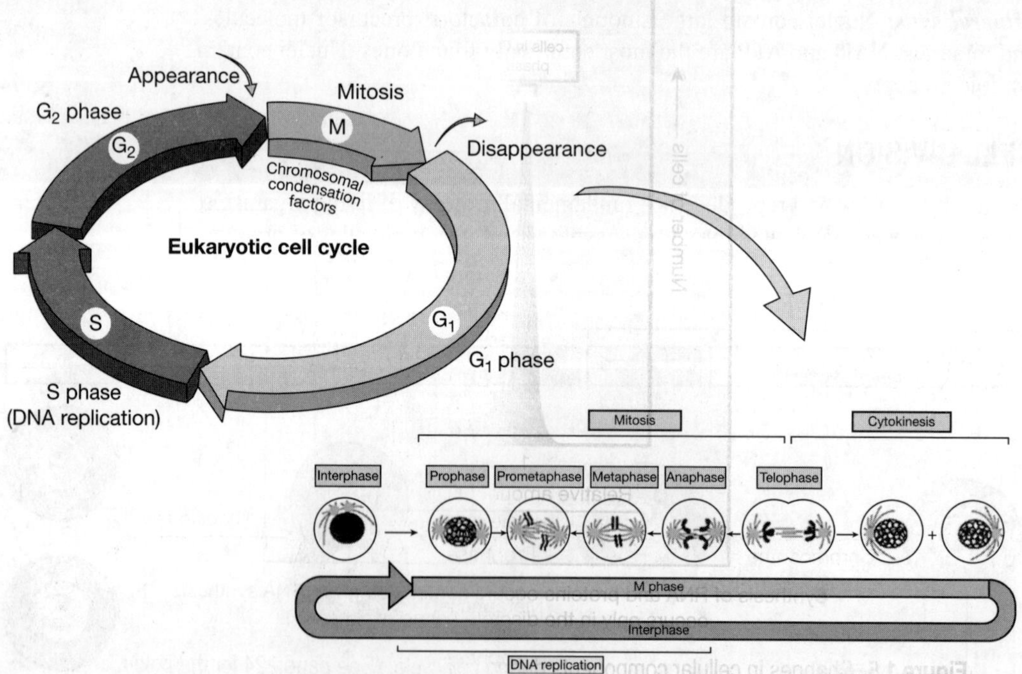

Figure 1.4 The eukaryotic cell cycle. (See page 223 for the colour image.)

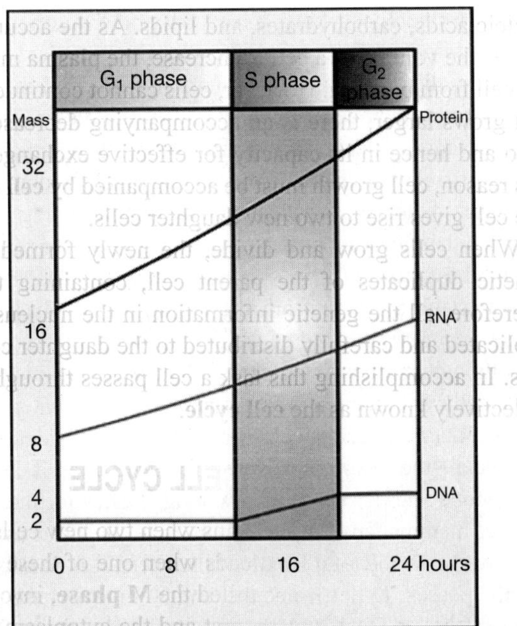

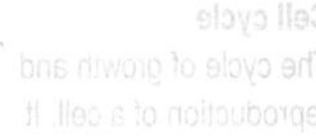

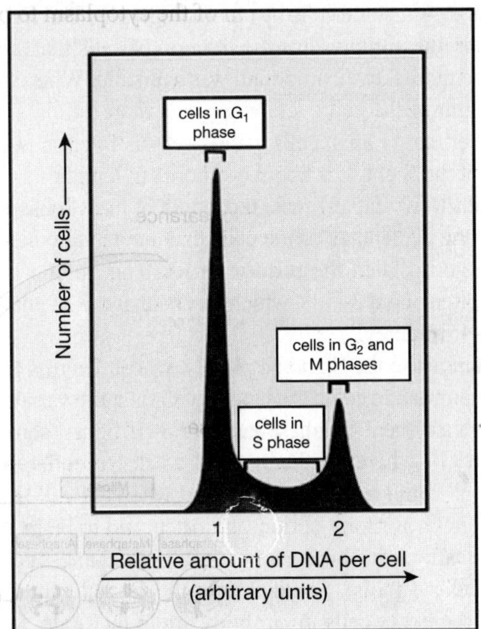

Synthesis of RNA and proteins occurs continuously, but DNA synthesis occurs only in the discrete period of S phase.

Figure 1.5 Changes in cellular components during cell cycle. (See page 224 for the colour image.)

Interphase
The preparatory phase
of cell cycle during
which the nucleus is not
undergoing division.

While visually striking, the events of the mitotic phase account for a relatively small portion of the total cell cycle. For a typical mammalian cell, the mitotic phase usually lasts less than an hour. Cells spend the majority of their time in the growth phase between divisions called **interphase**. Most cellular contents are synthesized continuously during interphase, so cell mass gradually increases as the cell approaches division. The amount of DNA doubles during interphase rather than the M phase. Subsequent experiments using radioactive DNA precursors revealed that DNA is synthesized during a defined period of interphase, which was named the **S phase** (S for synthesis) (Figure 1.5). A time gap called the G_1 **phase** separates the S phase from the preceding M phase, and a second gap, the G_2 **phase**, separates the end of the S phase from the beginning of the next M phase.

Although the cells of a multicellular organism divide at varying rates, most studies of the cell cycle involve cells growing in culture where the length of the cycle tends to be similar for different cell types. One can easily determine the overall length of the cell cycle—the *generation time*—for cultured cells by counting the cells under a microscope and determining how long it takes for the cell population to double. In cultured mammalian cells, for example, the total cycle usually takes about 18–24 hours. Once we know the total length of the cycle, it is possible to determine the length of specific phases. To determine the length of the S phase, we can expose cells to radioactively labelled DNA precursors (usually ^{3}H—thymidine) for a short period of time and then examine the cells by autoradiography. The fraction of cells with silver grains over their nuclei represents the fraction of cells that were somewhere in the S phase when the radioactive compound was available. When we multiply this fraction by the total length of the cell cycle, the result is an estimate of the average length of the S phase. For mammalian cells in culture, this fraction is often around 0.33, which indicates that the S phase is about 6–8 hours in length.

Similarly, we can estimate the length of the M phase by multiplying the generation time by the percentage of the cells that are actually in mitosis at any given time. This percentage is called the **mitotic index**. The mitotic index for cultured mammalian cells is often about 3–5%, which means that the M phase lasts less than an hour (usually 30–45 minutes).

In contrast to the S and M phases, whose lengths tend to be quite similar for different mammalian cells, the length of G_1 is quite variable, depending on the cell type. Although a typical G_1 phase lasts for 8–10 hours, some cells spend only minutes or hours in G_1, whereas others spend weeks, months, or years. During G_1, a major "decision" is made as to whether and when the cell is to divide again. Cells that are arrested in G_1 for long periods are often said to be in a G_0 **state** (where they remain metabolically active but no longer proliferate unless called on to do so by appropriate extracellular signals). Some cells in the G_0 state are destined never to divide again; most of the nerve cells in our body are in this state. In some cells, a similar kind of arrest also occurs in G_2. In general, however, G_2 is shorter than G_1 and is more uniform in duration among different cell types, usually lasting 4–6 hours.

For a typically rapidly dividing human cell, with a total cycle time of 24 hours, the G_1 phase might last about 11 hours, the S phase about 8 hours, the G_2 about 4 hours and the M phase about 1 hour (Figure 1.6).

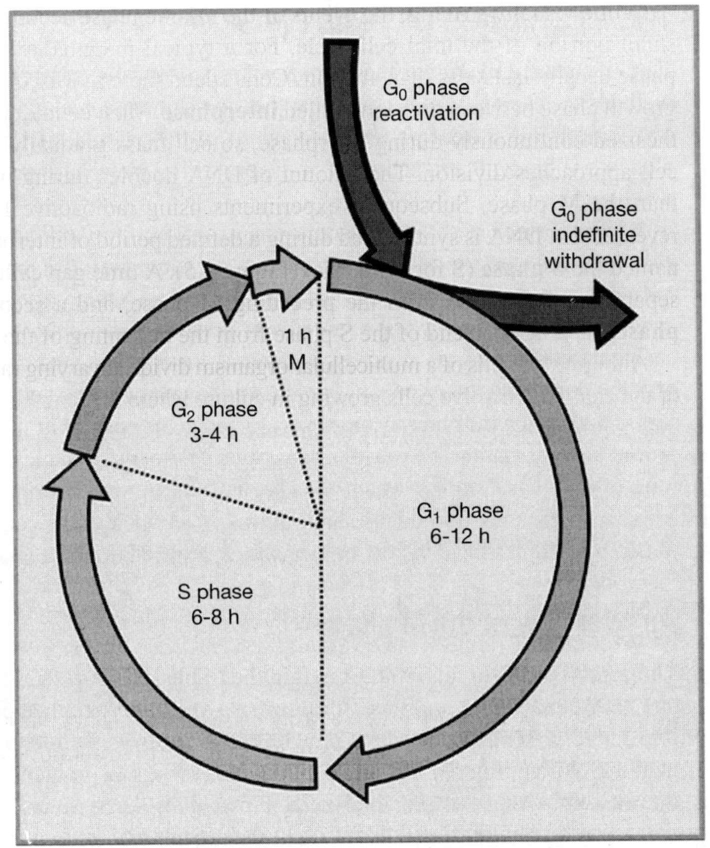

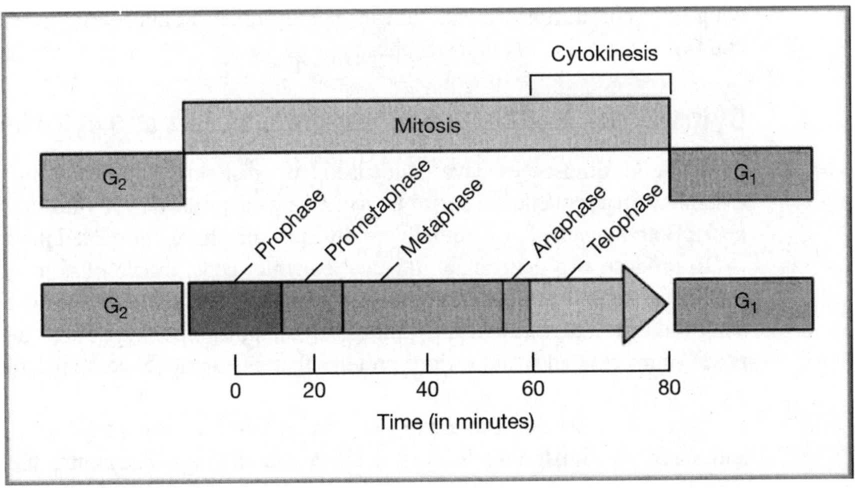

Figure 1.6 Duration of the cell cycle. (See page 225 for the colour image.)

THE MECHANICS OF CELL DIVISION

The mechanical events of the M phase (or cell division phase) of the cell cycle includes the various stages of nuclear division (mitosis), and cytoplasmic division (cytokinesis). In a brief period the contents of the parental cell, which were doubled by the biosynthetic activities of the preceding interphase, are segregated into two daughter cells.

Mitosis begins with chromosome condensation: the duplicated DNA strands, packaged into elongated chromosomes, condense into the much more compact chromosomes required for their segregation. The nuclear lamina dissociates into lamin subunits. The nuclear envelope then breaks down, and the replicated chromosomes, each consisting of a pair of *sister chromatids*, become attached to the microtubules of the *mitotic spindle*. As mitosis proceeds, the cell pauses briefly in a state called *metaphase*, when the chromosomes are aligned at the equator of the mitotic spindle, poised for segregation. The sudden separation of sister chromatids marks the beginning of *anaphase*, during which the chromosomes move to opposite poles of the spindle, where they decondense and reform intact nuclei. The cell is then pinched in two by cytoplasmic division, or *cytokinesis*, and cell division is complete.

An overview of the M phase

The central problem for a mitotic cell in the M phase is how to accurately separate and distribute (*segregate*) its chromosomes, which were replicated in the preceding S phase, so that each new daughter cell receives an identical copy of the genome. With minor variations, all eukaryotes solve this problem in a similar way: they assemble specialized cytoskeletal machines—first to pull the duplicated chromosome sets apart and then to split the cytoplasm into two halves. Before the duplicated chromosomes can be separated and distributed equally to the two daughter cells during mitosis, however, they must be appropriately configured, and this process begins in the S phase.

Cytoskeletal machines perform both mitosis and cytokinesis

After the chromosomes have condensed, two distinct cytoskeletal machines are assembled in a sequence to perform the mechanical processes of mitosis and cytokinesis. Both machines disassemble rapidly after they have completed their tasks.

To produce two genetically identical daughter cells, the cell has to separate its replicated chromosomes and allocate one copy to each daughter cell. In all eukaryotic cells, this task is performed during mitosis by a bipolar *mitotic spindle*, which is composed of microtubules and various proteins that interact with them, including *microtubule-dependent motor proteins*.

Different cytoskeletal structures are responsible for cytokinesis. In animal cells and many unicellular eukaryotes, it is the *contractile ring*. The contractile ring contains both actin and myosin filaments and is formed around the equator of the cell, just under the plasma membrane; as the ring contracts, it pulls the membrane inward, thereby dividing the cell into two.

Two mechanisms help ensure that mitosis always precedes cytokinesis

In most animal cells, the M phase takes only about an hour—a small fraction of the total cell-cycle time, which often lasts from 12 to 24 hours. The rest of the cycle is occupied by **interphase**. Under the microscope, interphase appears as a deceptively uneventful interlude, in which the cell simply continues to grow in size. Other techniques, however, reveal that interphase is actually a busy time for a proliferating cell, during which elaborate preparations for cell division are occurring in a tightly ordered sequence. Two critical preparatory events that are completed during interphase are DNA replication and duplication of the *centrosome*.

Cyclical oscillations in the activities of the cyclin-dependent kinases (CDKs) and of proteolytic complexes drive the cell cycle forward. CDKs trigger various steps of the cycle either by directly phosphorylating structural or regulatory proteins or by activating other protein kinases to do so. The proteolytic complexes activate specific steps in the cycle by degrading key cell-cycle proteins such as cyclins and CDK inhibitor proteins. The activation of CDKs and proteolytic complexes triggers cell-cycle transitions that are normally points of no return. Thus, a signal from M-CDK to enter the M phase results in chromosome condensation, nuclear envelope breakdown, and a dramatic change in microtubule dynamics, all triggered by the phosphorylation of regulatory proteins that control these processes.

It is crucial that the two major events of the M phase—nuclear division (mitosis) and cytoplasmic division (cytokinesis)—occur in the correct sequence. It would be catastrophic if cytokinesis occurred before all of the chromosomes had segregated during mitosis. At least two mechanisms seem to prevent this catastrophe. First, the cell-cycle control system that activates proteins required for mitosis is thought to inactivate some of the proteins required for cytokinesis; presumably for this reason, cytokinesis cannot occur until M-CDK is inactivated at the end of mitosis. Second, after the mitotic spindle has segregated the two sets of chromosomes to opposite poles of the cell, the residual central region of the spindle is required to maintain a functional contractile ring. Thus, until the spindle has separated the chromosomes and formed a *central spindle*, the ring cannot divide the cytoplasm in two.

Centrosome
A small region near the nucleus in the cytoplasm of a cell containing centrioles.

MITOSIS IN DETAIL

The first five stages of the M phase constitute **mitosis**, which was originally defined as the period in which the chromosomes are visibly condensed. **Cytokinesis** occurs in the sixth stage, which overlaps with the end of mitosis. These six stages form a dynamic sequence, in which many independent cycles, involving the chromosomes, cytoskeleton, and centrosomes, have to be coordinated in order to produce two genetically identical daughter cells.

The five stages of mitosis—*prophase, prometaphase, metaphase, anaphase,* and *telophase*—occur in strict sequential order, while cytokinesis begins in anaphase and continues through telophase (Figure 1.7). During prophase, the replicated chromosomes condense in step with the reorganization of the cytoskeleton.

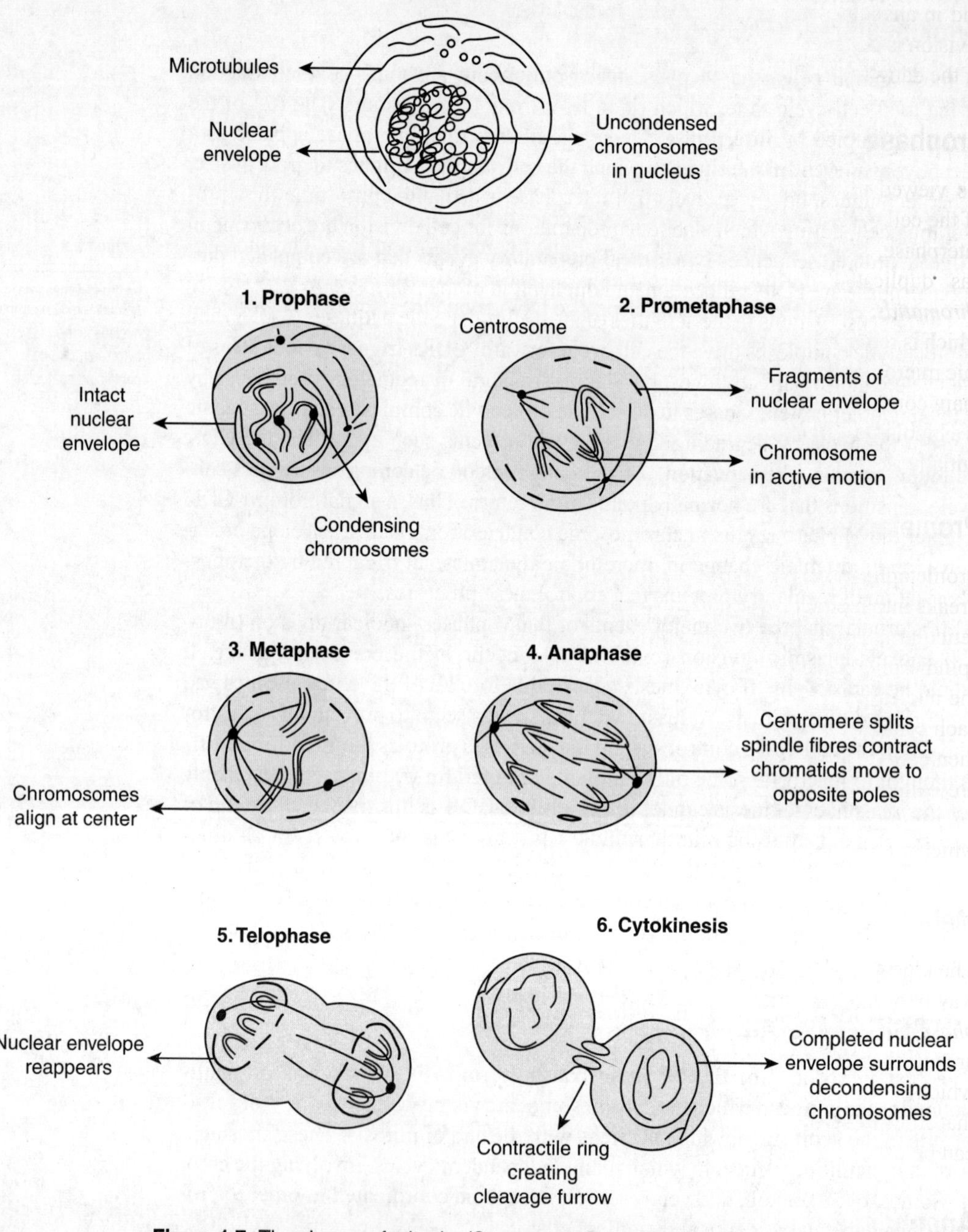

Figure 1.7 The phases of mitosis. (See page 226 for the colour image.)

In metaphase, the chromosomes are aligned at the equator of the mitotic spindle, and in anaphase they are segregated to the two poles of the spindle. Cytoplasmic division is complete by the end of telophase, and the nucleus and cytoplasm of each of the daughter cells then return to interphase, signaling the end of the M phase.

Prophase

As viewed in the microscope, the transition from the G_2 phase to the M phase of the cell cycle is not a sharply defined event. The chromatin, which is diffused in interphase, slowly condenses into well-defined chromosomes. Each chromosome has duplicated during the preceding S phase and consists of two sister *chromatids*; each of these contains a specific DNA sequence known as *centromere*, which is required for proper segregation. Towards the end of prophase, the cytoplasmic microtubules that are a part of the interphase cytoskeleton disassemble, and the main component of the mitotic apparatus, the *mitotic spindle*, begins to form. This is a bipolar structure composed of microtubules and associated proteins. The spindle initially assembles outside the nucleus between separating centrosomes.

Centromere
A specialized structure on the chromosome, appearing during cell division as the constricted central region where the two chromatids are held together.

Prometaphase

Prometaphase starts abruptly with the disruption of the nuclear envelope, which breaks into membrane vesicles that are indistinguishable from bits of endoplasmic reticulum. These vesicles remain visible around the spindle during mitosis. The spindle microtubules, which have been lying outside the nucleus, can now enter the nuclear region. Specialized protein complexes called *kinetochores* mature on each centromere and get attached to some of the spindle microtubules, which are then called *kinetochore microtubules*. The remaining microtubules in the spindle are called *polar microtubules*, while those outside the spindle are called *astral microtubules*. The kinetochore microtubules exert tension on the chromosomes, which are thereby thrown into agitated motion.

Metaphase

The kinetochore microtubules eventually align the chromosomes in one plane half way between the spindle poles. Each chromosome is held in tension at this *metaphase plate* by the paired kinetochores and their associated microtubules, which are attached to opposite poles of the spindle. The cell seems to pass at metaphase, which occupies about 20 minutes out of the hour or so required for mitosis. Agents that interphase with the functioning of the spindle, such as the drug **colchicine**, can be used to generate metaphase-arrested cells.

Colchicines
An alkaloid used to inhibit mitosis.

Anaphase

Triggered by a specific signal, anaphase begins abruptly as the paired kinetochores on each chromosome separate, allowing each chromatid (now called a chromosome) to be pulled slowly toward the spindle pole it faces. All of the newly separated chromosomes move at the same speed, typically about 1 µm per minute.

Two categories of movement can be distinguished. During *anaphase A*, kinetochore microtubules shorten as the chromosomes approach the poles. During *anaphase B*, the *polar microtubules* elongate and the two poles of the spindle move farther apart. Anaphase typically lasts only a few minutes.

Telophase

In telophase, the separated daughter chromosomes arrive at the poles and the kinetochore microtubules disappear. The polar microtubules elongate still more, and a new nuclear envelope re-forms around each group of daughter chromosomes. The condensed chromatin expands, the nucleoli reappear and mitosis is at an end.

Cytokinesis

The cytoplasm divides by a process known as *cleavage*, which usually starts during anaphase. In an animal cell, the membrane around the middle of the cell, perpendicular to the spindle axis and between the daughter nuclei, is drawn inward to form a *cleavage furrow*, which gradually deepens until it encounters the narrow remains of the mitotic spindle between the two nuclei. This thin bridge, or *mid body*, may persist for sometime before it narrows and finally breaks at each end, leaving two separate daughter cells.

The important features of the cell cycle are summarized in Table 1.1.

Table 1.1 Features of the cell cycle

Stage	Major Features
G_0 phase	Stable, non-dividing period of variable length
Interphase	
G_1 phase	Growth and development of the cell; G_1/S checkpoint
S phase	Synthesis of DNA
G_2 phase	Preparation for division; G_2/S checkpoint
M phase	
Prophase	Chromosome condenses and mitotic spindle forms
Prometaphase	Nuclear envelope disintegrates, spindle microtubules anchor to kinetochores
Metaphase	Chromosomes align on the metaphase plate
Anaphase	Sister chromatids separate, becoming individual chromosomes that migrate towards spindle poles
Telophase	Chromosomes arrive at spindle poles, the nuclear envelope reforms, and the condensed chromosomes relax
Cytokinesis	Cytoplasm divides

MEIOSIS

Introduction

The realization that germ cells are haploid led to the theory that they must be formed by a special kind of nuclear division in which the chromosome complement is precisely halved. This type of division is called meiosis. Meiosis involves two divisions rather than one. Thus, when an egg cell and sperm cell unite to form a zygote, the chromosomes from both the cells combine to form the diploid zygote.

Two cell divisions occur in meiosis. Each meiotic division has been divided into stages. It is broadly divided into two stages (Figure 1.8):

- Meiosis I
- Meiosis II

Meiosis I: This stage is also called reduction division because two haploid cells are formed from a diploid cell. The diploid cells are the oogonia in females and the spermatogonia in males.

Meiosis II: After meiosis I a second meiosis takes place where each haploid cell is replicated.

Meiosis I

Interphase I

This is the first stage of meiosis. During this phase important processes such as replication of chromosomal DNA occurs.

Prophase I

It is a complex phase and involves many key events. This phase begins as the chromatin strands coil and condense causing them to become visible as chromosomes. Synapsis occurs here and it is at this stage that the homologous chromosomes pair up. This pairing of homologous chromosomes is an important part of this cycle and differentiates it from mitosis. As prophase I continues, the chromatids of the two chromosomes intertwine. Each pair of intertwined homologous chromosomes is called a bivalent or a tetrad.

A second prominent feature of prophase I is the formation of chiasmata. These denote the points at which the homologous chromosomes are joined and where genetic information is exchanged. This process is called crossing over and results in the formation of chromosomes that contain combinations of parts of the original chromosomes.

Leptotene

The first stage of prophase I is the *leptotene* stage, also known as *leptonema*, from Greek words meaning "thin threads." In this stage of prophase I, individual

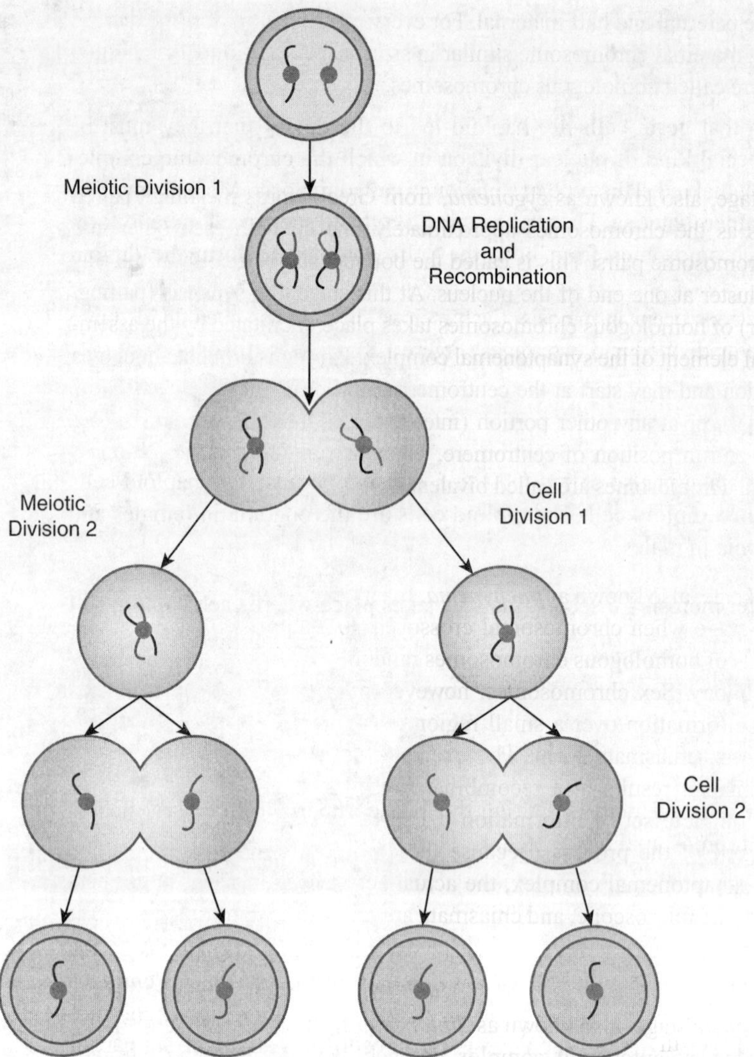

Figure 1.8 Meiosis I and II. (See page 227 for the colour image.)

chromosomes—each consisting of two sister chromatids—change from the diffused state they exist in during the cell's period of growth and gene expression, and condense into visible strands within the nucleus. However, the two sister chromatids are still so tightly bound that they are indistinguishable from one another. During leptotene, lateral elements of the synaptonemal complex assemble. Leptotene is of very short duration and progressive condensation and coiling of chromosome fibres takes place.

Chromosomes assume a long thread-like shape; they contract and become thick. At the beginning chromosomes are present in diploid number as in mitotic prophase. Each chromosome is made up of only one chromatid, and half of the total chromosome are paternal and half maternal. For every paternal chromosome there is a corresponding maternal chromosome similar in size, shape and nature of inherited characters and are called homologous chromosomes.

Zygotene

The *zygotene* stage, also known as *zygonema*, from Greek words meaning "paired threads," occurs as the chromosomes approximately line up with each other into homologous chromosome pairs. This is called the bouquet stage because of the way the telomeres cluster at one end of the nucleus. At this stage, the synapsis (pairing/coming together) of homologous chromosomes takes place, facilitated by the assembly of the central element of the synaptonemal complex. Pairing is brought about by a zipper-like fashion and may start at the centromere (procentric), at the chromosome ends (proterminal), or at any other portion (intermediate). Individuals of a pair are equal in length and in position of centromere. Thus, pairing is highly specific and exact. The paired chromosomes are called bivalent or tetrad chromosome.

Pachytene

The *pachytene* stage, also known as *pachynema*, from Greek words meaning "thick threads" is the stage when chromosomal crossover (crossing over) occurs. Non-sister chromatids of homologous chromosomes randomly exchange segments over regions of homology. Sex chromosomes, however, are not wholly identical, and only exchange information over a small region of homology. At the sites where exchange happens, chiasmata form. The exchange of information between the non-sister chromatids results in a recombination of information; each chromosome has the complete set of information it had before, and there are no gaps formed as a result of the process. Because the chromosomes cannot be distinguished in the synaptonemal complex, the actual act of crossing over is not perceivable through the microscope, and chiasmata are not visible until the next stage.

Diplotene

During the *diplotene* stage, also known as *diplonema*, from Greek words meaning "two threads," the synaptonemal complex degrades and homologous chromosomes separate from one another. The chromosomes themselves uncoil, allowing transcription of DNA. However, the homologous chromosomes of each bivalent remain tightly bound at chiasmata, the regions where crossing-over occurred. The chiasmata remain on the chromosomes until they are severed in anaphase I.

In human fetal oogenesis all developing oocytes develop to this stage and stop before birth. This suspended state remains so until puberty.

Diakinesis

Chromosomes condense further during the *diakinesis* stage, from Greek words meaning "moving through." This is the first point in meiosis where the four parts of the tetrads are actually visible. Sites of crossing over entangle together, effectively overlapping, making chiasmata clearly visible. Other than this observation, the rest of

Zygotene
Second stage of prophase, during which strands of homologous chromosomes line up and become pairs.

Pachytene
Third stage of prophase, during which each chromosome pair separates into sister chromatids with some breakage and crossing over of genes.

Diplotene
Late stage of prophase, in which the chromatid pairs of the tetrads begin to separate and chiasmata can be seen.

Diakinesis
Last stage of prophase, in which the nucleolus and nuclear envelope disappear, spindle fibres form, and chromosomes shorten in preparation for anaphase.

the stage closely resembles prometaphase of mitosis; the nucleoli disappear, the nuclear membrane disintegrates into vesicles, and the meiotic spindle begins to form.

Metaphase I

This stage follows prophase I and is characterized by the completion of spindle formation and the arrangement of the tetrads (which are still attached at the chiasmata) in the equatorial plane. The two centromeres of the bivalents lie on opposite sides of the equatorial plane.

Anaphase I

During this stage the chiasmata disappear and the homologous chromosomes are pulled by the spindle fibres to the opposite poles of the cell. However, here the centromeres do not duplicate and divide like in mitosis so only half the original number of chromosomes migrate towards each pole.

Telophase I

This stage begins when the chromosomes reach the opposite poles of the cell. The chromosomes uncoil slightly and a new nuclear membrane begins to form. The two daughter cells thus formed contain the haploid number of chromosomes. Cytokinesis occurs during this phase and thus the cytoplasm is divided equally among the two daughter cells.

Meiosis II

Interphase II

This is a very brief phase. The differentiating feature between this phase and interphase I of meiosis and the interphase of mitosis is that in interphase II no DNA replication occurs.

Prophase II

This stage is quite similar to that of the mitotic prophase except that the nucleus contains only a haploid set of chromosomes. The chromosomes thicken as they coil, the nuclear membrane disappears, and the new spindle fibres are being formed.

Metaphase II

In this phase the spindle fibres pull the chromosomes into alignment at the equatorial plane.

Anaphase II

This stage resembles the mitotic anaphase in that the centromeres split and each carries a single chromatid towards the pole of the cell. The chromatids have separated but may not be identical because of the crossing over that has already occurred and this differentiates it from mitosis.

Telophase II

This stage begins when the chromosomes reach the opposite poles of the cell. There they begin to uncoil. New nuclear membranes are formed around each group of chromosomes and cytokinesis occurs.

CHARACTERISTICS AND STRUCTURE OF DNA AND CHROMOSOMES—DNA PACKAGING AND CHROMOSOME CONDENSATION

Structure of chromosomes

The chromosomes of eukaryotic cells are larger and more complex than those found in prokaryotes. Although linear, the DNA molecules in eukaryotic chromosomes are highly folded and condensed; if stretched out, some human chromosomes would be several centimeters long—thousands of times longer than the span of a typical nucleus. To package such a tremendous length of DNA into this small volume, each DNA molecule is coiled again and again and tightly packed around histone proteins, forming rod-shaped chromosomes. Most of the time the chromosomes are thin and difficult to observe, but before cell division, they condense further into thick, readily observed structures; it is at this stage that chromosomes are usually studied (Figure 1.9).

A functional chromosome has three essential elements: a centromere, a pair of telomeres, and origins of replication. The *centromere* is the attachment point for *spindle microtubules*, which are the filaments responsible for moving chromosomes during cell division. The centromere appears as a constricted region that often stains less strongly than does the rest of the chromosome. Before cell division, a protein complex called the *kinetochore* assembles on the centromere, to which spindle microtubules later attach. Chromosomes without a centromere cannot be drawn into the newly formed nuclei; these chromosomes are lost, often with catastrophic consequences to the cell. On the basis of the location of the centromere, chromosomes are classified into four types:

- Metacentric
- Submetacentric
- Acrocentric
- Telocentric

One of the two arms of a chromosome (the short arm of a submetacentric or acrocentric chromosome) is denoted as the letter p and the other arm is denoted as q.

Telomeres are the structural ends of a chromosome. They serve to conserve and stabilize the chromosome ends and prevent loss of chromosome ends during cell division and DNA repair. When a chromosome breaks, producing new ends, these ends have an affinity to stick together, and this result in chromosome is degradation at the newly broken ends. Telomeres provide chromosome stability. Recent research evidences suggest that telomeres also participate in limiting cell division and may play important roles in aging and cancer.

Chromosome
Thread-like bodies consisting of chromatin, which carry the genes in a linear order.

Microtubule
A hollow cylindrical structure in the cytoplasm involved in intracellular shape and transport.

Telomere
Segment of DNA that occurs at the ends of chromosomes.

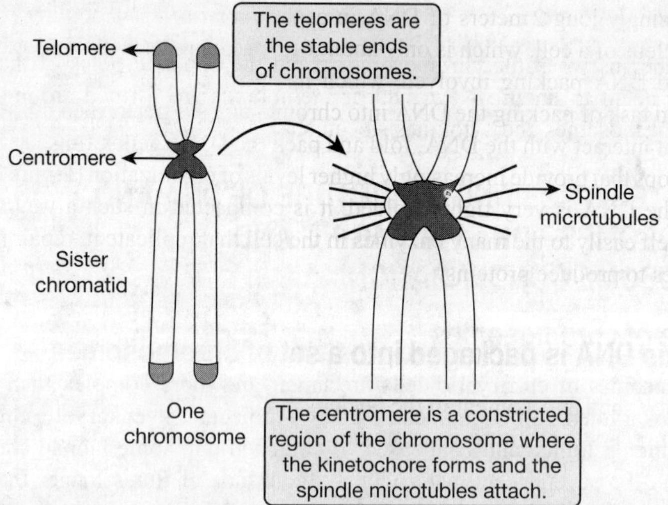

Figure 1.9 Structure of a eukaryotic chromosome. (See page 228 for the colour image.)

Chromosomal DNA and its packaging in the chromatin fibre

The total genetic content (in whole) is referred to as the genome of an organism. The genomes of eukaryotes are chromosomes that contain the genes and other accessory molecules. The DNA present on chromosomes carries genes that code for all the proteins that make up an organism.

The number of chromosomes and DNA molecules changes in the course of the cell cycle. The number of chromosomes per cell equals the number of functional centromeres, and the number of DNA molecules per cell equals the number of chromatids (Figure 1.10).

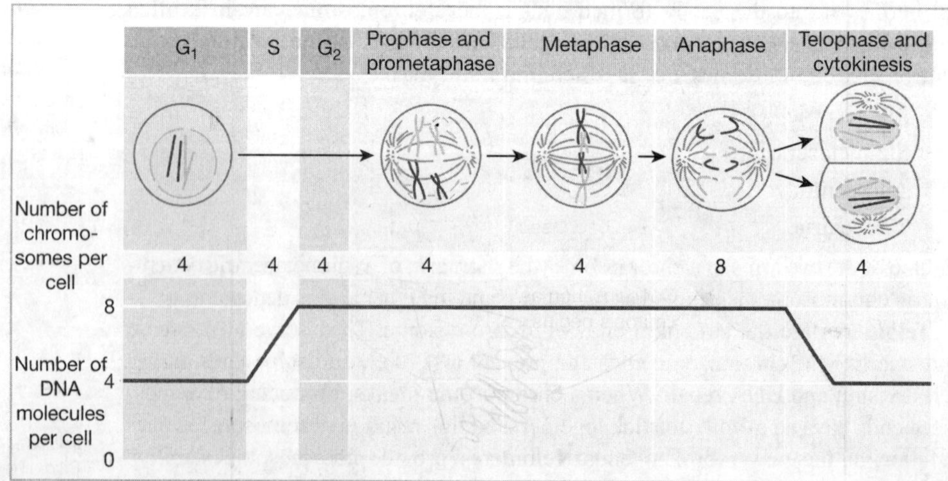

Figure 1.10 The number of chromosomes and DNA molecules changes in the course of the cell cycle. (See page 228 for the colour image.)

An amazingly long 2 meters of DNA in each human cell is smoothly packed into the nucleus of a cell, which is only about 6 µm in diameter. This demonstrates the intricate DNA packing involved, which has evolved over species, and this multifaceted task of packing the DNA into chromosomes is performed by specific proteins that interact with the DNA, fold and pack the DNA, generating a series of coils and loops that provide increasingly higher levels of organization (Figure 1.11). Although the DNA is very tightly folded, it is compacted in such a way that it presents itself easily to the many enzymes in the cell that replicate it, repair it, and use its genes to produce proteins.

Eukaryotic DNA is packaged into a set of chromosomes

In eukaryotes, the DNA content in the nucleus is distributed between the different **chromosomes** that constitute its genome. For example, the human genome—approximately 3.2×10^9 nucleotide—is distributed over 24 different chromosomes (Chromosomes 1-22, X and Y). Each chromosome consists of a single, long linear DNA molecule bound with proteins that fold and pack the DNA thread into a more compact structure. The complex of DNA and protein in its uncondensed form is called *chromatin*, which undergoes the process of condensation with the help of chromosome condensation factors during cell division (Figure 1.12).

Also, the processes of DNA replication, cell cycle checkpoint regulation, gene expression, and DNA repair are also governed and facilitated by specific proteins.

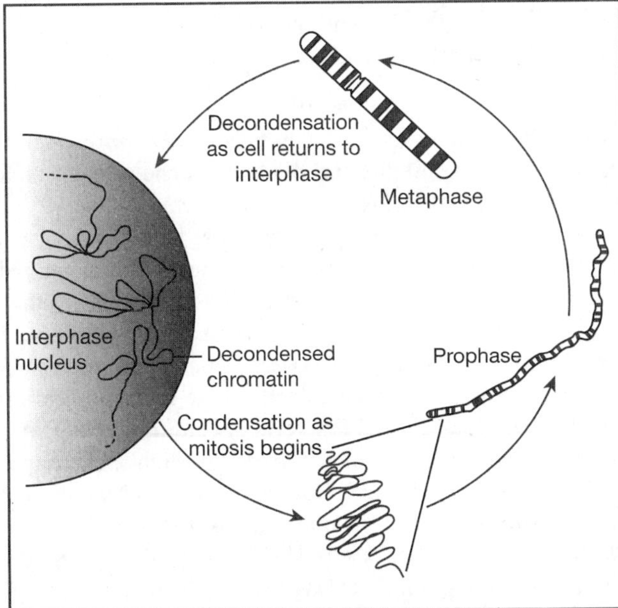

Figure 1.11 Cycle of condensation and decondensation and levels of chromatin packing. (See page 229 for the colour image.)

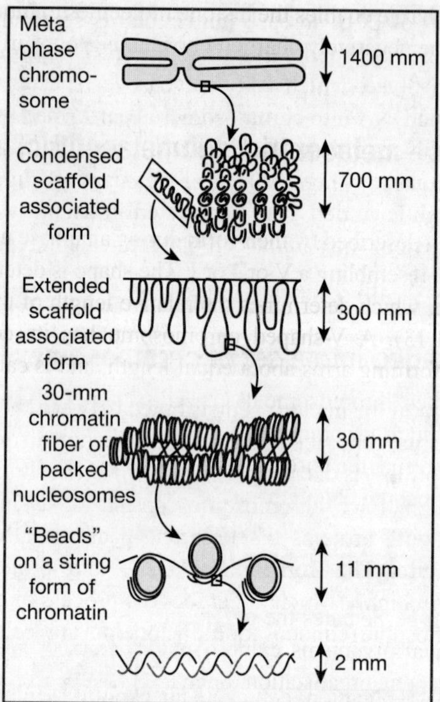

Figure 1.12 Organization of DNA into chromosomes. (See page 229 for the colour image.)

Nucleosomes are the basic unit of eukaryotic chromosome structure

The proteins that mediate DNA compaction and organization into chromosomes are classified as: the *histones* and the *non-histone chromosomal proteins*. The functional complex/unit of both histone and non-histone proteins along with the nuclear DNA of eukaryotic cells is termed as *chromatin*.

Histones are responsible for the first and most basic level of chromosome organization, the nucleosome. When interphase nuclei are examined under an electron microscope, the chromatin exhibits itself as a fibre. When this chromatin is examined when it is partially unfolded, it appears as a stretch of "beads on a string", where the string is the DNA and each bead is a nucleosome. A nucleo-some consists of DNA wound around a protein core formed from histones. The "beads on a string" characterizes the first level of chromosomal DNA packing.

Each nucleosome unit consists of a complex of eight histone proteins; two molecules each of histones H2A, H2B, H3, and H4 and double-stranded DNA that is 146 nucleotide pairs long. The *histone octamer* forms a protein core around which the double-stranded DNA is wound. This step of nucleosome formation condenses the DNA to one-third of its original length and serves as an important step in DNA packing.

Histones are small proteins that contain between 100 and 200 amino acids. A total of 20–30% of the amino acids are lysine and arginine, both of which have a

Histones
Small simple proteins that are found in association with the DNA in chromatin and contain a high proportion of basic amino acids.

Nucleosome
The repeating subunits of chromatin occurring at intervals along a strand of DNA consisting of DNA coiled around histones.

Deoxyribonucleic acid (DNA)
A nucleic acid that is the main constituent of the chromosomes of all organisms.

positive charge. The positive charge enables the histone molecules to bind to DNA by electrostatic attraction to the negatively charged phosphate groups in the sugar phosphate backbone of the DNA.

Forms of chromosomes—metacentric, submetacentric, and acrocentric

Chromosomes are conveniently described by their form during anaphase movement. Three distinct shapes are seen, resembling a V or J or I. The shape is determined by the position of the centromere, which determines the relative length of the lagging chromosome arms (Figure 1.13). A V-shaped chromosome has its centromere approximately in the middle, forming arms about equal length, and is called **meta-centric** chromosome. A J-shaped chromosome has an off-center centromere, forming arms of unequal length; such chromosomes are **submetacentric**. When the centromere is very close to one end, the chromosome appears I-shaped at anaphase because the arms are grossly unequal in length; such a chromosome is **acrocentric**.

Metacentric
A chromosome whose centromere is centrally located, creating two equal chromosome arms.

Submetacentric
The centromere is situated in such a way that one chromosome arm is shorter than the other.

Acrocentric
Centromere is closer to one end than to the other, creating two unequal arms.

CHROMOSOMES AND SEX DETERMINATION

Reproduction is a process that perpetuates the organism and over a period of time results in speciation. Biological organisms exhibit sexual and asexual modes of reproduction based on their genetic organization. Sexual reproduction involves two individuals who are sexually distinct and are referred to as male and female. Among most eukaryotes, sexual reproduction consists of two processes that lead to an alternation of haploid and diploid cells: meiosis produces haploid gametes, and fertilization produces a diploid zygote. The processes of meiosis and fertilization help in restoring the genetic constitution of an organism and in turn maintaining the gene pool. The fundamental difference between males and females is in the gamete they produce and its size. The mechanism by which sex is established is termed **sex determination**. The term **sex** refers to sexual phenotype of an individual. Sex determination in turn is governed by inheritance of chromosomes, which direct the determination of sex of the organism. Sex is determined by a pair of chromosomes known as the **sex chromosomes**, which differ between males and females. The non-sex chromosomes, which do not differ between males and females, are called **autosomes**.

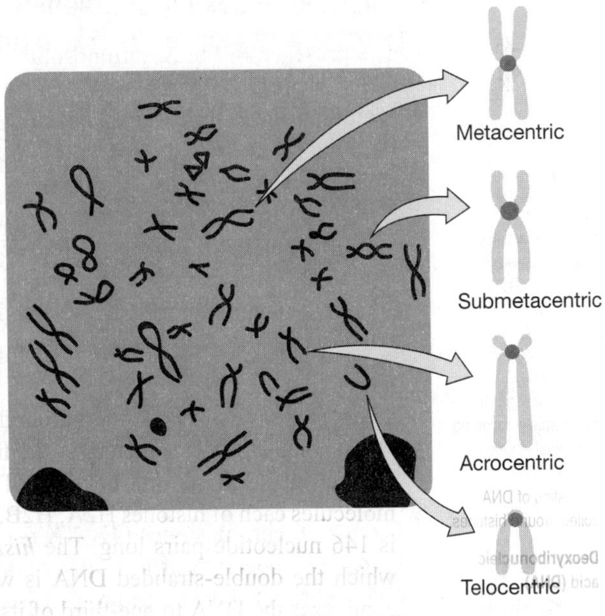

Figure 1.13 Forms of chromosomes. (See page 230 for the colour image.)

XX–XY sex determination in humans

Autosomes
Any chromosome other than a sex chromosome.

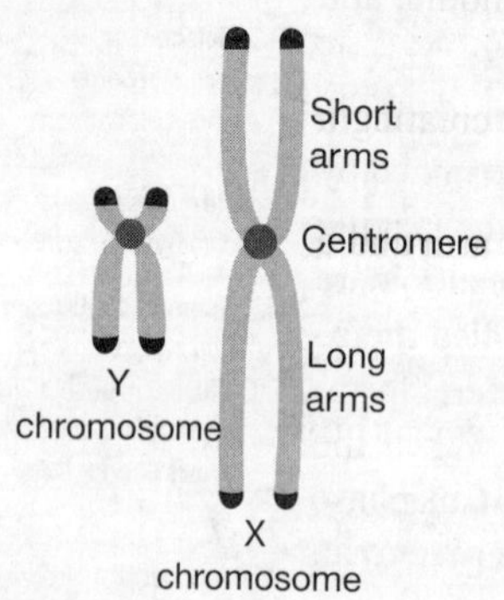

Figure 1.14 X and Y chromosomes in humans.

In many species, the cells of males and females have the same number of chromosomes, but the cells of females have two X chromosomes (XX), and the cells of males have a single X chromosome and a smaller sex chromosome called the Y chromosome (XY). In humans and many other organisms, the Y chromosome is acrocentric (Figure 1.14).

In this type of sex-determining system, the male is the heterogametic sex—half of his gametes have an X chromosome and half have a Y chromosome. The female is the homogametic sex—all her egg cells contain a single X chromosome. Many organisms, including some plants, insects, and reptiles, and all mammals (including humans), have the XX–XY sex-determining system.

Although the X and Y chromosomes are not generally homologous, they do pair and segregate into different cells in meiosis. They can pair because these chromosomes are homologous at small regions called the **pseudoautosomal regions** in which they carry the same genes. Genes found in these regions will display the same pattern of inheritance as that of genes located on autosomal chromosomes. In humans, there are pseudoautosomal regions at both tips of the X and Y chromosomes.

The role of sex chromosomes in phenotype and fertility

The presence of the X chromosome determines compatibility with life. At least one copy of the X chromosome (as in males) is required for fundamental human anatomic and physiological development. The X chromosome contains genes essential for both the sexes (male and female).

Females contain two X chromosomes (of which one is partly inactivated—**X inactivation** for dosage compensation with males).

X inactivation
Process by which one of the two copies of the X chromosomes present in females is inactivated.

Fertility of both males and females is determined by the X and Y chromosomes. The presence of two X chromosomes is required for a female to be fertile **(45, XO—Turner** female is infertile due to absence of one X chromosome) and ovulate regularly with the production of female sex hormones. Additional copies of the X chromosomes hinder normal development in both males and females and result in physical and mental abnormalities.

The Y chromosome codes for "maleness" and is responsible for the development of secondary sexual characteristics in males. The presence of a single Y chromosome expresses the male phenotype; even in the presence of more than one/two X chromosomes **(47, XXY—Klinefilter** is phenotypically a male irrespective of presence of female sexual characteristics because of the presence of two X chromosomes). The absence/loss of the Y chromosome results in a female phenotype.

OVERVIEW OF CHROMOSOME MORPHOLOGY

Anatomically, each functional chromosome has a centromere, where spindle fibers attach, and two telomeres that stabilize the chromosome. Chromosomes are classified into four basic types (based on the position of the centromere):

1. **Metacentric:** The centromere is located approximately in the middle, and so the chromosome has two arms of equal length.

2. **Sub metacentric:** The centromere is displaced toward one end, creating a long arm and a short arm.

3. **Acrocentric:** The centromere is near one end, producing a long arm and a knob, or satellite, at the other.

4. **Telocentric:** The centromere is at or very near the end of the chromosome (*humans do not have telocentric chromosomes*).

On human chromosomes, the short arm is denoted by the letter p (*petite* meaning small/short), and the long arm by the letter q.

The complete set of chromosomes that an organism possesses is called its *karyotype* and is usually presented as a picture of metaphase chromosomes lined up in descending order of their size. Karyotypes are established from mitotic cells of white blood cells, bone marrow cells, or cells from meristematic tissues of plants. After treatment with colchicines/colcemid (spindle inhibitor) that prevents them from entering anaphase, the cells are chemically fixed, spread on a microscope slide, stained, and photographed. The photograph is then enlarged, and the individual chromosomes are cut out and arranged in a karyotype. For human chromosomes, karyotypes are often routinely prepared by automated machines.

Types of chromosome mutations

Chromosome mutations can be grouped into two basic categories.

1. Structural abnormalities: Chromosome rearrangements
2. Numerical abnormalities: Aneuploids and polyploids

Chromosome rearrangements alter the structure of chromosomes; for example, a region of a chromosome might be duplicated, deleted, or inverted. In **aneuploidy**, the *number* of chromosomes is altered: one or more individual chromosomes are added or deleted. In **polyploidy**, one or more sets of chromosomes are present. A polyploid is any organism that has more than two sets of chromosomes ($3n$, $4n$, $5n$, or more).

Note: Humans are *diploid* and possess $2n$ number of chromosomes.

Structural chromosomal abnormalities

Chromosome rearrangements

Chromosome rearrangements are mutations that change the structure of individual chromosomes. The four basic types of rearrangements are *duplications, deletions, inversions, and translocations* (Figure 1.15).

Mutation
A sudden change in the structure of the genes or chromosomes of an organism.

Table 1.2 Types of chromosome mutations

Chromosome Rearrangement	Change in Chromosome Structure
Duplication	Duplication of a chromosome segment
Deletion	Deletion of a chromosome segment
Inversion	Chromosome segment inverted to 180 degrees
Paracentric inversion	Inversion that does not include the centromere in the inverted region
Pericentric inversion	Inversion that includes the centromere in the inverted region
Translocation	Movement of a chromosome segment to a non-homologous chromosome or region of the same chromosome
Nonreciprocal translocation	Movement of a chromosome segment to a non-homologous chromosome or region of the same chromosome without reciprocal exchange
Reciprocal translocation	Exchange between segments of non-homologous chromosomes or regions of the same chromosome
Aneuploidy	Change in number of individual chromosomes
Nullisomy	Loss of both members of a homologous pair
Monosomy	Loss of one member of a homologous pair
Trisomy	Gain of one chromosome, resulting in three homologous chromosomes
Tetrasomy	Gain of two homologous chromosomes, resulting in four homologous chromosomes
Polyploidy	Addition of entire chromosome sets
Autopolyploidy	Polyploidy in which extra chromosome sets are derived from the same species
Allopolyploidy	Polyploidy in which extra chromosome sets are derived from two or more species

Duplications

A **chromosome duplication** is a mutation in which part of the chromosome has been doubled. Let us consider a chromosome with segments AB•CDEFG, in which • represents the centromere. A duplication might include the EF segments, giving rise to a chromosome with segments AB•CDEFEFG. This type of duplication, in which the duplicated region is immediately adjacent to the original segment, is called a **tandem duplication**. If the duplicated segment is located some distance from the original segment, either on the same chromosome or on a different one, this type is called a **displaced duplication**. An example of a displaced duplication would be AB•CDEFGEF. A duplication can either be in the same orientation as the original sequence, as in the two preceding examples, or be inverted: AB•CDEFFEG. When the duplication is inverted, it is called a **reverse duplication**.

In humans, duplication of chromosomes 4, 7 and 9 have exhibited typical clinical features. However, they have not been characterized as a defined genetic disorder.

Duplication 4, short arm: Small head, short neck, low hairline, growth, and mental retardation

Duplication 4, long arm: Small head, sloping forehead, hand abnormalities

Duplication 7, long arm: Delayed development, asymmetry of the head, fuzzy scalp, small nose, low-set ears

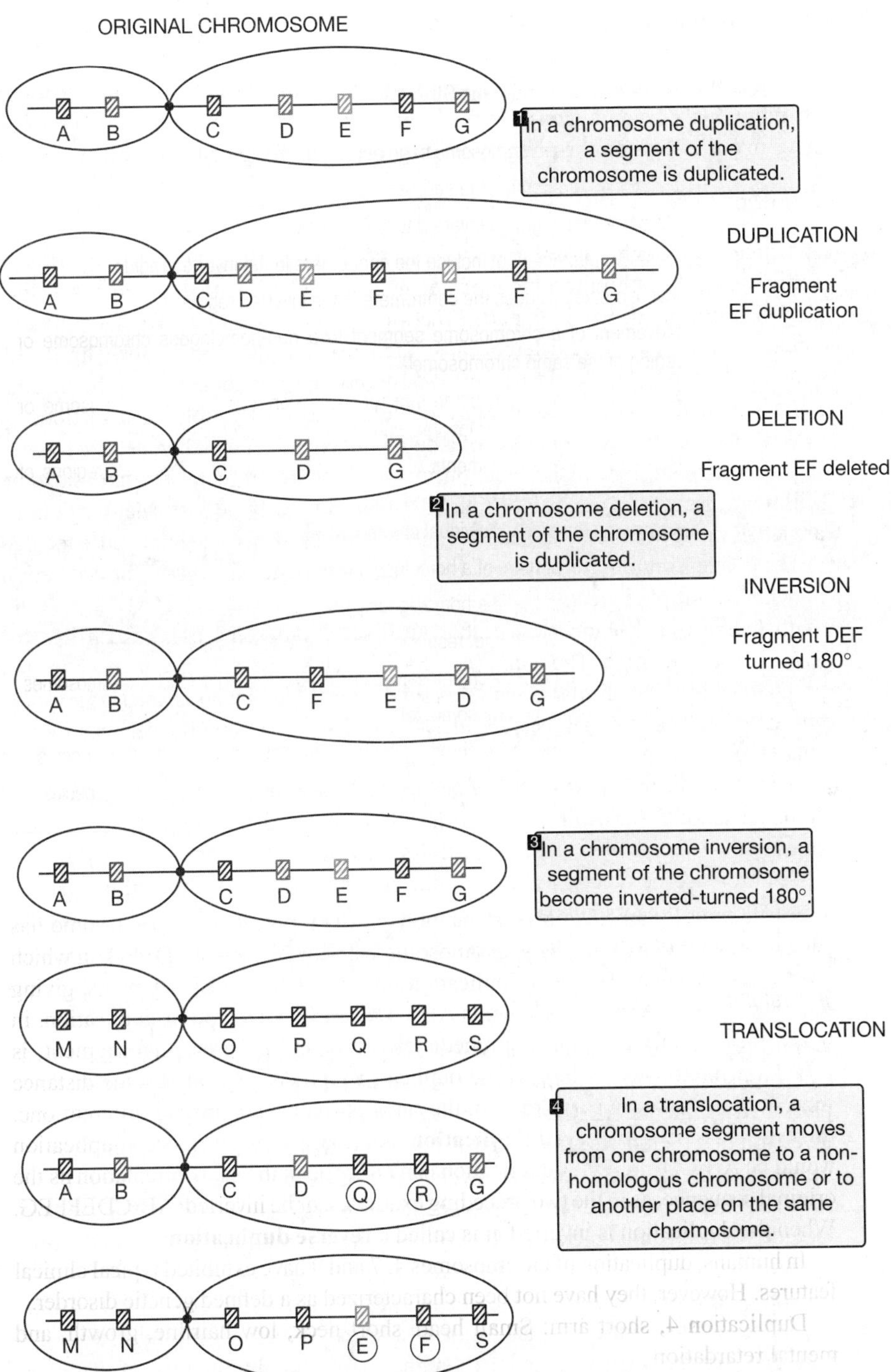

Figure 1.15 Structural chromosomal abnormalities. (See page 231 for the colour image.)

Duplication 9, short arm: Characteristic face, variable mental retardation, high and broad forehead, hand abnormalities

A chromosome duplication is a mutation that doubles part of a chromosome. In individuals heterozygous for a chromosome duplication, duplications often have major effects on the phenotype, possibly by altering gene dosage.

Deletions

A second type of chromosome rearrangement is a **deletion**, the loss of a chromosome segment. A chromosome with segments AB•CDEFG that undergoes a deletion of segment EF would generate the mutated chromosome AB•CDG. A large deletion can be easily detected because the chromosome is noticeably shortened. Smaller deletions, referred to as *microdeletions*, are not noticeable at the cytogenetic level and require molecular or molecular cytogenetic tools for detection.

The phenotypic consequences of a deletion depend on which genes are located in the deleted region. If the deletion includes the centromere, the chromosome will not segregate in meiosis or mitosis and will usually be lost. Many deletions are lethal in the homozygous state because all copies of any essential genes located in the deleted region are missing. Even individuals heterozygous for a deletion may have multiple defects.

In humans, a deletion on the short arm of chromosome 5 is responsible for *Cri-du-chat* Syndrome. The name (French for "cry of the cat") is derived from the peculiar, catlike cry of infants with this syndrome. A child who is heterozygous for this deletion has a small head, widely spaced eyes, a round face, and mental retardation.

The deletion of a part of the short arm of chromosome 4 results in another human disorder—the Wolf–Hirschhorn syndrome—which is characterized by seizures and by severe mental and growth retardation.

A chromosome deletion is a mutation in which a part of the chromosome is lost. Deletions do not undergo reverse mutation. They cause recessive genes on the undeleted chromosome to be expressed and cause imbalances in gene products.

Inversions

A third type of chromosome rearrangement is a **chromosome inversion**, in which a chromosome segment is inverted—turned 180 degrees. If a chromosome originally had segments AB•CDEFG, then chromosome AB•CFEDG represents an inversion that includes segments DEF. For an inversion to take place, the chromosome must break in two places. Inversions that do not include the centromere, such as AB•CFEDG, are termed **paracentric inversions**, whereas inversions that include the centromere, such as ADC•BEFG, are termed **pericentric inversions**.

Individuals with inversions have neither lost nor gained any genetic material; just the gene order has been altered. Nevertheless, these mutations often have pronounced phenotypic effects. An inversion may break a gene into two parts, with one part moving to a new location and destroying the function of that gene. Even when the chromosome breaks are between genes, phenotypic effects may arise from the inverted gene order in an inversion. Many genes are regulated in a position-dependent manner; if their positions are altered by an inversion, they may be expressed at inappropriate times or in inappropriate tissues. This outcome is referred to as a **position effect**.

In an inversion, a segment of a chromosome is inverted. Inversions cause breaks in some genes and may move others to new locations. When crossing over takes place within the inverted region, non-viable gametes are usually produced, resulting in a depression in observed recombination frequencies.

Translocations

A **translocation** entails the movement of genetic material between non-homologous chromosomes or within the same chromosome. In **non-reciprocal translocations**, genetic material moves from one chromosome to another without any reciprocal exchange. Consider the following two non-homologous chromosomes: AB•CDEFG and MN•OPQRS. If chromosome segment EF moves from the first chromosome to the second without any transfer of segments from the second chromosome to the first, a non-reciprocal translocation has taken place, producing chromosomes AB•CDG and MN•OPEFQRS. More commonly, there is a two-way exchange of segments between the chromosomes, resulting in a **reciprocal translocation**. A reciprocal translocation between chromosomes AB•CDEFG and MN•OPQRS might give rise to chromosomes AB•CDQRG and MN•OPEFS. Translocations can affect a phenotype in several ways.

First, they may create new linkage relations that affect gene expression (a position effect): genes translocated to new locations may come under the control of different regulatory sequences or other genes that affect their expression—an example is found in Burkitt lymphoma. Second, the chromosomal breaks that bring about translocations may take place within a gene and disrupt its function.

Deletions frequently accompany translocations. In a **Robertsonian translocation**, for example, the long arms of two acrocentric chromosomes become joined to a common centromere through a translocation, generating a metacentric chromosome with two long arms and another chromosome with two very short arms. The smaller chromosome often fails to segregate, leading to an overall reduction in chromosome number. Robertsonian translocations are the cause of some cases of Down Syndrome.

Translocations can play an important role in the evolution of karyotypes. Chimpanzees, gorillas, and orangutans all have 48 chromosomes, whereas humans have 46. Human chromosome 2 is a large, metacentric chromosome with G-banding patterns that match those found on two different acrocentric chromosomes of the apes. Apparently, a Robertsonian translocation took place in a human ancestor, creating a large metacentric chromosome from the two long arms of the ancestral acrocentric chromosomes and a small chromosome consisting of the two short arms. The small chromosome was subsequently lost, leading to the reduced human chromosome number.

In translocations, parts of chromosomes move to other non-homologous chromosomes or other regions of the same chromosome. Translocations may affect the phenotype by causing genes to move to new locations, where they come under the influence of new regulatory sequences or by breaking genes and disrupting their function.

Numerical chromosomal abnormalities

In addition to chromosome rearrangements, chromosome mutations also include changes in the *number* of chromosomes. Variations in chromosome number can be classified into two basic types: changes in the number of individual chromosomes (aneuploidy) and changes in the number of chromosome sets (polyploidy).

Aneuploidy

Aneuploidy can arise in several ways. First, a chromosome may be lost in the course of mitosis or meiosis if, for example, its centromere is deleted. *The loss of the centromere* prevents the spindle fibers from attaching; so the chromosome fails to move to the spindle pole and does not become incorporated into a nucleus after cell division. Second, the small chromosome generated by a Robertsonian translocation may be lost in mitosis or meiosis. Third, aneuploids may arise through *non-disjunction*, the failure of homologous chromosomes or sister chromatids to separate in meiosis or mitosis. Non-disjunction leads to some gametes or cells that contain an extra chromosome and others that are missing a chromosome.

Types of Aneuploidy

The four types of relatively common aneuploid conditions in diploid individuals are as follows:

- Nullisomy
- Monosomy
- Trisomy
- Tetrasomy

1. **Nullisomy** is the loss of both members of a homologous pair of chromosomes.
2. **Monosomy** is the loss of a single chromosome. A monosomic person has 45 chromosomes.
3. **Trisomy** is the gain of a single chromosome. A trisomic person has 47 chromosomes. The gain of a chromosome means that there are three homologous copies of one chromosome.
4. **Tetrasomy** is the gain of two homologous chromosomes. A tetrasomic person has 48 chromosomes. Tetrasomy is not the gain of *any* two extra chromosomes, but rather the gain of two homologous chromosomes; so there will be four homologous copies of a particular chromosome.

Aneuploidy, the loss or gain of one or more individual chromosomes, may arise from the loss of a chromosome subsequent to translocation or from non-disjunction in meiosis or mitosis. It disrupts gene dosage and often has severe phenotypic effects.

Monosomy X (45, XO)
Turner – An abnormal congenital condition resulting from a defect on or absence of the second sex chromosome, characterized by retarded growth of the gonads.

Klinefeilter Syndrome (47, XXY)
An abnormal condition in which at least one extra X chromosome is present in a male, characterized by reduced or absent sperm production, small testicles, and in some cases enlarged breasts.

Aneuploidy in humans

Aneuploidy in humans usually produces serious developmental problems that lead to spontaneous abortion (miscarriage). In fact, as many as 50% of all spontaneously aborted fetuses carry chromosome defects, and a third or more of all conceptions spontaneously abort in early pregnancy. Only about 2% of all fetuses with a chromosome defect survive to birth.

Sex-chromosome aneuploids: The most common aneuploidy seen in living humans has to do with the sex chromosomes. As is true of all mammals, aneuploidy of the human sex chromosomes is better tolerated than aneuploidy of autosomal chromosomes. Turner Syndrome and Klinefelter Syndrome result from aneuploidy of the sex chromosomes.

Autosomal aneuploids: Autosomal aneuploids resulting in live births are less common than sex-chromosome aneuploids in humans, probably because there is no mechanism of dosage compensation for autosomal chromosomes. Most autosomal aneuploids are spontaneously aborted, with the exception of aneuploids of some of the small autosomes.

Because these chromosomes are small and carry fewer genes, the presence of extra copies is less detrimental. For example, the most common autosomal aneuploidy in humans is **trisomy 21**, also called **Down Syndrome**. Few autosomal aneuploids besides trisomy 21 result in human live births. **Trisomy 18**, also known as **Edward Syndrome**, arises with a frequency of approximately 1 in 8000 live births. Babies with Edward Syndrome are severely retarded and have low-set ears, a short neck, deformed feet, clenched fingers, heart problems, and other disabilities. Few live for more than a year after birth. **Trisomy 13** has a frequency of about 1 in 15,000 live births and produces features that are collectively known as **Patau Syndrome**. Characteristics of this condition include severe mental retardation, a small head, sloping forehead, small eyes, cleft lip and palate, extra fingers and toes, and numerous other problems. About half of children with trisomy 13 die within the first month of life, and 95% die by the age of 3. Rarer is **trisomy 8**, which arises with a frequency of about 1 in 25,000 to 50,000 live births. This aneuploid is characterized by mental retardation, contracted fingers and toes, lowest malformed ears, and a prominent forehead. Many who have this condition have normal life expectancy.

Trisomy 21 (47, XX, +21/47, XY, +21)
Down – A genetic disorder, associated with the presence of an extra chromosome 21, characterized by a mild to severe mental impairment, weak muscle tone, shorter stature, and a flattened facial profile.

Trisomy 18 (47, XX, +18/47, XY, +18)
Edward – A congenital condition characterized by mental retardation and craniofacial, cardiac, gastrointestinal, and genitourinary abnormalities, caused by the presence of an extra chromosome 18.

Trisomy 13 (47, XX, +13/47, XY, +13)
Patau – A syndrome associated by the presence of an extra chromosome 13, characterized by mental retardation, cardiac problem, and multiple deformities.

Polyploidy

Most eukaryotic organisms are diploid ($2n$) for most of their life cycles, possessing two sets of chromosomes. Occasionally, whole sets of chromosomes fail to separate in meiosis or mitosis, leading to polyploidy, the presence of more than two genomic sets of chromosomes. Polyploids include *triploids* ($3n$), *tetraploids* ($4n$), *pentaploids* ($5n$), and even higher numbers of chromosome sets. Polyploidy is common in plants and is a major mechanism by which new plant species have evolved. Approximately 40% of all flowering-plant species and from 70 to 80% of grasses are polyploids. They include a number of agriculturally important plants, such as wheat, oats, cotton, potatoes, and sugar cane. Polyploidy is less common in animals, but is found in some invertebrates, fishes, salamanders, frogs, and lizards.

Polylploidy is generally not seen in humans; however, certain cancerous conditions result in polyploidy state.

Polyploidy is the presence of extra chromosome sets. Autopolyploids possess extra chromosome sets from the same species; allopolyploids possess extra chromosome sets from two or more species. Problems in chromosome pairing and segregation often lead to sterility in autopolyploids, but many allopolyploids are fertile.

Chromosome mutations and cancer

Most tumors contain cells with chromosome mutations. Some types of tumors are consistently associated with *specific* chromosome mutations, suggesting that in these cases the specific chromosome mutation played a vital role in the development of the cancer. However, many cancers are not associated with specific types of chromosome abnormalities, and individual *gene* mutations are now known to contribute towards many types of cancer. However, chromosome instability is a hallmark of cancer cells, causing them to accumulate chromosome mutations, which then affect individual genes that contribute to the cancer process. Thus, chromosome mutations appear to both *cause* and *be a result* of cancer. At least three types of chromosome rearrangements—deletions, inversions, and translocations—are associated with certain types of cancer. Deletions may result in the loss of one or more genes that normally control cell division. When these tumor-suppressor genes are lost, cell division is not regulated and cancer may result. Inversions and translocations contribute towards cancer in several ways. First, the chromosomal breakpoints that accompany these mutations may lie within tumor-suppressor genes, disrupting their function and leading to uncontrolled cell proliferation.

Second, translocations and inversions may bring together sequences from two different genes, generating a fused protein that stimulates some aspect of the cancer process. Such fusions are seen in most cases of chronic myeloid leukemia, a fatal form of leukemia affecting bone marrow cells. About 90% of patients with chronic myeloid leukemia have a reciprocal translocation between the long arm of chromosome 22 and the tip of the long arm of chromosome 9. This translocation produces a shortened chromosome 22, called the Philadelphia chromosome because it was first discovered in Philadelphia. At the end of a normal chromosome 9 is a potential cancer-causing gene called *c-ABL*. As a result of the translocation, part of the *c-ABL* gene is fused with the *BCR* gene from chromosome 22. The protein produced by this *BCR–c-ABL* fusion gene is much more active than the protein produced by the normal *c-ABL* gene; the fusion protein stimulates increased, unregulated cell division and eventually leads to leukemia.

A third mechanism by which chromosome rearrangements may produce cancer is by the transfer of a potential cancer-causing gene to a new location, where it is activated by different regulatory sequences. Burkitt lymphoma is a cancer of the B cells, the lymphocytes that produce antibodies.

Many people having Burkitt lymphoma possess a reciprocal translocation between chromosome 8 and chromosomes 2, 14, or 22, each of which carries genes for immunological proteins.

Most tumors contain a variety of types of chromosome mutations. Some tumors are associated with specific deletions, inversions, and translocations. Deletions can eliminate or inactivate genes that control the cell cycle; inversions and translocations can cause breaks in genes that suppress tumors, fuse genes to produce cancer-causing proteins, or move genes to new locations, where they are under the influence of different regulatory sequences.

PRINCIPLES OF GENETICS: MENDELIAN PRINCIPLES
Early life of Johann Gregor Mendel (1822–1884)

Gregor Mendel was born in Czech Republic. His parents were poor farmers and could not afford good education for an academically bright Mendel. He was admitted to the Augustinian monastery in Brno in 1843. The monastery funded the formal education of Mendel and after graduating he was ordained a priest and appointed to a teaching position in a local school. He excelled at teaching, and the abbot of the monastery recommended him for further study at the University of Vienna, which he attended from 1851 to 1853. There, Mendel took courses in mathematics, chemistry, entomology, paleontology, botany, and plant physiology. Mendel was known for his scientific enquiry, systematic observation and documentation and meticulous mathematical calculations. His degree in botany and plant physiology along with mathematics and chemistry helped him successfully complete his genetic experiments and arrive at genetic concepts, which the rest of the scientific world could catch up only 40 years after his demise.

After his study in Vienna, Mendel returned to Brno, where he taught at a school and began his experimental work with pea plants. He conducted breeding experiments from 1856 to 1863 and presented his results publicly at meetings of the Brno Natural Science Society in 1865. Mendel's paper "Experiments in Plant Hybridization" was published in 1866. In spite of widespread interest in heredity, the effect of his research on the scientific community was minimal. The scientific community failed to appreciate his hard work and understand his basic principles of inheritance. A highly depressed and demotivated Mendel took up more administrative responsibilities in the monastery and this brought an end to his teaching and experiments in genetics. He died at the age of 61 on January 6, 1884, unrecognized for his contribution to genetics.

The significance of Mendel's discovery was unappreciated until 1900, when three botanists—Hugo de Vries, Erich von Tschermak, and Carl Correns—independently began conducting similar experiments with plants and arrived at results and conclusions exactly similar to those of Mendel. Referring Mendel's paper, they interpreted their results in terms of his principles and threw light on his path-breaking discovery. Sadly Mendel never saw that the whole world stands up for his contribution to genetics and today the scientific community has aptly honoured him as the "father of genetics" for his pioneering work.

MENDEL'S EXPERIMENTAL ORGANISM: THE PEA PLANT

Mendel's experiments in genetics were successful for several reasons. First, was the choice of the experimental organism, the pea plant *Pisum sativum*. The pea plant presented evident advantages:

1. Easy to cultivate (short generation time): Had he chosen an organism with a longer generation time, rabbits/horses he might have never completed his experiments in his life time.

2. Pea plants produce many offspring (seeds): This allowed Mendel to carefully observe and analyse the differences in the offspring and make a mathematical calculation of the same. He observed consistent mathematical ratios in his experiments, and the ratios remained the same for different traits. This gave him statistically significant values. Had he chosen a higher organism whose gestational age and offspring ratio was low, he would have taken much longer to arrive at his results.

3. Pea plant is a pure breeding variety: It varied in different characters and was genetically pure. This helped Mendel perform experiments with plants of variable, however known, genetic makeup. The genes coding for the characters were not linked. Linked genes would have greatly affected the phenotypic ratio and interfered in Mendel's conclusions. (At that time, even the term gene was not coined, and the concept of genes and linked genes were totally unfamiliar).

4. Pea plant demonstrated seven contrasting characters that were phenotypically distinguishable: He chose characters that existed in two easily differentiated forms, such as white versus red flower colour, round versus wrinkled seeds, and inflated versus constricted pods.

Mendel was successful because he adopted a professional experimental approach. He was a perfect researcher. He designed hypotheses based on his preliminary observations and conducted additional crosses to test his hypothesis. He repeated experiments to test consistency in results and made a careful observation of the phenotypes and recorded all the mathematical values with respect to phenotypes observed. He paid attention to small details in appearance of the patterns of inheritance and computed the ratios. He never manipulated his mathematical data to obtain results he expected. He was extremely patient in maintaining his greenhouse of pea plants, grooming them regularly, and conducting his experiments systematically for almost 10 years before attempting to publish his results.

In order to understand Mendel's experiments and his results, it is important to understand a few related genetic terminologies. They are described in Table 1.3.

Table 1.3 Genetic terminologies

Gene	A genetic factor (region of DNA) that helps determine a characteristic/feature.
Allele	One of two or more alternate forms of a gene.
Locus	Specific place on a chromosome occupied by an allele/gene.
Genotype	Set of alleles that an individual possesses/genetic constitution of a gene.
Heterozygote	An individual possessing two different alleles at a locus. *Example*: Aa.
Homozygote	An individual possessing two of the same alleles at a locus. *Example*: AA or aa.
Phenotype	The appearance or manifestation of a character. External expression the character—tall or dwarf. Phenotype results from the genotype.
Character	An attribute or trait.
Dominant	The character that masks the expression of the recessive trait. Expresses in both homozygous and heterozygous condition.
Recessive	The character that can express only in the absence of the dominant allele and expression takes place only in homozygous condition.

MENDEL'S EXPERIMENT: MONOHYBRID AND DIHYBRID CROSSES

Mendel exploited the seven contrasting characters (Table 1.4) of the pea plant to perform his monohybrid and dihybrid crosses and propose the laws of inheritance based on his observations and results (Figure 1.16).

Table 1.4 Seven contrasting characters of *Pisum sativum*

Character	Dominant Form	Recessive Form
Stem length	Tall	Short
Flower color	Red	White
Flower position	Axial (along the stem)	Terminal (at the tip of the stem)
Seed color	Yellow	Green
Seed (endosperm) shape	Round	Wrinkled
Pod color	Green	Yellow
Pod shape	Inflated	Constricted

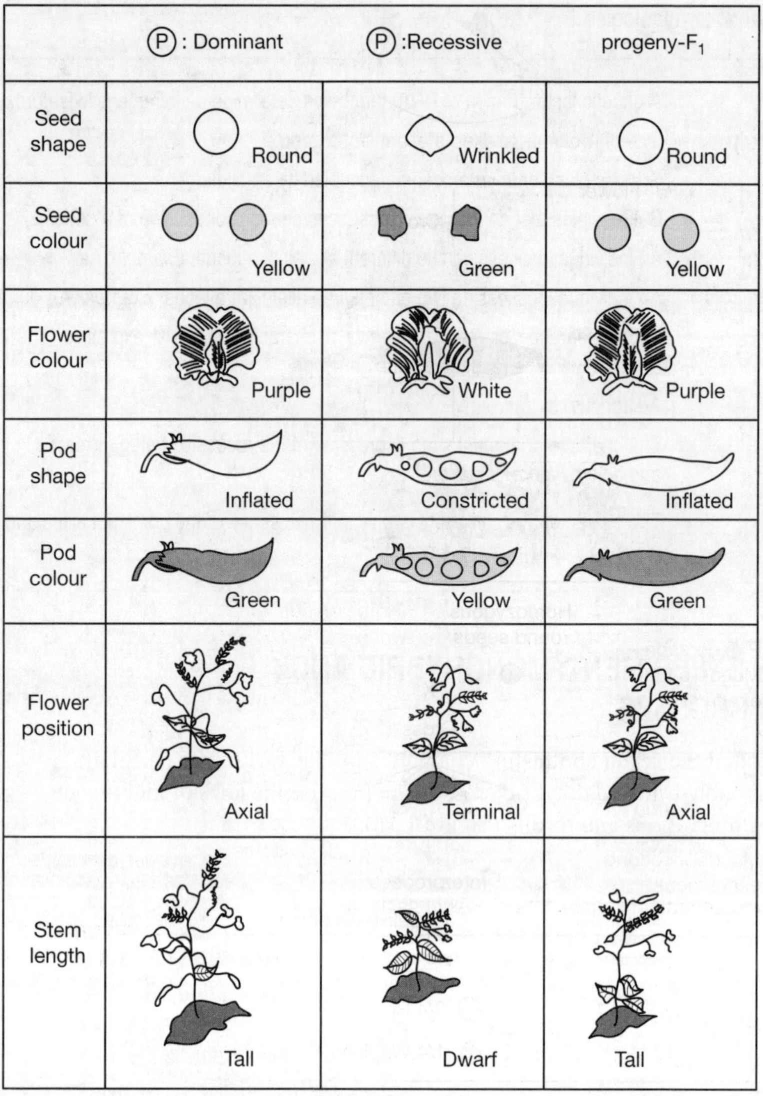

	P : Dominant	P : Recessive	progeny-F$_1$
Seed shape	Round	Wrinkled	Round
Seed colour	Yellow	Green	Yellow
Flower colour	Purple	White	Purple
Pod shape	Inflated	Constricted	Inflated
Pod colour	Green	Yellow	Green
Flower position	Axial	Terminal	Axial
Stem length	Tall	Dwarf	Tall

Figure 1.16 Seven contrasting characters of Mendel's experimental organism. (See page 232 for the colour image.)

Monohybrid
The offspring of individuals that differ with respect to a particular gene pair.

Monohybrid cross

Mendel began his experiments by studying **monohybrid crosses**—those between parents that differed in a single characteristic (example: shape of the seed) (Figure 1.17). Mendel crossed a pea plant homozygous for round seeds with one that was homozygous for wrinkled seed. This first generation of a cross is the **P** (parental) **generation**. After crossing the two varieties in the P generation,

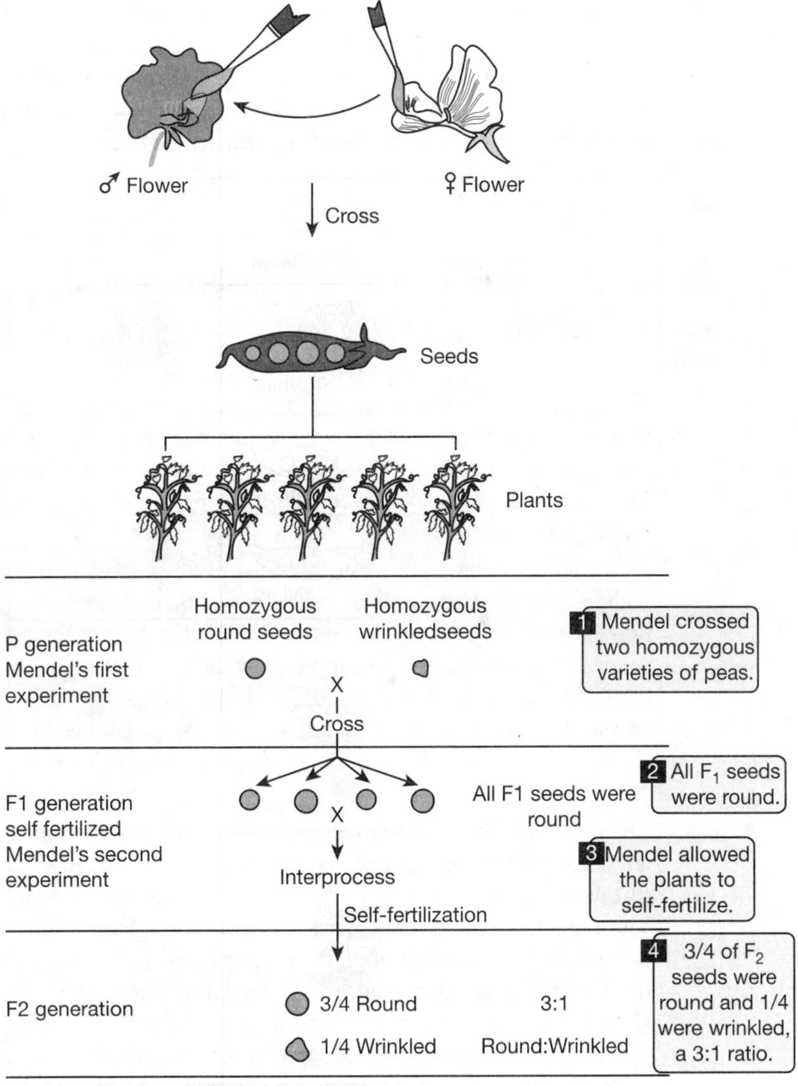

Figure 1.17 Monohybrid cross. (See page 233 for the colour image.)

Mendel observed the offspring that resulted from the cross. The offspring from the parents in the P generation are the **F1** (first filial) **generation**.

When Mendel examined the F1 of this cross, he found that they expressed only one of the phenotypes present in the parental generation, i.e. all the F1 seeds were round. The wrinkled character disappeared in F1.

Inquisitive to explore the results of F1, he planted the F1 seeds, cultivated the plants that germinated from them, and allowed the plants to self-fertilize, producing a second generation (the **F2 generation**). Both the traits (round and wrinkled) from the P generation emerged in the F2; Mendel counted 5474 round seeds and

1850 wrinkled seeds in the F2 generation. He observed that the number of the round and wrinkled seeds constituted approximately a 3:1 ratio; that is, about 75% (3/4) of the F2 seeds were round and 25% (1/4) were wrinkled.

Mendel conducted monohybrid crosses for all seven of the characteristics that he studied in pea plants, and in all of the crosses he obtained the same result: all of the F1 resembled only one of the two parents, but both parental traits emerged in the F2 in a ratio of **3:1**.

Mendel's conclusions from the monohybrid cross

Mendel arrived at several important conclusions from the results of his monohybrid crosses.

1. Though the F1 offspring display the phenotype of only one parent, they must have inherited genetic factors from both parents because they transmit both phenotypes to the F2 generation. The expression of round and wrinkled in the F2 can be explained only if the F1 had inherited the genetic factors coding for both the characters from the parents.

2. He concluded that each plant must therefore possess two genetic factors coding for a character. The genetic factors that Mendel discovered (today known as alleles) are, by convention, denoted by letters; the allele for round seeds (dominant trait) is usually represented by R (*capital letter*), and the allele for wrinkled seeds (recessive trait) by r (*small letter*). The plants in the P generation of Mendel's cross possessed two identical alleles (homozygous): RR in the round-seeded parent and rr in the wrinkled-seeded parent.

3. The next conclusion of Mendel was that during gamete formation, the two alleles in each plant separate and one allele enters one gamete. During fertilization, two gametes (one from each parent) fuse to produce a zygote. Thus, the genotype of the offspring is established by the equal contribution of both the parents. Therefore, the F1 plants have inherited an R allele from the round-seeded plant and an r allele from the wrinkled-seeded plant. However, only the trait encoded by the round allele (R) was *observed* in the F1, since all the F1 progeny had round seeds. Those traits that were expressed in the F1 heterozygous offspring were termed as **dominant**, and those traits that disappeared in the F1 heterozygous offspring he called **recessive**. When dominant and recessive alleles are present together, the recessive allele is masked or suppressed. The principle of dominance was an important conclusion that Mendel derived from his monohybrid crosses.

4. The final conclusion of Mendel from the monohybrid cross was that the two alleles of an individual plant separate with equal probability into the gametes. When plants of the F1 (with genotype Rr) produced gametes, half of the gametes received the R allele for round seeds and half received the r allele for wrinkled seeds. The gametes then paired randomly to produce the following genotypes in equal proportions among the F2: RR, Rr, rR, rr. Because round (R) is dominant over wrinkled (r), there were three round

progeny in the F2 (*RR*, *Rr*, *rR*) and one wrinkled progeny (*rr*) in the F2. This 3:1 ratio of round to wrinkled progeny that Mendel observed in the F2 could occur only if the two alleles of a genotype separated into the gametes with equal probability.

The conclusions that Mendel developed about inheritance from his monohybrid crosses have been formulated into

1. Principle of segregation
2. Concept of dominance

The **principle of segregation** (Mendel's first law) states that each individual diploid organism possesses two alleles for any particular characteristic. These two alleles segregate (separate) during gamete formation, and one allele goes into each gamete. Furthermore, the two alleles segregate into gametes in equal proportions.

The **concept of dominance** states that when two different alleles (dominant and recessive) are present in a genotype, only the trait of the dominant allele is observed in the phenotype.

Dihybrid cross and the principle of independent assortment

Apart from his work on monohybrid crosses, Mendel also crossed varieties of peas that differed in *two* characteristics (**dihybrid crosses**) (Figure 1.18). For example, he took one homozygous variety of pea that produced round seeds and yellow endosperm; another homozygous variety that produced wrinkled seeds and green endosperm. When he crossed the two, all the F1 progeny had **round seeds and yellow endosperm** (dominant trait).

He then self-fertilized the F1 and obtained the following progeny in the F2: 315 round, yellow seeds; 101 wrinkled, yellow seeds; 108 round, green seeds; and 32 wrinkled, green seeds. Mendel recognized that these traits appeared approximately in a **9:3:3:1** ratio; that is, of the

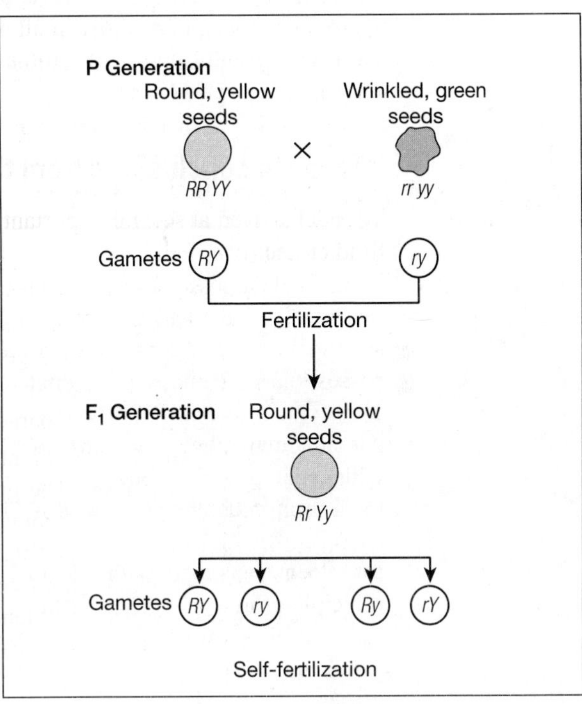

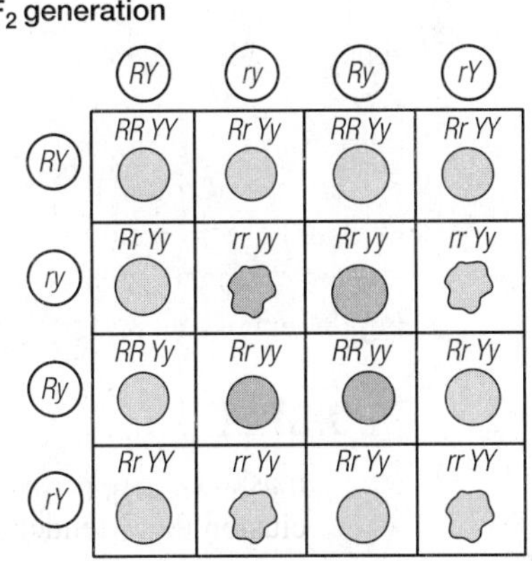

Figure 1.18 Dihybrid cross. (See page 234 for the colour image.)

Dihybrid
The offspring of parents differing in two specific pairs of genes.

progeny were round and yellow, were wrinkled and yellow, were round and green, and were wrinkled and green.

Mendel carried out a number of dihybrid crosses for pairs of characteristics and always obtained a 9:3:3:1 ratio in the F2 generation. Mendel recognized in his dihybrid crosses: the **principle of independent assortment** (Mendel's second law). This principle states that alleles at different loci separate independently of one another.

The principle of independent assortment is an extension of the principle of segregation. The principle of segregation states that the two alleles of a locus separate when gametes are formed; the principle of independent assortment states that, when these two alleles separate, their separation is independent of the separation of alleles at *other* loci.

Each plant possesses two alleles coding for each characteristic, so the parental plants must have had genotypes *RRYY* and *rryy*. According to the principle of segregation, the alleles for each locus separate, and one allele for each locus passes to each gamete. The gametes produced by the round, yellow parent therefore contain alleles *RY*, whereas the gametes produced by the wrinkled, green parent contain alleles *ry*. These two types of gametes unite to produce the F1, all with genotype *RrYy*. Because round is dominant over wrinkled and yellow is dominant over green, the phenotype of the F1 generation will be round and yellow.

When Mendel self-fertilized the F1 plants to produce the F2, the alleles for each locus separated, with one allele going into each gamete. This is where the principle of independent assortment becomes important. Each pair of alleles can separate in two ways: (1) *R* separates with *Y* and *r* separates with *y* to produce gametes *RY* and *ry* or (2) *R* separates with *y* and *r* separates with *Y* to produce gametes *Ry* and *rY*.

The principle of independent assortment shows us that the alleles at each locus separate independently; thus, both kinds of separation occur equally and all four types of gametes (*RY*, *ry*, *Ry*, and *rY*) are produced in equal proportions. When these four types of gametes are combined to produce the F2 generation, the progeny consist of round and yellow, wrinkled and yellow, round and green, and wrinkled and green, resulting in a 9:3:3:1 phenotypic ratio.

Note: Punnett square—The Punnett square is a short-hand method of predicting the genotypic and phenotypic ratios of progeny from a genetic cross.

PEDIGREE

Pedigree
A table/chart recording family history using standard pictorial representation.

An important tool used by geneticists to study human inheritance is the pedigree. A **pedigree** is a pictorial representation of a family history; a family tree that outlines the inheritance of characteristics. The symbols commonly used in pedigrees are summarized in Figure 1.19.

Inheritance
The process of genetic transmission of traits from parents to offspring.

PATTERNS OF INHERITANCE IN HUMANS

The human genome is vast and complex and this increases the complexity in analysing and understanding human genetic diseases. This also emphasizes the importance of analysing and exploring human heredity. This field has evolved with the contribution by renowned geneticists who have developed tools and techniques, which have helped the scientific community understand human biology and genetics dynamically.

Males in a pedigree are represented by squares, females by circles. A horizontal line drawn between two symbols representing a man and a woman indicates a mating; children are connected to their parents by vertical lines extending below the parents. Persons who exhibit the genetic trait (affected individuals) are represented by filled circles and squares. Unaffected persons are represented by open circles and squares. Each generation in a pedigree is identified by a Roman numeral; within each generation, family members are assigned Arabic numerals, and children in each family are listed in birth order from left to right. Deceased family members are indicated by a slash through the circle or square. Twins are represented by diagonal lines extending from a common point (non-identical twins). When a particular characteristic or disease is observed in a person, a geneticist studies the family of this affected person and draws a pedigree. The person from whom the pedigree is initiated is called the **proband/consultand** and is usually designated by an arrow.

Pedigree is a fundamental technique used in genetic counselling and genetic testing services to identify and understand the mode of inheritance and transmission of a genetic trait, calculate the recurrence risk, and document the personal family history along with medical history of the proband. Pedigree helps in identifying autosomal recessive traits through consanguinity.

Transmission of characters from one generation to another is termed as heredity as this transmission takes place through genes present on chromosomes. Human chromosomes are broadly classified as autosomes and sex chromosomes and hence the inheritance of genes on the autosomes is termed as autosomal inheritance and the inheritance of the genes on the sex chromosomes are termed as sex-linked inheritance.

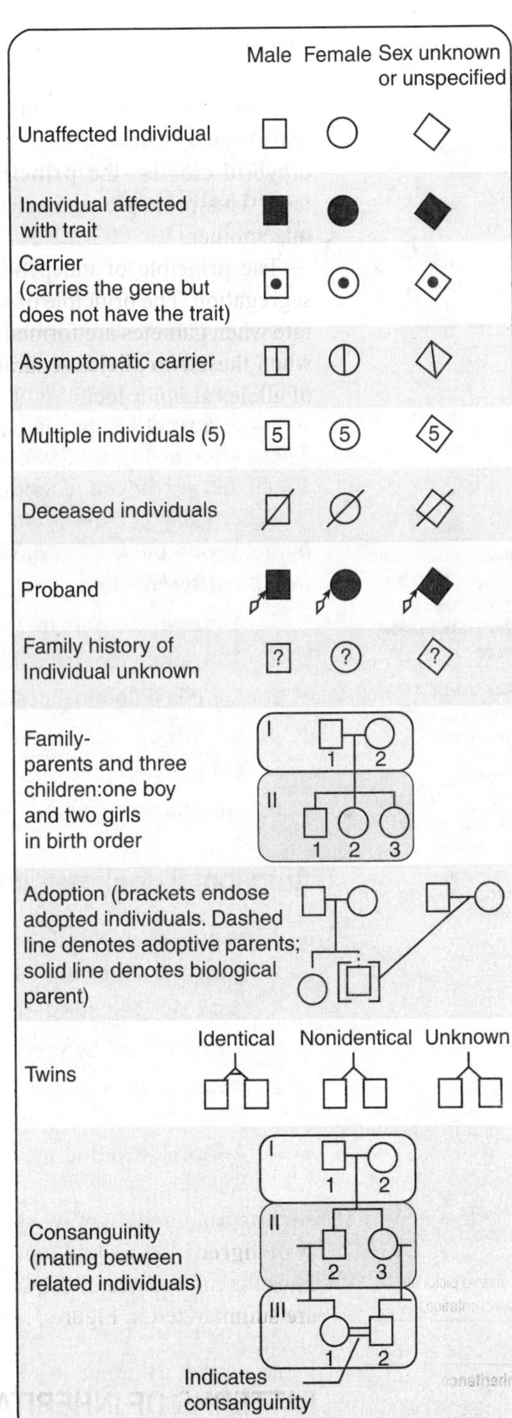

Figure 1.19 Pedigree notations. (See page 235 for the colour image.)

Females posses the karyotype 46,XX [23 pairs of chromosomes; where 22 pairs are autosomes and 1 pair are sex chromosomes (XX)].

Males posses the karyotype 46,XY [23 pairs of chromosomes; where 22 pairs are autosomes and 1 pair are sex chromosomes (XY)].

During gamete formation (spermatogenesis/oogenesis), the diploid state of the parent cell is halved (reductional division; meiosis) and the gamete contains 23,X/23, Y (sperms), while the ovum contributes only 23, X (since females are homozygous for the X chromosome.

Autosomes are common to both males and females and hence autosomal inheritance is expressed in both the sexes with equal frequency, whereas sex-linked inheritance is dominated by the inheritance of the alternate sex chromosomes X and Y, and their transmission through the germ cells (sperm/ovum) is based on the law of segregation and independent assortment as directed by Mendel's laws. There also exists the phenomenon of dominance and recessiveness in both autosomal and sex-linked inheritance,

Refer Chapter 5 on Mendelian inheritance for dominance, recessiveness and homozygous and heterozygous alleles.

The different patterns of inheritance in humans are as follows:

1. Autosomal dominant inheritance
2. Autosomal recessive inheritance
3. X-Linked dominant inheritance
4. X-Linked recessive inheritance
5. Mitochondrial inheritance
6. Multifactorial inheritance

Proband/Consultand
A patient who is the initial member of a family to come under study.

Autosomal
Pertaining to autosomal chromosome.

Sex-linked
Determined by a gene located in a sex chromosome.

Autosomal dominant inheritance

1. Expresses in both sexes with equal frequency (autosomal).
2. Both sexes transmit the trait to their offspring.
3. Does not skip generations.
4. Characterized by vertical transmission.
5. Presence of a single defective allele is sufficient for disease expression (dominant).
6. Affected offspring must have an affected parent, unless they possess a new mutation.
7. When one parent is affected (heterozygous) and the other parent is unaffected, approximately ½ (50%) of the offspring will be affected.
8. All the offspring of a homozygous parent are affected (100% penetrance).
9. Unaffected parents do not transmit the trait.

Examples: Huntington's Disease, polydactyly, familial hypercholesterolemia, achondroplasia.

Pedigree depicting autosomal dominant inheritance is represented in Figure 1.20.

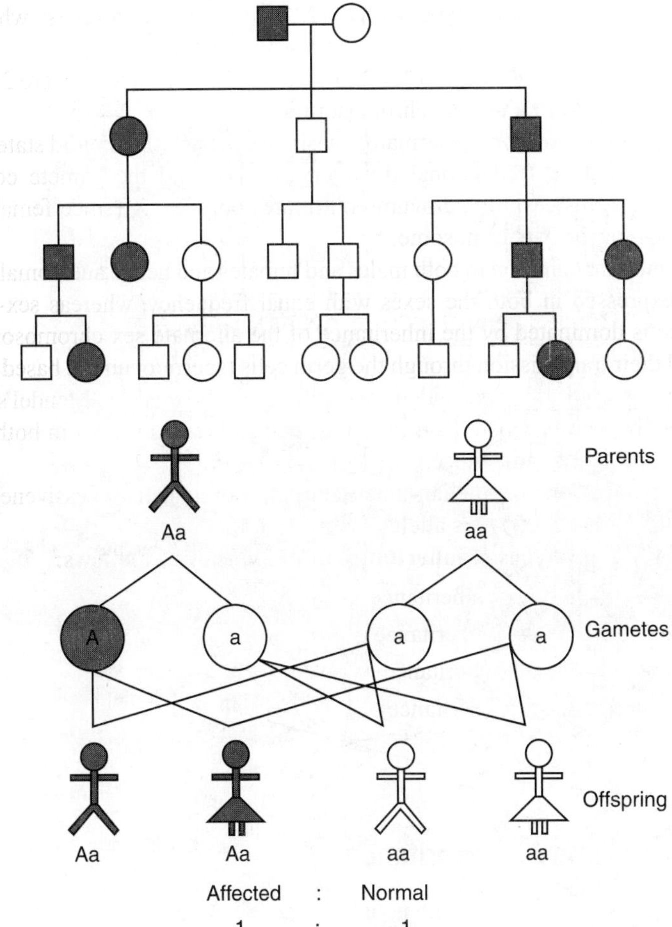

Figure 1.20 Autosomal dominant inheritance. (See page 236 for the colour image.)

Autosomal recessive inheritance

1. Expresses in both sexes with equal frequency (autosomal).
2. Trait tends to skip generations.
3. Characterized by horizontal transmission.
4. Presence of both the defective alleles is required for disease expression (recessive).
5. Affected offspring are usually born to unaffected parents (carriers).
6. When both parents are heterozygous, approximately ¼ (25%) of the offspring will be affected.
7. Appears more frequently among the children of consanguineous marriages.

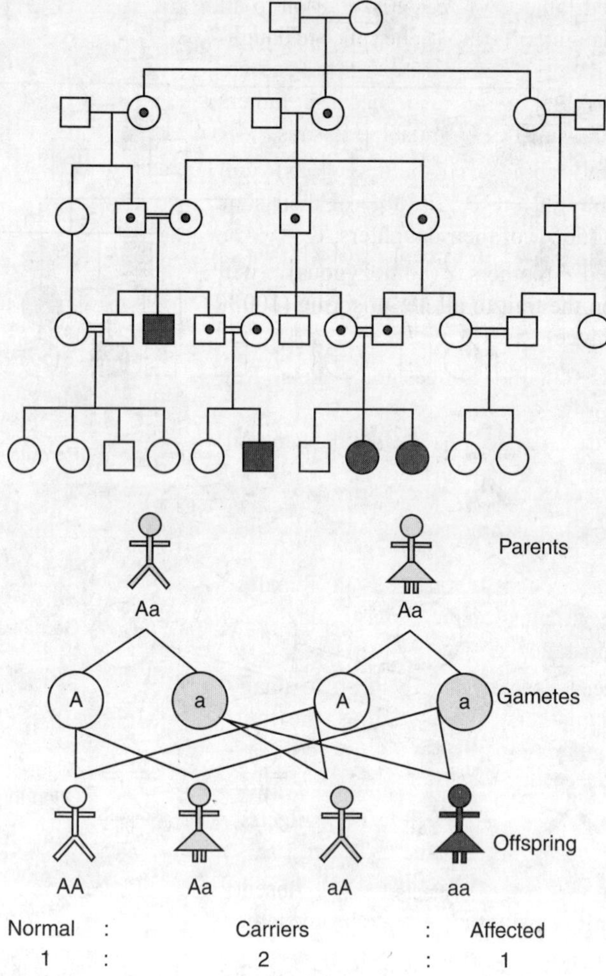

Figure 1.21 Autosomal recessive inheritance. (See page 237 for the colour image.)

Examples: Most human metabolic diseases, Tay–Sachs disease, thalassemia, cystic fibrosis, sickle cell anaemia.

Pedigree depicting autosomal recessive inheritance is represented in Figure 1.21.

X-linked dominant inheritance

1. Both males and females are affected; often females are more affected than males.
2. Does not skip generations.
3. Affected sons must have an affected mother (males receive their X chromosome only from their mother); affected daughters must have either an affected mother or an affected father (females receive a copy of X from both the parents).

4. Affected fathers will pass the trait on to all their daughters (100% penetrance to daughters, since it's a dominant trait). Sons are not affected in this case because fathers don't transmit X chromosome to sons.

5. Affected mothers (if heterozygous) will pass the trait on to ½ (50%) of their sons and ½ (50%) of their daughters.

6. Affected mothers (homozygous) will pass on the trait to all her offspring (100% penetrance)

Examples: Vitamin D-resistant rickets, Rett Syndrome, Goltz Syndrome.

Pedigree depicting X-linked dominant inheritance is represented in Figure 1.22.

X-linked recessive inheritance

1. Males are more affected than females (since males have only one X chromosome).

2. Affected sons are usually born to unaffected mothers (carriers); thus, the trait skips generations.

3. A carrier (heterozygous) mother produces approximately ½ (50%) affected sons.

4. Father to son transmission is absent (fathers transmit only the Y chromosome to their sons).

5. All daughters of affected fathers are carriers.

Examples: Duchene muscular dystrophy, hemophilia, fragile X syndrome, Lesch Nyhan Syndrome.

Pedigree depicting X-linked recessive inheritance is represented in Figure 1.23.

Y-linked inheritance

1. Only males are affected.

2. Characterized by father to son transmission (also known as **holandric** inheritance).

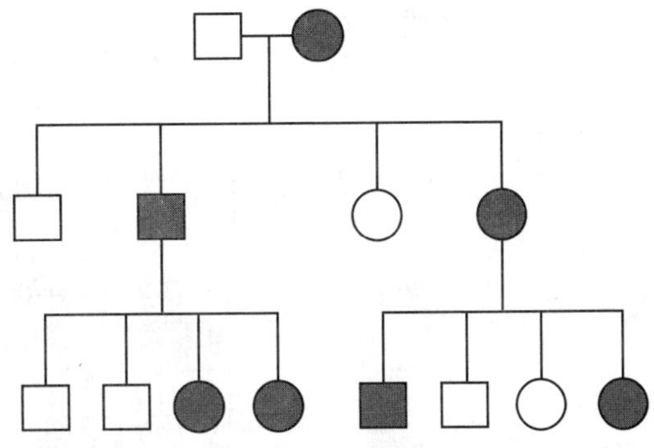

Figure 1.22 X-linked dominant inheritance. (See page 237 for the colour image.)

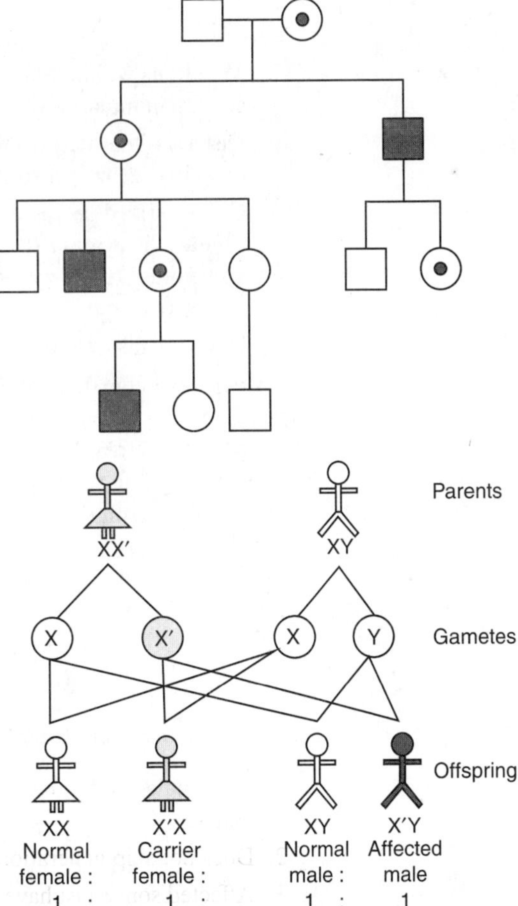

Figure 1.23 X-linked recessive inheritance. (See page 238 for the colour image.)

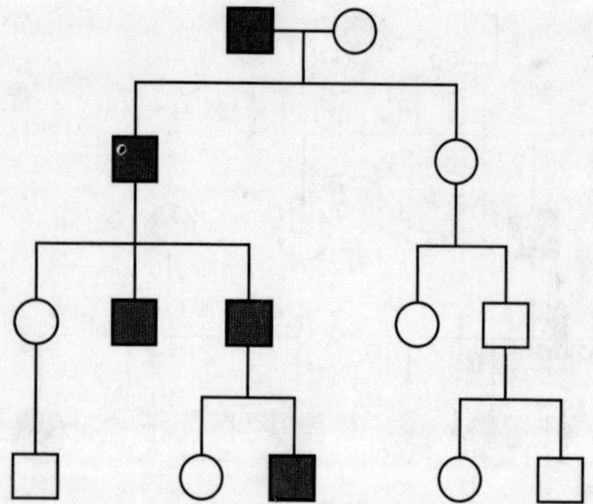

Figure 1.24 Y-linked inheritance. (See page 238 for the colour image.)

3. Does not skip generations.

Examples: Baldness, hairy ears, webbed toes, porcupine skin.

Pedigree depicting Y-linked inheritance is represented in Figure 1.24.

Mitochondrial inheritance

1. The mitochondria (power house of the cell) are autonomous organelles that contain their own DNA. This mitochondrial DNA consists of 16 569 base pairs that constitute 37 genes. There is some difference in the genetic code between the nuclear and mitochondrial genomes, and mitochondrial DNA is almost exclusively coding, with the genes containing no intervening sequences.

2. Mutations within mitochondrial DNA appear to be 5 or 10 times more common than mutations in nuclear DNA.

3. Diseases inherited from mutated mitochondrial genes are known as mitochondrial genetic disorders.

4. Characterized by maternal transmission (during fertilization, the ova contributes the cytoplasm along with cell organelles. The mitochondria are also transmitted to the zygote from the mother; the sperm contributes only the nucleus).

5. Descendants of affected fathers are unaffected.

Examples: Leber hereditary optic neuropathy (LHON), myoclonic epilepsy with ragged red fibres (MERRF), mitochondrial myopathy with encephalopathy, lactic acidosis, stroke-like episodes (MELAS), and progressive external ophthalmoplegia including Kaerns–Sayre Syndrome.

Pedigree depicting mitochondrial inheritance is represented in Figure 1.25.

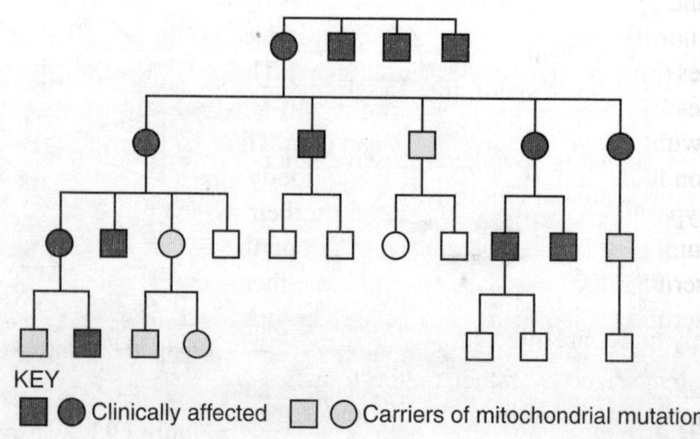

Figure 1.25 Mitochondrial inheritance. (See page 239 for the colour image.)

Multifactorial inheritance

1. The phenomenon of multifactorial inheritance implies that a disease is caused by the interaction of several genetic and environmental factors.
2. Members of family affected with a multifactorial disorder have a genetic predisposition to develop the disorder in combination with lifestyle (environmental factors).

Examples: Diabetes, cancer, coronary heart disease, schizophrenia.

MULTIPLE ALLELES AND BLOOD GROUPS

Mendelian genetics designates that genetic systems consist of two alleles. In Mendel's experiment with peas, for instance, one allele coded for round seeds and another for wrinkled seeds; in cats, one allele produced a black coat and another produced a gray coat. For some loci, more than two alleles are present within a group of individuals—the locus has **multiple alleles** (multiple alleles may also be referred to as an *allelic series*). Although there may be more than two alleles present within a *group*, the genotype of each diploid *individual* still consists of only two alleles. The inheritance of characteristics encoded by multiple alleles is no different from the inheritance of characteristics encoded by two alleles, except that a greater variety of genotypes and phenotypes are possible.

Multiple alleles
Three or more alternative forms of a gene existing in a population.

The classic example of multiple human alleles is in the ABO blood group, which Karl Landsteiner discovered in 1900. This is the best known of all the red-cell antigen systems primarily because of its importance in blood trans-fusions.

THE ABO BLOOD GROUP

There are four blood-type phenotypes produced by three alleles. The three common alleles for the ABO blood group locus are: *I*A, which codes for the A antigen; *I*B, which codes for the B antigen; and *i*, which codes for no antigen (O).

Antigen
Any substance that can stimulate the production of antibodies and combine specifically with them.

The *I*A and *I*B alleles are responsible for the production of the A and B antigens found on the surface of the erythrocytes (red blood cells). Antigens are substances, normally foreign to the body, that induce the immune system to produce antibodies (proteins that bind to the antigens). The ABO system is unusual because antibodies can be present (for example, anti-B antibodies can exist in a type A person) without prior exposure to the antigen. Thus, people with a particular ABO antigen on their red cells will have the antibody against the other antigen in their serum: type A persons have A antigen on their red cells and anti-B antibody in their serum; type B persons have B antigen on their red cells and anti-A antibody in their serum; type O persons do not have either antigen but have both antibodies in their serum; and type AB persons have both A and B antigens and form neither anti-A or anti-B antibodies in their serum.

Antibody
A protein substance produced in the blood or tissues in response to a specific antigen, forming the basis of immunity.

We can represent the dominance relations among the ABO alleles as follows: *I*A _ *i*, *I*B _ *i*, *I*A _ *I*B. The *I*A and *I*B alleles are both dominant over *i* and are codominant with each other; the AB phenotype is due to the presence of an *I*A

Pheno type	Geno type	Antigen type	Antibodies made by body	Blood-recipient reactions to donor-blood antibodies			
				A (B anti bodies)	B (A anti bodies)	AB (no anti bodies)	O (A and B antibodies)
A	I^AI^A or I^Ai	A	B				
B	I^BI^B or I^Bi	B	A				
AB	I^AI^B	A and B	None				
O	ii	None	A and B				

Red blood cells that do not react with the recipient antibody remain evently disposed. Donor blood and recipient blood are compatiable.

Blood cells that react with the recipient antibody clump together. Donor blood and recipient blood are not compatible.

Type O donors can donate to any recipient: they are universal donors.

Type AB recipients can accept blood from any donor: they are universal recipients

Blood Type Corresponding to Antigens on Red Blood Cells	Antibodies in Serum	Genotype	Reaction of Red Cells to Anti-A Antibodies	Reaction of Red Cells to Anti-B Antibodies
O	Anti-A and anti-B	ii	–	–
A	Anti-B	I^AI^A or I^Ai	+	–
B	Anti-A	I^BI^B or I^Bi	–	+
AB	None	I^AI^B	+	+

Figure 1.26 ABO blood group system—Genotypes and phenotypes. (See page 239 for the colour image.)

allele and an *I*B allele, which results in the production of A and B antigens on red blood cells. An individual with genotype *ii* produces neither antigen and has blood type O. The six common genotypes at this locus and their phenotypes are shown in Figure 1.26.

FUNCTION OF *I*A, *I*B AND *I* ALLELES OF THE ABO GENE

The *I*A and *I*B alleles, coding for glycosyl transferase enzymes, each cause a different modification to the terminal sugars of a mucopolysaccharide (H structure) found on the surface of red blood cells (Figure 1.27). They are codominant because both modifications (antigens) are present in a heterozygote. In fact, whichever enzyme (product of the *I*A or *I*B allele) reaches the H structure first will modify it. Once modified, the H structure will not respond to the other enzyme. Therefore, both A and B antigens will be produced in the heterozygote in roughly equal proportions. The *i* allele causes no change to the

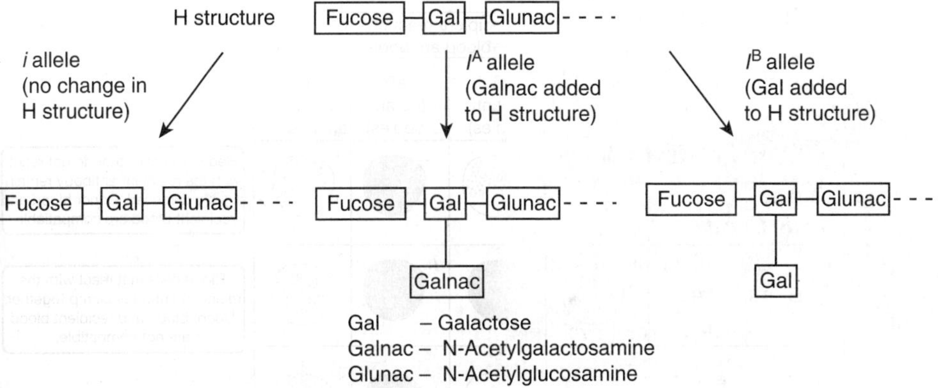

Figure 1.27 Function of *IA*, *IB* and *I* alleles of the ABO gene.

H structure: because of a mutation it produces a non-functioning enzyme. The *i* allele and its phenotype are recessive; the presence of the *IA* or *IB* allele, or both, will modify the H product, thus masking the fact that the *i* allele was ever there.

Adverse reactions to blood transfusions primarily occur because the antibodies in the recipient's serum react with the antigens on the donor's red blood cells. Thus, type A persons cannot donate blood to type B persons. Type B persons have anti-A antibody, which reacts with the A antigen on the donor red cells and causes the cells to clump. Since both *IA* and *IB* are dominant to the *i* allele, this system not only shows multiple allelism, it also demonstrates both codominance and simple dominance.

According to the American Red Cross, 46% of blood donors in the United States are type O, 40% are type A, 10% are type B, and 4% are type AB. Many other genes also have multiple alleles.

Codominance
Two different alleles that are fully expressed in a heterozygous individual.

OTHER GENETIC SYSTEMS THAT EXHIBIT MULTIPLE ALLELISM

In some plants, such as red clover, there is a gene, the S gene, with several hundred alleles that prevent self-fertilization. This means that a pollen grain is not capable of forming a successful pollen tube in the style if the pollen grain or its parent plant has a self-incompatibility allele that is also present in the plant to be fertilized. Thus, pollen grains from a flower falling on its own stigma are rejected. Only a pollen grain with either a different self-incompatibility allele or from a parent plant with different self-incompatibility alleles is capable of fertilization; this avoids inbreeding. Thus, over evolutionary time, there has been selection for many alleles of this gene.

Recent research has indicated that the products of the *S* alleles are ribonuclease enzymes, enzymes that destroy RNA. Researchers are interested in discovering the molecular mechanisms for this pollen rejection.

In *Drosophila*, numerous alleles of the white-eye gene exist, and people (humans) have numerous hemoglobin alleles. In fact, multiple alleles are more of a rule rather than the exception/deviation.

More than two alleles (multiple alleles) may be present within a group of individuals, although each diploid individual still has only two alleles at that locus.

REVIEW QUESTION

Essay Question

1. Explain in detail with diagrams the difference between prokaryotic and eukaryotic cell.
2. Explain the cell cycle in detail with appropriate diagrams.
3. Explain the M phase in detail with relevant illustrations.
4. Explain the process of cytokinesis.
5. Describe the organization of genetic material in chromosomes in detail with relevant diagrams. Add a note on DNA packaging.
6. Describe the structure of chromosomes. Add a note on sex chromosomes and the different forms/anatomy of chromosomes.
7. Define mutation. Explain the different structural chromosomal abnormalities in detail with illustrative diagrams.
8. Describe the various numerical chromosomal abnormalities with clinical examples.
9. Explain the laws of dominance and segregation using a monohybrid cross.
10. Explain dihybrid cross using a Punnett square and add a note on the principle of independent assortment.
11. Explain the advantages of the experimental organism of Mendel. Add a note on Mendel's early life.
12. Define pedigree. Explain its application in genetic counselling in brief.
13. Compare autosomal and sex-linked inheritance with relevant pedigree and examples.
14. Explain the multiple allele system with a classic example. Add a note on the function of the three alleles of the ABO gene.

Short Notes

1. Write short notes on the following:
   (a) Mitosis
   (b) Interphase
   (c) Cytokinesis
   (d) Cleavage furrow
   (e) Metaphase
   (f) Centromere
   (g) Centrosomes
   (h) Spindle fibres
   (i) Eukaryotic cell

  (j) Nucleus
  (k) Cell organelles
2. Write short notes on the following:
  (a) Chromosome structure
  (b) Nucleosomes
  (c) Histones
  (d) Sex chromosomes
  (e) Forms of chromosomes
  (f) Sex determination in humans
3. Write short notes on the following:
  (a) Mutation
  (b) Chromosomal rearrangement
  (c) Aneuploidy
  (d) Numerical chromosomal abnormalities
  (e) Duplication
  (f) Deletion
  (g) Inversion
  (h) Translocation
  (i) Polyploidy
4. Write short notes on the following:
  (a) Mendel's experimental organism
  (b) Seven contrasting traits of *Pisum sativum* in Mendel's experiments
  (c) Monohybrid ratio
  (d) Dihybrid ratio
  (e) Punnett square
  (f) Law of independent assortment
  (g) Law of segregation
5. Write short notes on the following:
  (a) Draw 10 pedigree notations with appropriate explanations.
  (b) Autosomal dominant inheritance—features and examples.
  (c) Autosomal recessive inheritance—features and examples.
  (d) Holandric inheritance—features and examples.
  (e) Mitochondrial inheritance—features and examples.
  (f) Sex-linked inheritance—features and examples.
  (g) Multifactorial inheritance—features and examples.
6. Write short notes on the following:
  (a) Multiple alleles
  (b) ABO blood group system—genotypes and phenotypes
  (c) Function of ABO gene and its alleles

2

Explain Maternal, Prenatal and Genetic Influences on Development of Defects and Diseases

INFECTIONS DURING PREGNANCY

Bacterial infections

Bacterial infections are a part of our life, either as a symbiotic partner or as a pathological agent (Figure 2.1). Pregnant women are susceptible to infections during pregnancy and her immune system works in focus by upregulation to fight infections and down regulation to prevent foetal rejection. These two processes coexist; however, they do not counteract each other. The bacterial infections most often associated with pregnancy are urinary tract infections, genital tract infections, and pulmonary and some other rarer cases of dermatological and central nervous system involvements.

The growing foetus is a potential target that requires the mother's immune system to remain intact to protect itself from bacterial infections. A pregnant woman has defined immunological barriers that are different from a non-pregnant woman. Under normal physiological conditions the endometrial cavity has no normal flora. Only when the functional tissue undergoes changes in mucosal integrity and the presence of blood and necrotic deciduas can it sustain bacterial colonization. The foetus has its own innate immune system: that of amniotic fluid, which surrounds the foetus. It has bacteriostatic properties, which inhibit bacterial growth. Amniotic fluid has been shown to be ineffective in suppressing the growth of common organisms in premature gestations; however, at term it can suppress the growth of bacteria for up to 32 hours.

One of the risks associated with bacterial infections is preterm labour. The cascade of events that have been hypothesized to cause premature labour consists of bacteria-releasing endotoxins (lipopolysaccharides) or exotoxins that initiate cytokine and interleukin responses. These responses in turn affect the decidua, membranes, or prostaglandin production that leads to uterine contractions. With these contractions come cervical dilation and a potential opening for more microbes into the uterus. Other risks associated with bacterial infection include maternal or neonatal sepsis, foetal distress, and foetal demise.

The bacteria may enter the amniotic cavity by the following pathways:

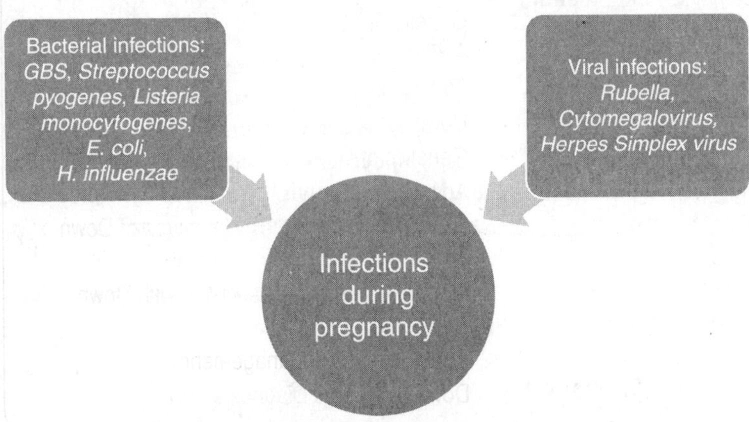

Figure 2.1 Common infections during pregnancy—bacterial and viral.

1. Ascending from either the cervix or vagina.
2. Hematogenous spread with transplacental passage, usually associated with maternal bacteremia.
3. Entry through the fallopian tubes or peritoneal cavity.
4. Nosocomial through amniocentesis or chorionic villus sampling.

The most common of these pathways is ascending infection. The most prevalent bacteria associated with maternal or foetal risks during gestation include many exogenous and endogenous organisms.

Exogenous pathogens include *Chlamydia trachomatis*, *Bordetella pertussis*, *Calmymmatobacterium granulomatis*, *Hemophilus ducreyi* (Chancroid), *Hemophilus influenza*, *Listeria monocytogenes*, *Neissiera gonorrhoeae*, *Salmonella typhi*, and Group A β -hemolytic streptococci (*Streptococcus pyogenes*).

Endogenous pathogens include Bacteroidacea, Clostridia, *Escherichia coli*, *Gardnerella vaginallis* (*Hemophilus vaginallis*), *Proteus*, *Staphylococcus aureus*, *Staphylococcus epidermidis*, and Group B hemolytic streptococci.

Group B beta-hemolytic streptococci (GBS)

Group B beta-hemolytic streptococci (GBS) are gram-positive cocci that grow in chains. They lack a protein, which exists on the Group A streptococci, and hence demonstrates a different degree of virulence. GBS is a normal constituent of the vaginal flora and the gastrointestinal tract. Foecal colonization exceeds any other colonization rates. Between 14 and 25% of pregnant women may be continually, intermittently, or transiently colonized. GBS is rarely a cause of maternal morbidity. It is, however, the most common cause of neonatal sepsis, meningitis, and pneumonia.

Group A beta-hemolytic streptococcus (*Streptococcus pyogenes*)

Streptococcus pyogenes is a gram-positive cocci. Its capsule contains hyaluronic acid, which lyses endothelium cells, and it has the M protein to interfere with phagocytic cells. Infections are associated with puerperal sepsis, prepubertal vulvovaginitis, endometritis–salpingitis–peritonitis, and necrotizing fascitis. In gravid women *Streptococcus pyogenes* can be present as part of the normal vaginal flora; however, infections can occur if there is a break in the mucosal epithelial barrier. Clinically, it presents as a high maternal fever and uterine tenderness. Other evidence of infection of the uterus and pelvis can include leukocytosis, tachycardia, edematous soft uterus, and a serosanguinous vaginal discharge. Maternal septicemia will occur before foetal involvement occurs, but with ruptured membranes, it can ascend to infect the foetus, amniotic fluid, and chorion. Treatment includes penicillin, ampicillin, or vancomycin.

Listeria monocytogenes

Listeria monocytogenes is a gram-positive, catalase-positive bacillus in the corynebacteriaceae family. Infections occur more frequently in pregnant women compared to the general population at a rate of 12 per 100,000. The gastrointestinal tract is the most likely usual reservoir for *Listeria monocytogenes*. The depressed cell-mediated immunity during pregnancy may be responsible for the unusual high incidence in pregnant women. Maternal infections can present as a mononucleosis-like syndrome with a short duration. However, foetal death may occur. Contaminated food may be a likely source. If Listeria chorioamnionitis is diagnosed preterm, in utero therapy with high-dose penicillin or trimethoprim-sulfamethoxazole should be attempted in order to avoid the high risk of preterm delivery. Preterm labour occurs in 50% of cases. Treatment may include ampicillin with clavulanic acid, erythromycin, or trimethoprim-sulfamethoxazole. The most effective strategy to prevent this disease is to eliminate the most likely source; contaminated food.

Haemophilus influenzae

Haemophilus influenzae is a gram-negative capsulated coccus that forms short chains. Its prevalence is low, but it has a high infectious rate. Infections associated with this organism include meningitis, epiglotitis, pneumonia, otitis, and bronchitis. There is a higher correlation with postpartum maternal infections than neonatal disease. Treatment includes cefotaxime, ceftriaxone, or trimethoprim-sulfamethoxazole.

Escherichia coli

Escherichia coli is a motile gram-negative bacillus, which is part of the normal flora of the intestine and vagina. It is by far, the most common cause of urinary tract infections (UTI) and neonatal sepsis with an incidence is 0.5–1.5 cases per 1000 live births. It is also associated with chorioamnionitis, postpartum endometritis, and septic abortions, often a part of a polymicrobial infection. UTIs in pregnancy are associated with pyelonephritis and preterm labor. They have also been known to increase IgM lymphoblastic responses in neonates. Treatment is with cephalosporins, trimethoprim-sulfamethaxazole, ampicillin with clavulanic acid, or gentamicin, depending on the site.

Viral infections

Viruses are ubiquitous in our surroundings, producing a range of clinical manifestations when infecting humans. Viral agents also infect the pregnant human host and such infections traverse the maternal–placental barrier to result in a variety of outcomes for the foetus. These outcomes vary depending on the specific viral agent, the period of gestation at which the infection occurs, the maternal immune status, and the mechanism of action of the virus on the foetal host. The impact of a maternal viral infection on the foetus ranges from abortion, stillbirth, preterm labour and delivery, physical defects, intrauterine growth disturbances, and the postnatal persistence of infection. Many viral agents have been reported to affect the developing foetus in utero, transmission occurring by the transplacental passage of the virus during the period of maternal viremia. Ascending infection from the lower genital tract or local extension from adjacent upper genital or gastrointestinal tract infections are also portals of entry for viruses to the foetoplacental unit.

The mechanisms by which viral agents may produce adverse effects on the foetus include placental dysfunction secondary to maternal infection (fever, toxins, altered placental circulation, thrombosis, or placentitis producing hypoxia with altered cell growth and subsequent foetal damage), chromosomal damage, cellular necrosis, and antigen–antibody formation.

Rubella

The rubella virus produces an acute, contagious exanthem that usually occurs in epidemics. A single-stranded RNA Togavirus, the rubella virus, is spread by nasopharyngeal droplets from which the virus implants and multiplies in the respiratory epithelium, with an incubation period of 14–21 days. The typical maculopapular rash and generalized lymphadenopathy of rubella infection is preceded by a short period of prodromal symptomatology with malaise, fever, headache, conjunctivitis, and pharyngitis. The duration of the rash is usually 3 days, commencing on the face and migrating caudally.

It is the potential teratogenic effect of the rubella virus in pregnancy that produces most concern. Intrauterine transmission of the virus occurs after primary infection of the mother. The gestational age of the foetus at the time of maternal infection is the principal factor determining pregnancy outcome. Defects attributable to rubella result from infections occurring before 16 weeks of gestation. Infections beyond 16–20 weeks of gestation do not appear to result in congenital anomalies, probably because of foetal structural development and developing immunologic competence. The frequency of foetal rubella infection after clinical maternal infection is more than 80 % during the first 12 weeks of pregnancy, 54 % at 13–14 weeks, and 25 % at the end of the second trimester.

Cytomegalovirus

Cytomegalovirus (CMV) is a double-stranded DNA herpes virus and is highly species specific. The Herpesvirus family is characterized by latency and reactivation phenomena. CMV is not highly contagious; it spreads by close contact with infected secretions. CMV may be excreted in the urine and bodily secretions of those infected, and viral transmission to an uninfected host occurs by close body contact. Human blood, marrow, or organs may be a source of infection if received from a seropositive donor.

The newborn may be congenitally infected by the transplacental passage of virus from mother to foetus in utero or the virus may be perinatally acquired from contact with maternal genital tract secretions or breast milk. The severity of congenital infection appears to be related to the gestational age at the time of exposure to the virus. Infection occurs with similar frequency in all trimesters although in the first half of pregnancy the risk of significant foetal anomalies is greater. The overall rate of vertical transmission for CMV is in the order of 35–40 %.

Herpes simplex virus

Herpes simplex virus (HSV), a double-stranded DNA virus, produces a range of infections. HSV type 2 is most often associated with genital herpes infection. The herpes virus has the ability to reactivate intermittently after a primary infection, between periods of latency in the body. The sites of latency are the central nervous system sensory ganglia. Most herpes infections in pregnancy represent recurrent disease, with the recurrence rate increasing as gestation advances. HSV damages the neonate mainly through *intrapartum* infections, but can also cause congenital disease. Congenital HSV is a distinct entity and is not related to perinatally acquired HSV occurring around the time of birth. There is an associated increase in spontaneous abortions and stillbirths with primary HSV infections, especially in the first half of pregnancy.

The foetal effects that have been reported include cutaneous defects (scars, calcifications, vesicles), microcephaly, hydranencephaly, cerebral and cerebellar necrosis, intracranial calcification, microphthalmia, hepatosplenomegaly, chorioretinitis, and bone anomalies. Primary HSV infection in early pregnancy has been associated with as high as a 10% incidence of central nervous system and musculoskeletal defects in the foetus. The transplacental transmission of HSV and secondary foetal infection may produce a severe in utero infection leading to foetal death.

CONSANGUINITY ATOPY

When partners are related to each other by blood, it increases the likelihood of having children with certain birth defects. There are a number of harmful or lethal genetic mutations that follow autosomal recessive inheritance and since consanguineous couples have a higher proportion of their genes in common, they are more likely to carry the same rare genetic mutation. A genetic counsellor can assess family medical histories, ethnicity, and coefficient of relationship for such couples, educate them about their risks, and offer genetic testing when appropriate.

CONSANGUINEOUS MARRIAGE AND RISK OF INHERITING GENETIC DISORDER

Consanguinity is an important indication used for genetic assessment because of the increased risk of autosomal recessive disorders occurring in the children born to consanguineous couples. In marriages between first cousins the probability that the child inherits the same recessive gene from both parents that originated from one of the common grandparents is 1 in 64. A different recessive gene may similarly be transmitted from the other common grandparent so that the risk of homozygosity for a recessive disorder in the child is 1 in 32. If everyone carries two recessive genes, the risk would be 1 in 16.

Marriage between first cousins generally increases the risk of genetic abnormality and mortality in offspring by 3–5% compared with that in the general population.

The increased risk associated with marriage between second cousins is around 1%. Marriage between first and second-degree relatives is almost universally illegal, although marriages between uncles and nieces occur in some Asian countries. Marriage between third-degree relatives (between cousins or half uncles and nieces) is more common (Figure 2.2).

The offspring of incestuous relationships are at high risk of severe abnormality, mental retardation, and childhood death. Only about half of the children born to couples who are first-degree relatives are normal, and this has important implications for decisions about termination of pregnancy or subsequent adoption.

Refer to Autosomal Recessive Inheritance for mode of inheritance of genetic disorders in consanguineous marriages.

A classic example of inheritance of genetic disorder due to consanguineous marriage is the family history of haemophilia expression in the Queen's family in England. So much so the disease was called a Royal Disease since it was observed only in members of the royal family. It was later attributed to the fact that haemophilia was a recessive disorder, and marriage between close relatives was very common in the Royal family. This in turn lead to an understanding that the disease-causing allele of haemophilia was circulating between members of the family (carriers) and when such carriers married their offspring expressed the disease condition. The pedigree below shows the inheritance of haemophilia in the Royal family (Figure 2.3). Note: the disease expression has disappeared after the end of consanguineous marriages.

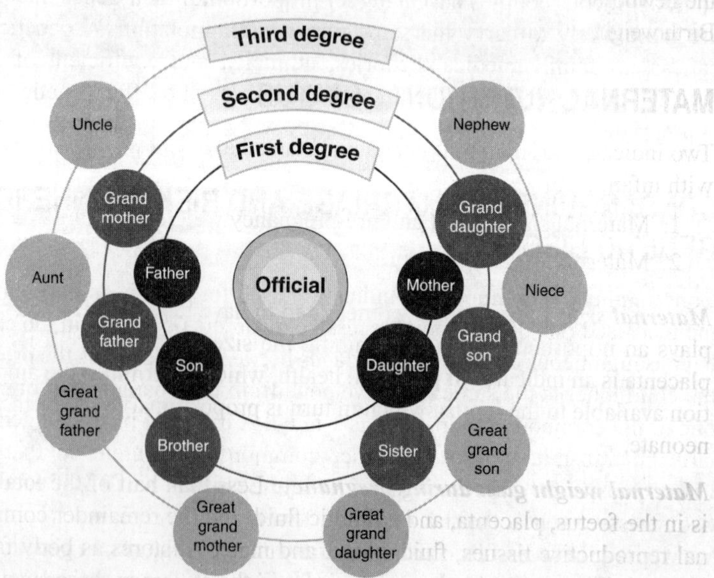

Figure 2.2 Degrees of consanguinity. (See page 243 for the colour image.)

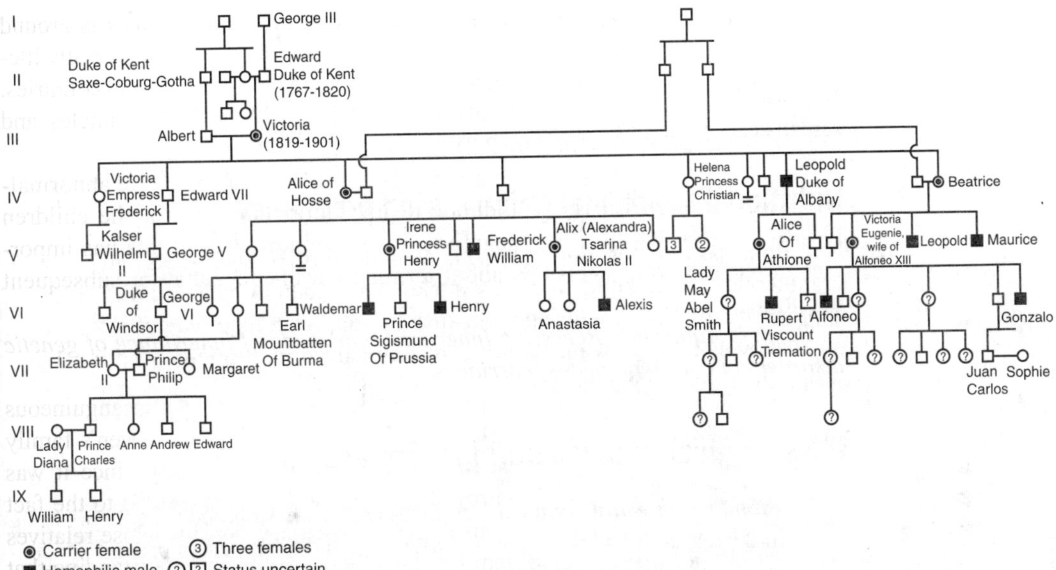

Figure 2.3 Pedigree showing haemophilia inheritance in the Royal family of England.

PRENATAL NUTRITION

Various factors determine the outcome of a pregnancy, including the nutritional status of the mother before conception and during pregnancy. Nutritional factors can affect the newborn's birth weight, risk of neural tube defect, and foetal alcohol syndrome. Birth weight is highly correlated with infant mortality and morbidity.

MATERNAL NUTRITIONAL STATUS

Two indicators of maternal nutritional status have consistently shown association with infant birth weight:

1. Maternal size (height and pre-pregnancy weight of the mother)
2. Maternal weight gain during pregnancy

Maternal size: Large stature women tend to have large babies, and maternal size plays an important role in determining the size of the placenta. The size of the placenta is an indicator of placental health, which determines the amount of nutrition available to the foetus, which in turn is proportional to the birth weight of the neonate.

Maternal weight gain during pregnancy: Less than half of the total weight gain is in the foetus, placenta, and amniotic fluid, and the remainder comprises maternal reproductive tissues, fluid, blood, and maternal stores as body fat. Gradually increasing amounts of sub-cutaneous fat in the abdomen, back, and thigh serves as an energy source for pregnancy and lactation.

In normal weight females, a weight gain of 26–35 lb during gestation is associated with optimal outcome.

Obesity: Risk of gestational diabetes, pregnancy-induced hypertension, and caesarean section increases in females who are obese.

Nutritional supplementation during pregnancy

Nutritional requirement during pregnancy in the form of energy, protein, vitamin, or minerals exceed the routine daily intake of a woman. A balanced diet results in appropriate weight gain during pregnancy by supplying required nutrients during pregnancy. Folate supplementation is recommended in all pre-conceptional prescriptions and during pregnancies.

Physiological changes during pregnancy

1. ***Blood volume and composition:*** 50% expansion of blood volume resulting in decreased hemoglobin, serum albumin, and other serum protein concentrations is observed during pregnancy.

2. ***Cardiovascular and pulmonary function:*** Cardiac output increases during pregnancy and cardiac size increases by 12%. Maternal oxygen requirements increase as the threshold for carbon dioxide decreases making the mother feel dyspenic (breathlessness)—as the growing uterus pushes the diaphragm upwards.

3. ***Gastrointestinal function:*** Nausea and vomiting, cravings, and aversion towards food are generally observed during pregnancy. Increased progesterone concentrations relax the uterine muscles to allow foetal growth but they decrease the gastrointestinal motility and increase the absorption of water resulting in constipation. The relaxation of the lower oesophageal sphincter and pressure on the stomach from the growing uterus often result in regurgitation and gastric reflux.

4. ***Renal function:*** Glomerular filtration rate (GFR) increases by 50% during pregnancy. The blood volume increases because of GFR with low serum creatinine and blood urea nitrogen concentrations. Renal tubular absorption decreases.

5. ***Placenta:*** The placenta is the site for hormone production for foetal growth and regulation. It is also the site for exchange of nutrients, oxygen, and waste products.

Nutritional requirements during pregnancy

1. ***Energy:*** Additional energy is required during pregnancy to meet the metabolic demands of pregnancy and foetal growth. The metabolism increases by 15% during pregnancy. The estimated average requirement of **carbohydrates** for pregnant women is 135 g/day and an adequate intake is 175 g/day. A requirement of 135–175 g/day is recommended to provide enough

calories, to avoid ketosis, and to maintain blood glucose levels during pregnancy.

2. *Protein:* Pregnant women have additional protein requirement to support the synthesis of maternal and foetal tissues. Protein use in pregnant women is about 70% same as those to foetus. Protein requirement increases throughout gestation and peaks during the third trimester.

3. *Fiber:* Consumption of whole grain breads, cereals, leafy green vegetables, and fresh and dried fruits during pregnancy is encouraged. The recommended fibre value is 28 g/day during pregnancy.

4. *Lipids:* The amount of fat in the diet should depend on energy requirements for proper weight gain.

5. *Vitamins and Minerals:*

   Folate: Folic acid supplementation is important to support maternal erythropoiesis, maternal and foetal placental growth, and to prevent neural tube defects.

   Vitamins: Vitamins B6 manages nausea and vomiting during pregnancy; vitamin D is important for calcium balance during pregnancy; and vitamins C, A, E, and K are required in adequate amounts for general nutritional requirements.

   Minerals: **Calcium** is important during pregnancy and lactation, **Iron** is important for oxygen delivery to the foetus, and deficiency leads to foetal hypoxia and maternal anaemia. **Zinc** supplementation avoids congenital abnormalities; **Magnesium** reduces the incidence of IUGR; **Sodium** is important for excretion, and maternal **Iodine** deficiency results in neonatal cretinism. Phosphorous, copper, and fluoride are also required in trace amounts.

6. *Fluids:* A total of 6–8 glasses of fluid intake is mandatory during pregnancy to avoid dehydration and to maintain the amniotic fluid index.

FOOD ALLERGIES

The term adverse reaction encompasses food intolerance and food hypersensitivity. Food intolerance is an adverse reaction to a food caused by toxic, pharmacologic, metabolic, idiosyncratic, or non-immunoglobulin E (IgE) reactions to food or chemical substances in the food. Food hypersensitivity or food allergy is an IgE mediated reaction that occurs when the immune system reacts to a normally harmless food macromolecule that the body has identified as non-self (antigen). IgE reactions usually occur instantly or within two hours of exposure, with severity ranging from mild to life threatening. Exposure includes inhalation, ingestion, and skin contact.

Symptoms

A wide range of symptoms has been attributed to food allergy. Skin, respiratory, cardiovascular, and gastrointestinal symptoms express during an allergic reaction (Table 2.1).

Table 2.1 Symptoms of food allergy

Gastrointestinal Manifestations:
Abdominal pain
Nausea
Vomiting
Diarrhoea
Gastrointestinal bleeding
Oral and pharyngeal pruritus

Cutaneous Manifestations:
Urticaria (hives)
Angioedema
Eczema
Erythema (skin reddening)
Itching
Flushing

Respiratory Manifestations:
Rhinitis
Asthma
Cough
Laryngeal edema
Airway tightening

Systemic Manifestations:
Anaphylaxis
Hypotension
Dysrhythmias

Controversial/Unproven Manifestations:
Behavioural disorders
Tension fatigue syndrome
Psychiatric disorders
Migraine headache

Some common food allergies

Carbohydrate (lactose) intolerance: Lactase deficiency is the most common enzyme deficiency worldwide. People who have a deficiency of the intestinal enzyme lactase have a decreased ability to digest lactose, a sugar in milk and milk products and experience symptoms of abdominal cramping, flatulence, and diarrhoea after its ingestion. Restriction of foods containing milk and milk products avoids the allergic reaction to a large extent.

Egg allergy: Many children and pregnant women are allergic to egg white, egg yolk, apovitellin, and other protein constituents of egg and show mild to severe cutaneous and gastrointestinal manifestations.

Peanut allergy: Ground nuts, peanut butter, beer nuts, peanut oil, mixed nuts, and products that contain peanuts have shown near fatal and fatal anaphylactic reactions.

Wheat allergy: Atta, bread flour, cake flour, wheat bran, whole wheat flour, wheat bread, and wheat flakes/pasta/flakes have shown allergic reactions similar to lactose intolerance and results in gastrointestinal manifestations.

Soy allergy: Soy flour, soy sauce/milk, curd, and soy products have proven to be allergic in many infants and children.

Diagnostic test available for food allergies

1. *Skin testing:* A drop of the antigen is placed on the skin, and the skin is scratched or punctured to allow penetration. This is a screening tool and cannot be relied upon as a diagnostic tool.
2. *Radioallergosorbent test (RAST):* Serum is mixed with food on a paper disk and then washed with radioactively labelled IgE.
3. *Enzyme-linked immunosorbent assay (ELISA):* Same as RAST; except non-radioactively labeled (enzyme) IgE is used.
4. *Sublingual testing:* Drops of allergen extract are placed under the tongue, and symptoms are recorded.
5. **Provocative testing and neutralization:** Subcutaneous injection of an allergen extract elicits symptoms; this is followed by the injection of a weaker or stronger preparation to neutralize the symptoms.

Treatment: Total avoidance of the food allergen is the only proven treatment for food allergy. However antihistamines are used to control allergies under unavoidable exposures.

ANEUPLOIDIES AND ADVANCED MATERNAL AGE

Aneuploidy is a numerical chromosomal abnormality that occurs as a consequence of non-disjunction. **Non-disjunction** is the failure of chromosome pairs to segregate properly during meiosis. Non-disjunction can occur during meiosis I or meiosis II or mitosis, and this results in imbalance in the diploid state of the cell. Such a cell is called an aneuploid cell.

Loss of a single chromosome (2n–1), in which the daughter cell(s) will have one chromosome missing from one of its pairs, is referred to as monosomy. Gaining a single chromosome, in which the daughter cell(s) will have one chromosome in addition to its pairs, is referred to as trisomy.

Advanced maternal age refers to any women aged 35 years or above at the expected date of delivery. As maternal age increases, the risk of birth defects (particularly chromosomal abnormalities) increases.

Older egg model: In advanced maternal age

The high percentage of trisomy 21 cases in which the abnormal gamete originated during maternal meiosis I suggests that maternal meiosis I is related to increased maternal age. One possibility is the "older egg" model, which suggests that older the oocyte, the greater the chances that the chromosomes will fail to disjoin correctly. Analysis of autosomal trisomies has implicated the number and/or placement of recombination events as a determinant of whether the chromosome pair will disjoin properly during two meiotic divisions. Older eggs may be less efficient to overcome a susceptibility to non-disjunction.

The number of oocytes that women will produce through her life time is predetermined when she is a foetus, and all the oocytes in a woman are as old as the woman herself. The oocytes are arrested in prophase of first meiotic division and produces to further stages during oogenesis after puberty. Thus, the older egg model suggests that the probability of error in meiosis could increase with the age of the egg (the age of the mother). Despite recognition of important associations between recombination and segregation in chromosomes, a full understanding of non-disjunction and maternal age continues to be elusive.

Trisomy

The most frequent numeric abnormality is trisomy, in which three copies of a given chromosome exist in the cell, instead of two, resulting in a total of 47 chromosomes per cell. For example, trisomy 21 implies that all cells of such individuals have three copies of chromosome 21. This is described by present nomenclature as 47,XX,+21 or 47,XY,+21. The most frequent cause of trisomy is non-disjunction, whereby the chromosome pair fails to separate during meiosis I or II. This results in one monosomic daughter cell having 45 chromosomes, a state usually incompatible with cellular viability, and the other daughter cell having an extra chromosome (trisomy). Non-disjunction is more frequent in maternal meiosis than in paternal meiosis. Maternal meiotic non-disjunction occurs with an exponentially increasing frequency with advancing maternal age. Conversely, paternal meiotic non-disjunction is not age related and thus may be found in offspring of younger parents. The most frequent autosomal trisomies found in liveborn infants (in decreasing order of frequency) are trisomy 21, 18, and 13, respectively. Other autosomal trisomies, such as trisomy 16 and 22, are commonly seen in spontaneous abortions but never in liveborn infants.

Monosomy

Monosomy is characterized by the presence of only one representative of a given chromosome pair in the cell. Most monosomies are embryologically lethal, the only exception known in humans is monosomy X (45,X; Turner syndrome).

Mosaicism

Non-disjunction can also occur in mitosis, and thus result in mosaicism, a situation where at least two cell lines are present: the original one, derived from the zygote, and the second, derived after the non-disjunction event. Not uncommonly, however, there are more than two cell lines present. The phenotypic expression of the mosaicism depends on the proportion of the different cell lines and their distribution in different tissues and organ systems. The phenotype in these cases is usually an intermediate between the normal and the fully aneuploid. Mosaicism for autosomal trisomy is relatively rare, although some well-described syndromes exist (i.e. mosaic trisomy 8). Mosaicism for sex chromosome aberrations however, is relatively common. These may sometimes be discovered only with the evaluation of infertility in the presence of premature ovarian failure and male infertility.

AUTOSOMAL ANEUPLOIDIES

Trisomy 21 (Down syndrome)

Down syndrome, is characterized by hypotonicity, brachycephaly with flat facies and mild microcephaly, upslanted palpebral fissures and speckling of the iris (Brushfield spots), small ears, short metacarpals and phalanges, hypoplasia of the midphalanx of the fifth digit with clinodactyly, single palmar crease, wide gap between the first and second toes, joint hypermobility, cardiac anomalies including endocardial cushion defect (A-V canal), ventricular septal defect (VSD), patent ductus arteriosus, increased incidence of leukemia (1%), gastrointestinal abnormalities including tracheo-esophageal fistulas and duodenal atresia, and mental deficiency. The intelligence quotient (IQ) is usually about 50 although it may approach 65–70 in some individuals. The major cause of early mortality is congenital heart disease. Trisomy 21 occurs in about 1 in 800 births. The incidence of trisomy 21 increases with advanced maternal age. Birth-prevalence rates of Down syndrome, plotted by maternal age, form a J-shaped curve, with women 20–24 years of age having the lowest prevalence rate (1/1,400 births). For women who are 35 years old, the rate is 1/350 births, and for women above 45 years the rate rises to 1/25 births. As many as 95% of Down syndrome cases are caused by trisomy 21, which typically results from non-disjunction during meiosis. About 3% are the result of Robertsonian translocations, of which half are inherited and half are de novo, and 2% have trisomy 21 mosaicism.

The risk ratio fact sheet for Down syndrome based on advanced maternal age is presented in Figure 2.4.

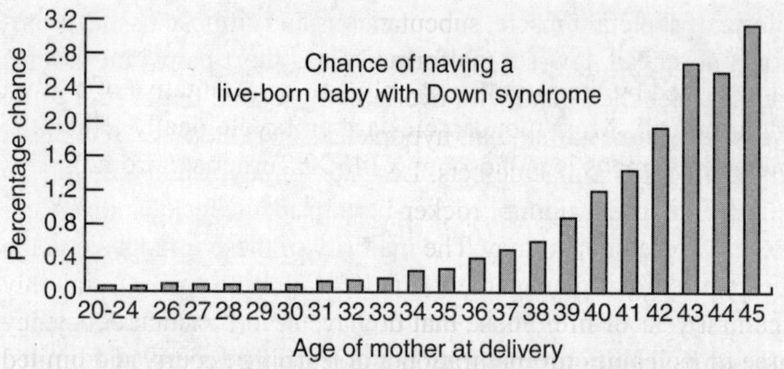

Age of mother at delivery	Chance of having a live-born baby with Down syndrome	Age of mother at delivery	Chance of having a live-born baby with Down syndrome
20-24 years	1 in 1411	35 years	1 in 338
25 years	1 in 1383	36 years	1 in 259
26 years	1 in 1187	37 years	1 in 201
27 years	1 in 1235	38 years	1 in 162
28 years	1 in 1147	39 years	1 in 113
29 years	1 in 1002	40 years	1 in 84
30 years	1 in 959	41 years	1 in 69
31 years	1 in 837	42 years	1 in 52
32 years	1 in 695	43 years	1 in 37
33 years	1 in 589	44 years	1 in 38
34 years	1 in 430	45 years	1 in 32

Figure 2.4 The risk ratio fact sheet for down syndrome based on advanced maternal age

Trisomy 18 (Edwards syndrome)

Trisomy 18 is the second most frequent autosomal chromosome abnormality. The majority of trisomy 18 cases are due to non-disjunction, and empirical recurrence risks for this disorder are less than 1%. More than 130 different structural abnormalities have been reported in patients with trisomy 18, including growth deficiency, hypoplasia of skeletal muscle, subcutaneous and adipose tissue, prominent occiput, narrow forehead, low-set malformed ears, short palpebral fissures and small oral opening, clenched hand with overlapping second finger over third, and fifth finger over forth, short hallux, nail hypoplasia, short sternum, redundant skin with mild hirsutism, and cardiac defects. Less commonly found are cleft lip and palate, hypoplastic to absent thumb, rocker-bottom feet, Meckel's diverticulum, omphalocele, and horse-shoe kidney. The majority of these infants die in the neonatal period despite optimal management due to "failure to thrive," and only 5–10% survive the first year of life. Those that do have severe mental deficiency though some degree of psychomotor maturation and learning occurs, and limited social interaction is possible.

Trisomy 13 (Patau syndrome)

This is the third most common autosomal trisomy occurring in about 1 in 5000 livebirths. Most cases are due to non-disjunction and advanced maternal age has been implicated. Recurrence risk is presumably low. Trisomy 13 is commonly associated with holoprosencephaly varying in severity from cyclopia or cebocephaly to less severe forms. Other manifestations include microcephaly with sloping forehead, capillary haemangiomata, localized scalp defects, microphthalmia, colobomata, cleft lip and palate, polydactyly, narrow hyperconvex fingernails, cardiac defects, single umbilical artery, structural kidney malformations, and omphalocele. As with trisomy 18, most trisomy 13 conceptions result in miscarriage. Those that survive to term often succumb within the first days of life usually of complex heart disease, and only about 5% survive past the first 6 months. Survivors have severe mental deficiency, minor motor seizures with a hypsarrhythmic EEG pattern, and failure to thrive.

SEX CHROMOSOME ANEUPLOIDIES

There are four clearly defined syndromes associated with the sex chromosomes (X and Y). These include a monosomy X (Turner syndrome, 45,X), and three trisomies (47,XXY— Klinefelter syndrome, 47,XYY, and 47,XXX). The effects of these chromosomal aberrations on development have been prospectively studied in newborns with sex chromosome aneuploidies.

Monosomy X (Turner syndrome)

Monosomy X occurs most commonly because of non-disjunction. In the majority the single X chromosome is of maternal origin, suggesting that the non-disjunction event occurred in the father and is therefore unrelated to maternal age. With the advent of ultrasound, these foetuses are increasingly being recognized in utero, presenting with increased nuchal translucency in the first trimester and later with large cystic hygroma of the neck. The cause of the cystic hygroma is usually obstruction at the connection between the lymphatic and venous system at the jugular junction. In some foetuses with monosomy X, it may also be caused by coarctation of the aorta. Though the incidence of monosomy X in liveborn is rather low (1 in 5000 live female births), it is the single most common abnormality found in early spontaneous abortions, accounting for as many as 20 % of cytogenetically abnormal gestations. About 99 % of such foetuses abort spontaneously and only a minority survives to term. Individuals with Turner Syndrome may manifest a characteristic phenotype including swelling of hands and feet at birth, short stature with onset around 6 years of age, gonadal dysgenesis, webbed neck, low hairline, broad chest with widely spaced nipples, congenital heart disease including coarctation of the aorta, and horseshoe kidneys. If untreated, these individuals fail to develop secondary sexual characteristics in puberty and usually present with primary amenorrhea, and later complications of hypoestrogenism.

Hormone replacement therapy in the form of combination oestrogen and progesterone therapy may alleviate some of the growth deficiency, and induce secondary sexual maturation as well as menses. While some learning difficulties may be encountered, these individuals are intellectually normal and often lead normal and meaningful lives, although needing in some instances social support. Childbearing for these patients has now become possible using donated oocytes. Most patients with Turner Syndrome have 45,X; however, 50 % of patients have other karyotypes such as a mosaicism with only a proportion of cells being 45, X, structural abnormalities of the X chromosome, such as deletions of the long or short arm, isochromosomes of the long arm, or translocations.

47,XXY (Klinefelter syndrome)

Patients with 47,XXY have a normal male phenotype at birth and during childhood. At the onset of puberty, however, they appear relatively tall and thin, and in the absence of corrective hormonal therapy, demonstrate signs of hypogonadism, and gynaecomastia. Their testes remain small and they are almost invariably infertile. Although no major malformations are associated with this syndrome, patients usually have IQ scores that are 10–15 points lower than their siblings. In addition, there is an increased incidence of learning difficulties, immaturity, and emotional and behavioural problems. Klinefelter Syndrome is one of the most common causes of male infertility with an incidence of about 1 in 1000 liveborn males. It is estimated that about half of the conceptions with a 47,XXY karyotype are spontaneously aborted, despite the fact that the phenotype is rather benign. The non-disjunctional error appears to be paternal meiosis I in about 50 % of the cases, maternal meiosis I in about 33 %, and meiosis II in the remainder. About 15 % of Klinefelter Syndrome are mosaic, most commonly 47,XXY/46,XY. These are usually the result of mitotic non-disjunction in the early embryonic stages.

The other common forms of sex chromosome aneuploidy are 47,XYY in males, and 47,XXX in females. Much is known about the frequency of these genotypes but there is a biased association with phenotype. Thus, 47,XXY is present in about 1 per 1,000 males, the prevalence increasing with maternal age, although not as steeply as the common autosomal aneuploidies.

MATERNAL DRUG THERAPY

Overprescribing of drugs is a major problem in modern medicine, and unnecessary use of drugs is most dangerous in pregnancy. However, it is important to understand that modern drugs have made a major contribution to human health and even in pregnancy, drugs play an important role in treating maternal diseases and reducing pain in labour.

In an ideal situation, no medical treatment would be best in pregnancy; but the reality is that many women develop conditions requiring treatment during pregnancy. Therefore, an absolute ban on drug usage in pregnancy would not be practical. It is therefore the moral, social, and legal responsibility of the doctor and the patient to understand the risks and benefits of the concerned drug therapy module and use it judiciously.

Some medical disorders that require drug therapy during pregnancy:

1. *Hypertension:* Hypertension complicates up to 10% pregnancies and causes much maternal and foetal morbidity and its management challenges the physician. Hydralazine and Labetol are the drugs of choice prescribed for hypertensive pregnant women. Some women show adverse effects of headache, nausea, and vomiting. Foetal distress following parenteral hydrazine has been reported.

2. *Diabetes mellitus:* During normal pregnancy, maternal metabolism adjusts to provide nutrition for both the mother and the growing foetus. Increasing levels of oestrogen and progesterone in early pregnancy alters glucose homeostasis. There is heightened peripheral utilization of glucose causing reduction in maternal fasting glucose levels. Diabetes mellitus in pregnant women causes alterations in oxyhaemoglobin dissociation and ketoacidosis in mother, hyperglycemia and ketonemia in foetus and also reduces uteroplacental blood flow causing foetal hypoxia. Patients with poor glycemic control face hydramnios and foetal macrosomia. Foetal demise may also occur. Many cardiovascular, central nervous systems, skeletal, and gastrointestinal congenital abnormalities are observed in children born to diabetic mothers.

   Blood glucose levels monitored in combination with aggressive insulin therapy will help maintain normal maternal glycemic levels. Insulin therapy must be individualized with dosage determination tailored to diet and exercise. Diet therapy is important to successful regulation of maternal diabetes.

3. ***Thyroid disorders:*** A number of changes occur in the thyroid and measurement of thyroid hormones during pregnancy. The renal clearance of iodine is increased due to increased glomerular filtration rate during pregnancy. When iodine intake is marginal, it results in iodine deficiency due to increased iodine clearance. Iodine in the diet usually prevents this deficiency. Care should be taken to avoid excess iodine, which may result in neonatal goiter. A total of 95% of hyperthyroidism is due to Grave's disease, which ameliorates during pregnancy. Unregulated hyperthyroidism in mothers results in low birth of the foetus and foetal demise in most cases. Drugs prescribed include Propylthiouracil, Methimazole, and Propranolol. Side effects include rash, fever, and sore throat.

4. ***Cardiovascular disease:*** The cardiovascular system undergoes extensive alteration during pregnancy. Aortic dissection, pericardial disease, and dysrhythmias are a few heart diseases acquired during pregnancy. Medical therapy includes diuretics and steroids.

PRENATAL GENETIC TESTING AND DIAGNOSIS

Prenatal diagnosis has evolved into a multidisciplinary medical service, which works in collaboration with obstetrics, ultrasonography, clinical genetics, and laboratory services for the purpose of assessment, diagnosis, and genetic counselling. The purpose of prenatal diagnosis is not just to simply detect abnormalities in the foetal life and allow termination of pregnancy when the foetus is detected to have a defect. The goals of prenatal diagnosis are as follows:

1. To provide a range of informed choice to couples at a risk of having a child with an abnormality.
2. To provide reassurance and alleviate anxiety among high-risk groups.
3. To allow couples at high risk to continue their normal pregnancy (after testing), who might otherwise forego having children.
4. To allow couples the option of appropriate management while awaiting the birth of a child with a genetic disorder in terms of psychological support, pregnancy, and delivery management and postnatal care.
5. To enable prenatal treatment of the affected foetus (in utero foetal surgeries are promising).

INDICATIONS FOR PRENATAL DIAGNOSIS (PND)

1. Advanced maternal age
2. Previous child with a chromosomal abnormality
3. Presence of structural chromosomal abnormality in one of the parents
4. Family history of genetic disorder
5. Risk of neural tube defect

6. Family history of X-linked disorder
7. Abnormal results suggested by screening methods: ultrasound and triple test

METHODS OF PRENATAL DIAGNOSIS

The methods of PND, both invasive and non-invasive are given in Table 2.2. Both amniocentesis and chorionic villus sampling (CVS) are invasive procedures associated with a small risk of foetal loss. It is therefore indicated only for pregnant women who meet the indications outline above. In contrast, a combination of maternal serum screening (MSS)/Triple screening and ultrasonographic scanning can be used for foetal evaluation in low risk as well as in some high-risk pregnancies because both are non-invasive and without risk to the foetus.

PRINCIPLES OF SCREENING TESTS

The principle of screening for any disease/syndrome requires a basic understanding of the differences between diagnostic and screening tests. Diagnostic tests are designed to give a confirmatory result to the problem. Diagnostic tests are generally complex, require sophisticated analysis, and interpretation, and these tests tend to be expensive, and they are usually only advised to patients "at risk." On the other hand, screening tests are generally performed on healthy patients and are often offered to the general population. They are hence more affordable, easy to use, and are easily interpretable. Their function is to help define who, among the low-risk group, is in fact at high risk.

Table 2.3 highlights the differences between diagnostic and screening tests.

Table 2.2 Methods of PND

Invasive Testing

Amniocentesis

Chorionic villus sampling

Cordocentesis

Preimplantation genetic diagnosis

Non-invasive Testing

Maternal serum alpha fetoprotein (AFP)

Maternal serum screen

Ultrasonography

Isolation of fetal cells from maternal circulation

Table 2.3 Screening tests vs. diagnostic tests

Diagnostic Tests

Performed only on "at risk" population

Commonly expensive

Commonly have risk

Give definitive answer

Screening Tests

Offered to general population of patients

Healthy patients

Cheap

Easy

Reliable

Quick

Define "at risk" population

Do not give definitive answer

NON-INVASIVE TESTING

Ultrasound diagnosis of foetal anomalies

Some genetic conditions can be detected through direct visualization of the foetus (Figure 2.5). Such visualization is most commonly done with **ultrasonography**—usually referred to as ultrasound. In this technique, high-frequency sound is beamed into the uterus; when the sound waves encounter dense tissue, they bounce back and are transformed into an image.

Antenatal ultrasound scanning at about 18–20 weeks of gestation permits the detection of most major foetal structural anomalies. Ultrasound examinations that are restricted to the documentation of foetal life, foetal number, foetal presentation, gestational age, growth assessment, amniotic fluid volume assessment, and placental localization are considered incomplete. The employment of a systematic approach to the evaluation of the foetal anatomy is of paramount importance.

This is usually accomplished by the sequential study of the distinct regions of the foetal anatomy:

1. The head, spine, thorax, abdomen, and extremities: Examination of the foetal head is most often performed with transverse views at a minimum of three levels: the lateral ventricle, the biparietal diameter, and the cerebellum. At these planes, the foetal skull can be assessed.

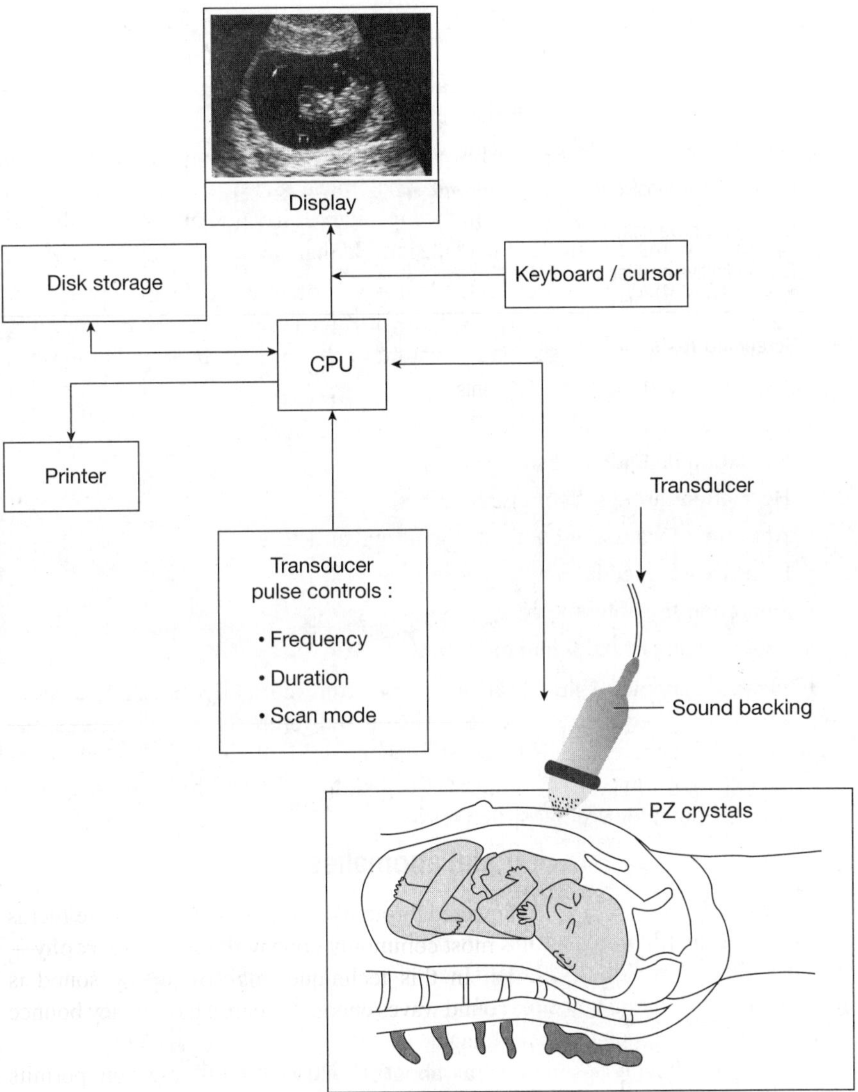

Figure 2.5 Ultrasound. (See page 240 for the colour image.)

2. The spine should be viewed in its entirety in a saggital plane. This is then complemented by a series of transverse sonograms to identify normal anterior and posterior ossification elements.

3. The position of the heart within the thorax should be noted, and an attempt should be made to obtain a four-chambered view. Atria and ventricles should be of equal and appropriate sizes, and the interventricular septum should be intact. Examination of the foetal outflow tracts increases the detection of heart anomalies.

4. In the region of the abdominal cavity, the foetal stomach and bladder should be visualized by 14 weeks of gestation; kidneys should be visualized by 16 weeks. A view of the umbilical cord insertion site is mandatory to determine whether the anterior abdominal wall is intact.

5. The long bones of at least the lower extremities should be visualized. Although not considered part of the *minimum* anatomical survey, an examination of all areas of the anatomy, including face, genitalia, all four extremities with their digits, and measurement of nuchal skinfold thickness, is desirable.

Sonographic examination of foetal anatomy is often more detailed when it is targeted to look for a certain anomaly. Many foetal anomalies can be grouped into the following categories based on the nature of the dysmorphology that permits sonographic detection:

- Absence of a structure normally present
- Dilatation behind an obstruction
- Herniation through a structural defect
- Abnormal location or contour of a normal structure
- Presence of an additional structure
- Abnormal foetal biometry
- Absent or abnormal foetal motion

A classic example of the absence of a structure normally detected by ultrasound is anencephaly, the absence of calvaria and forebrain. In these cases, the ultrasound clearly reveals the absence of echogenic skull bones and the presence of a heterogeneous mass of cystic tissue, called the area cerebrovasculosa, which replaces well-defined cerebral structures.

Maternal serum screening

In this screening test (which is not a diagnostic tool), maternal blood sample is collected, serum from blood is isolated, and biochemical marker levels are analyzed in the serum. Further diagnostic testing and counselling must be offered to women whose MSS test is positive. Also, women whose MSS test is negative must be aware that though their risk of having a child with Down syndrome, Trisomy 18, or NTDs is greatly reduced, it is not zero (the result is only a risk estimate).

When the foetus has an open NTD, the concentration of Alpha Feto Protein (AFP) is **higher** than normal in maternal serum as well as in the amniotic fluid. This observation is the basis for the use of MSAFP measurement at 16 weeks as a test for open NTDs. The combined use of MSAFP assay with detailed diagnostic ultrasound approaches accuracy of this test for the detection of open NTDs.

Triple screening

This test measures three blood markers, and this test is made available to most pregnant women at 15 to 20 weeks of gestation to identify those at increased risk for Down syndrome, Trisomy 18, and NTDs. The three serum components in this screening test include AFP, unconjugated estriol (uE3), and human chorionic gonadotropin (HCG).

In pregnancies with Down syndrome, the levels of AFP and uE3 are **reduced** in the maternal serum.

HCG in maternal serum is significantly **higher** than normal when the foetus has Down syndrome.

When the level of all the three biochemical markers is **low**, the risk for Trisomy 18 is significantly increased.

Foetal cell sorting

Prenatal tests that utilize only maternal blood are highly desirable because they are non-invasive and pose no risk to the foetus. During pregnancy, a few foetal cells are released into the mother's circulatory system, where they mix and circulate with her blood. Recent advances have made it possible to separate foetal cells from a maternal blood sample (a procedure called **foetal cell sorting**). With the use of lasers and automated cell-sorting machines, foetal cells can be detected and separated from maternal blood cells. The foetal cells obtained can be cultured for chromosome analysis or used as a source of foetal DNA for molecular testing.

INVASIVE TESTING

Amniocentesis

The diagnosis of genetic disorders in samples of amniotic fluid and cells was introduced in the early 1960s (Figure 2.6). The first diagnoses of foetal chromosome anomalies performed on amniocytes were shortly followed by the development of enzymatic assays for prenatal diagnosis of metabolic disorders (for example, galactosemia). The diagnostic accuracy and the relatively low risk of foetal or maternal compromise associated with amniocentesis established it as the basic procedure in modern prenatal diagnosis. Amniocentesis is considered frequently the "gold standard" to which other methods for prenatal diagnosis are compared.

It is a procedure for obtaining a sample of amniotic fluid from a pregnant woman. Amniotic fluid—the substance that fills the amniotic sac and surrounds the developing foetus—contains foetal cells that can be used for genetic testing. Amniocentesis is routinely performed as an outpatient procedure with the use of a local or no anesthetic. First, ultrasonography is used to locate the position of the foetus in the uterus. Next, a long, sterile needle is inserted through the abdominal wall into the amniotic sac, and a small amount of amniotic fluid is withdrawn through the needle. Foetal cells are separated from the amniotic fluid and are placed in a culture medium that stimulates them to grow and divide. Genetic tests are then performed on the cultured cells. Some laboratories use fluorescence in situ hybridization (FISH) with probes for chromosomes 13, 18, 21, X, and Y, diagnosing most

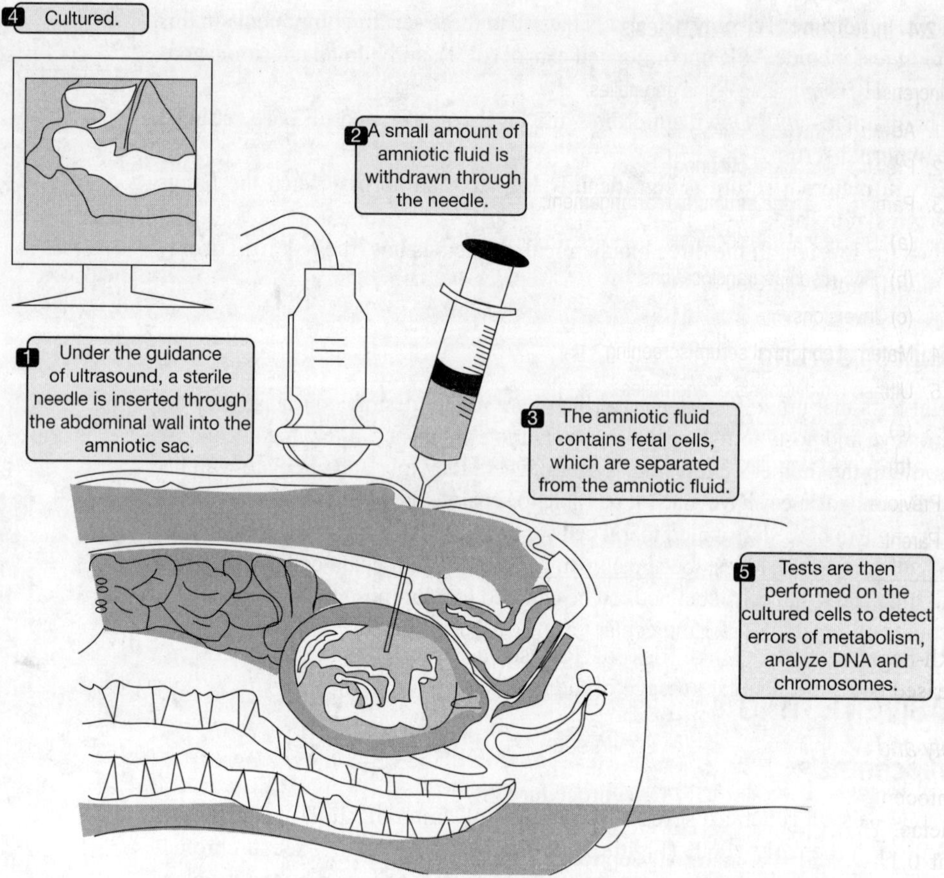

Figure 2.6 Amniocentesis. (See page 241 for the colour image.)

cases of potentially viable trisomies within 24 hours from sampling. FISH is applied to uncultured amniocytes, obviating the possibility of culture failure, a complication that affects about 1 in 700 amniotic fluid samplings in mid trimester. The use of FISH to diagnose numerical chromosome anomalies is very reliable and efficient in patients that need rapid results. In addition, FISH analysis can be used to identify microdeletions that cannot be diagnosed with standard cytogenetics, as in the Di George, Angelman, Prader Willi, or Smith Magenis Syndromes.

Indications for genetic amniocentesis are summarized in Table 2.4.

Amniocentesis should be performed by an obstetrician trained and experienced in the procedure. It should be preceded by genetic counselling, in which the family pedigree and genetic risk are evaluated, and the advantages and risks of the procedure are explained. A detailed ultrasound examination should assess gestational age, amniotic fluid volume, and foetal and placental location and should exclude gross foetal malformations. The patient's blood type and antibody status should be known prior to amniocentesis, and Rh-negative women with negative antibody screening should receive Rh immuno-prophylaxis after the procedure.

Table 2.4 Indications for amniocentesis

A. Increased risk for chromosome anomalies:
  1. Advanced maternal age
  2. Previous aneuploid offspring
  3. Parental balanced structural rearrangement:
      (a) Reciprocal translocations
      (b) Robertsonian translocations
      (c) Inversions
  4. Maternal abnormal serum screening
  5. Ultrasound diagnosis of anomalies
      (a) Major malformations
      (b) Minor anomalies
B. Previous offspring with NTD
C. Parents carriers of Mendelian traits

In Rh-negative patients, the risk of Rh isosensitization is probably slightly increased by transplacental passage of the needle.

Safety and complications of amniocentesis

Amniocentesis is a relatively safe procedure, with almost non-existent severe sequelae. The frequency of severe chorioamnionitis following amniocentesis is about 0.1%; however, maternal septicemia with pulmonary oedema and renal failure have been reported occasionally. Leakage of amniotic fluid is a relatively frequent complication, experienced by 1–2% of patients after amniocentesis, but is of minor clinical significance and usually resolves within 48–72 hours. Although rare, persistent and significant amniotic fluid leakage may however lead to oligohydramnion and may result in foetal pressure deformities and pulmonary hypoplasia. In experienced hands, the overall procedure-related pregnancy loss is 0.2–0.5% above the spontaneous pregnancy loss rate at 16 weeks gestation, the latter being estimated at 2–3%.

Chorionic villus sampling

A major disadvantage with amniocentesis is that it is routinely performed in about the 16th week of a pregnancy (Figure 2.7). The cells obtained with amniocentesis must then be cultured before genetic tests can be performed, requiring more time. For these reasons, genetic information about the foetus may not be available until the 17th or 18th week of pregnancy. By this stage, abortion carries a risk of complications and may be stressful for the parents. **Chorionic villus sampling** (CVS) can be performed earlier (between the 10th and 11th weeks of pregnancy) and collects more foetal tissue, which eliminates the necessity of culturing the cells.

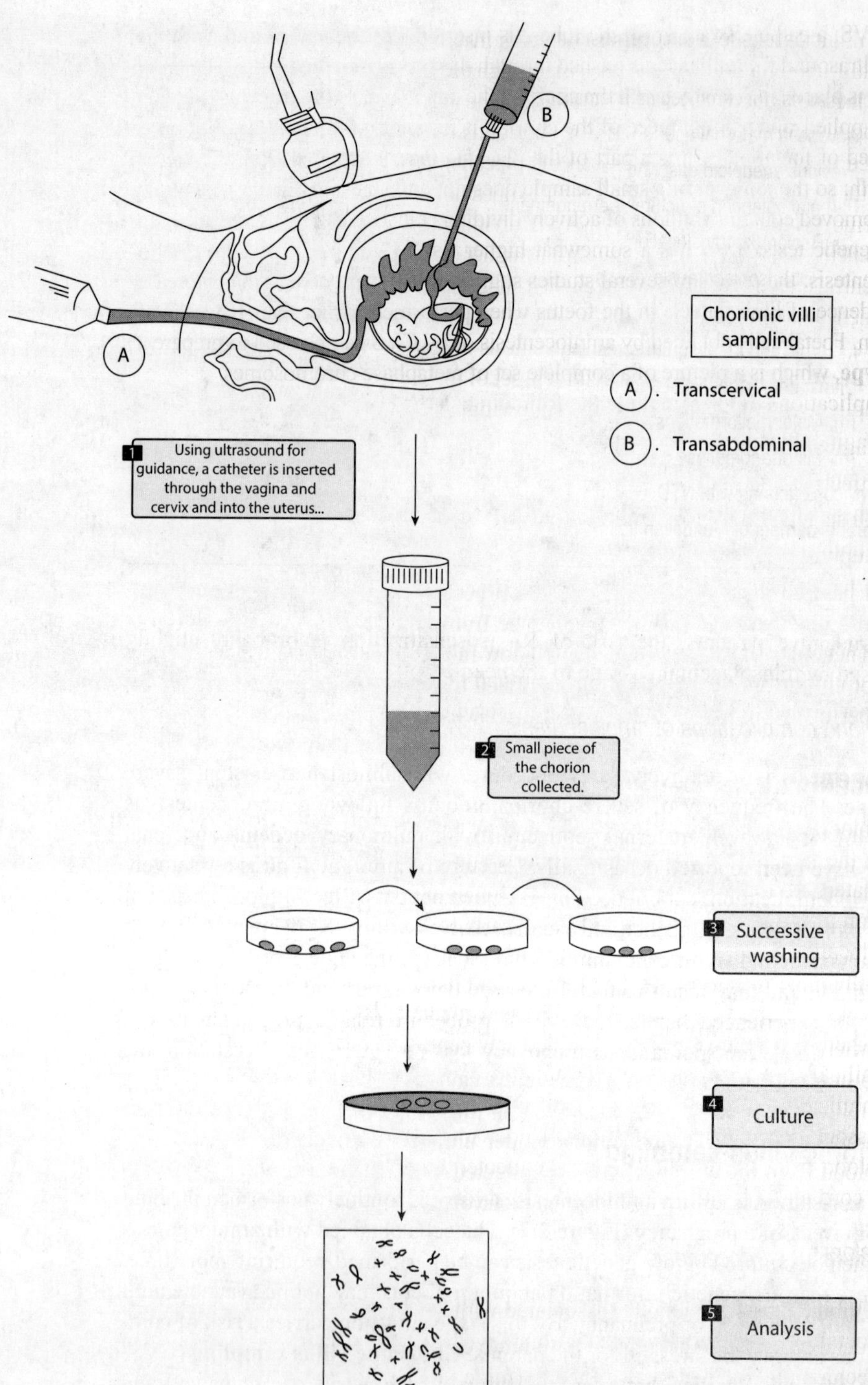

Figure 2.7 Chorionic villus sampling. (See page 242 for the colour image.)

In CVS, a catheter—a soft plastic tube—is inserted into the vagina and, with the use of ultrasound for guidance, is pushed through the cervix into the uterus. The tip of the tube is placed into contact with the chorion, the outer layer of the placenta. Suction is then applied, and a small piece of the chorion is removed. Although the chorion is composed of foetal cells, it is a part of the placenta that is expelled from the uterus after birth; so the removal of a small sample does not endanger the foetus. The tissue that is removed contains millions of actively dividing cells that can be used directly in many genetic tests. CVS has a somewhat higher risk of complication than that of amniocentesis; the results of several studies suggest that this procedure may increase the incidence of limb defects in the foetus when performed earlier than 10 weeks of gestation. Foetal cells obtained by amniocentesis or by CVS can be used to prepare a **karyotype**, which is a picture of a complete set of metaphase chromosomes.

Complications of CVS include the following:

1. Vaginal bleeding
2. Infection
3. Rh sensitization
4. Rupture of membranes

CVS has proved to be a relatively safe procedure with approximately 2–3% foetal loss in experienced centres. Evidence from multiple studies demonstrates the high accuracy of this technique, with a low rate of both maternal cell contamination or chromosomal abnormalities confined to the placenta. Technically, CVS can be performed transabdominally or transcervically.

Cordocentesis

Foetal blood sampling was first performed in the 1960s using a foetoscope to identify the targeted vessel. Foetoscopy was cumbersome and risky—the procedure-related loss rate exceeded 5%. Fortunately, the development of high-resolution ultrasound made it possible to clearly image the umbilical cord.

Cordocentesis can be performed as early as 12 weeks gestation, though it is technically more difficult prior to 20 weeks, and the loss rate is much higher prior to 16 weeks' gestation. The preferred location for cord puncture is the placental origin where it is relatively fixed. The first few centimeters of the foetal origin of the umbilical cord are innervated. Its puncture causes pain and should be avoided. The umbilical vein rather than the artery is the preferred target because of its lower association with complications. Under ultrasound guidance, a few ml of foetal blood from the umbilical cord is collected without causing foetal distress, and the cord blood is cultured in vitro and karyotype is prepared.

Risk factors for cordocentesis

1. Umbilical artery puncture (associated with bradycardia)
2. Foetal hypoxemia (associated with bradycardia)
3. Technique—freehand versus needle guide
4. Gestational age—prior to 20 weeks, both techniques

5. Number of punctures
6. Duration of procedure
7. Experience

Complications of cordocentesis

1. Bradycardia or asystole
2. Premature rupture of membranes
3. Premature labour
4. Umbilical haemorrhage
5. Placental haemorrhage
6. Chorioamnionitis
7. Umbilical thrombosis
8. Foetal to maternal haemorrhage

Protocols for culture and preparation of human chromosomes from amniotic fluid, chorionic villi, cord blood and peripheral blood along with Giemsa staining is given in annexure.

Preimplantation genetic diagnosis

Prenatal genetic tests provide today's couples with increasing amounts of information about the health of their future children. New reproductive technologies also provide couples with options for using this information. One of these technologies is in vitro fertilization. In this procedure, hormones are used to induce ovulation. The ovulated eggs are surgically removed from the surface of the ovary, placed in a laboratory dish, and fertilized with sperm. The resulting embryo is then implanted into the uterus. Genetic testing can be combined with in vitro fertilization to allow implantation of embryos that are free of a specific genetic defect. This technique called preimplantation genetic diagnosis allows couples undergoing IVF to avoid producing a child with a genetic disorder.

For example, when a woman is a carrier of an X-linked recessive disease, approximately half of her sons are expected to have the disease. Through in vitro fertilization and preimplantation testing, it is possible to select an embryo without the disorder for implantation in her uterus. The procedure includes the production of several single-celled embryos through artificial reproductive techniques like IVF. The embryos are allowed to divide several times until they reach the 8 or 16-cell stage. At this point, one cell is removed from each embryo and tested for the genetic abnormality. Removing a single cell at this early stage does not harm the embryo. After determination, a healthy embryo is selected and implanted in the woman's uterus.

Preimplantation genetic diagnosis requires the ability to conduct a genetic test on a single cell. Such testing is possible with the use of the polymerase chain

Table 2.5 Examples of genetic diseases and disorders that can be detected prenatally and the techniques

Disorder	Method of Detection
Chromosome abnormalities	Examination of a karyotype from cells obtained by amniocentesis or CVS
Cleft lip and palate	Ultrasound
Cystic fibrosis	DNA analysis of cells obtained by amnio / CVS
Haemophilia	Foetal blood sampling / DNA analysis
Lesch–Nyhan Syndrome	Biochemical tests on cells obtained by amniocentesis or CVS
Neural-tube defects	Initial screening with maternal blood test, followed by biochemical tests on amniotic fluid obtained by amniocentesis and ultrasound
Phenylketonuria	DNA analysis of cells obtained by amniocentesis or CVS
Sickle-cell anemia	Foetal blood sampling or DNA analysis of cells obtained by amniocentesis or CVS
Tay–Sachs disease	Biochemical tests on cells obtained by amniocentesis or CVS

reaction through which minute quantities of DNA can be amplified (replicated) quickly. After amplification of the cell's DNA, the DNA sequence is examined. Preimplantation diagnosis is still experimental and is available at only a few research centres. Its use raises a number of ethical concerns because it provides a means of actively selecting for or against certain genetic traits.

Examples of genetic diseases and disorders that can be detected prenatally and the techniques are described in Table 2.5.

Genetic testing is used to screen newborns for genetic diseases, detect persons who are heterozygous for recessive diseases, detect disease-causing alleles in those who have not yet developed symptoms of the disease, and detect defective alleles in unborn babies. Preimplantation genetic diagnosis combined with in vitro fertilization allows for selection of embryos that are free from specific genetic diseases.

EFFECT OF DRUGS, CHEMICALS AND RADIATION

Teratogens are agents (drugs, infections, chemicals, radiation) that cause birth defects. Understanding the action of teratogens has important implications for both clinical medicine and for biomedical and basic science. Identifying the teratogenic effects of drugs or environmental toxins have clear ramifications for public health, and understanding the mechanisms of teratogenicity can provide an insight into the underlying developmental pathways that have gone awry (Figure 2.8). The mechanism of teratogenesis is given in Table 2.6.

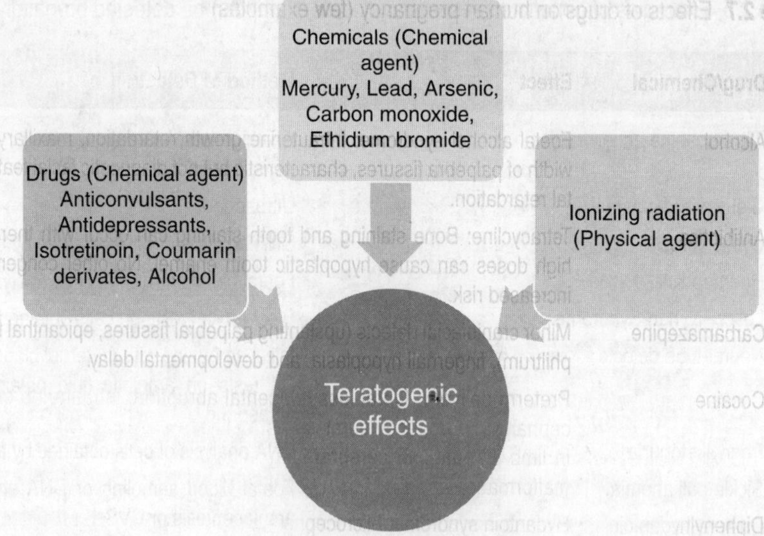

Figure 2.8 Teratogenic agents

Table 2.6 Mechanisms of teratogenesis

1. Cell death or mitotic delay beyond the restorative capacity of the embryo or foetus.
2. Inhibition of cell migration, differentiation and cell communication.
3. Interference with histogenesis by processes such as cell depletion, necrosis, calcification, or scarring.
4. Biologic and pharmacological receptor-mediated developmental effects.
5. Metabolic inhibition or nutritional deficiencies.
6. Physical constraint, vascular disruption, inflammatory lesions, and amniotic band syndrome.
7. Interference with nutritional support of the embryo due to abnormalities of yolk sac or chorioplacental transport.

Effect of drugs

A common concern of expectant couples is the potential of birth defects from the prescription of drugs. There is limited and often conflicting data with regard to the teratogenicity of most drugs. Limitation of unnecessary drug exposure during pregnancy and avoidance of the known teratogens will minimize drug-induced malformations. The effects of a few drugs on human pregnancy are given in Table 2.7.

Anticonvulsant drugs

Epileptic women have increased incidence of congenital anomalies. Recent research suggests that the pathophysiology of congenital malformation associated with epilepsy is a combination of exposure to anticonvulsant medication in an

Table 2.7 Effects of drugs on human pregnancy (few examples)

Drug/Chemical	Effect
Alcohol	Foetal alcohol syndrome: Intrauterine growth retardation, maxillary hypoplasia, reduction in width of palpebra fissures, characteristic but not diagnostic facial features, microcephaly, mental retardation.
Antibiotics	Tetracycline: Bone staining and tooth staining can occur with therapeutic doses. Persistent high doses can cause hypoplastic tooth enamel. No other congenital malformations are at increased risk.
Carbamazepine	Minor craniofacial defects (upslanting palpebral fissures, epicanthal folds, short nose with long philtrum), fingernail hypoplasia, and developmental delay.
Cocaine	Preterm delivery; foetal loss; placental abruption; intrauterine growth retardation; microcephaly; neurobehavioural abnormalities; vascular disruptive phenomena resulting in limb amputation, cerebral infarctions, and certain types of visceral and urinary tract malformations.
Diphenylhydantoin	Hydantoin syndrome: Microcephaly, mental retardation, cleft lip/palate, hypoplastic nails, and distal phalanges; characteristic, but not diagnostic facial features.
Thalidomide	Thalidomide syndrome: Limb reduction defects (preaxial preferential effects, phocomelia), facial hemangioma, esophageal or duodenal atresia, anomalies of external ears, eyes, kidneys, and heart, increased incidence of neonatal and infant mortality. There appears to be an increased risk of abortion.
Toluene	Intrauterine growth retardation; craniofacial anomalies; microcephaly. It is likely that high exposures from abuse or intoxication increase the risk of teratogenesis.
Thyroid	Foetal hypothyroidism or goiter with variable neurologic and aural damage. Maternal hypothyroidism is associated with an increase in infertility and abortion.
Cyclophosphamide	Growth retardation, ectrodactyly, syndactyly, cardiovascular anomalies, and other minor anomalies.

individual who may be "genetically" susceptible. An enzyme deficiency may be responsible for certain malformations seen with anticonvulsant use. The enzyme, epoxide hydrolase, is required to metabolize intermediary oxidative metabolites of anticonvulsants that utilize the arene oxide pathway. Epoxide hydrolase is regulated by a single gene, which has two allelic forms. Thus, it would appear that in foetuses homozygous for the recessive allele would have a lower enzyme activity and therefore be at a greater risk of malformation from anticonvulsant use. Multiple drug therapy appears to increase the risk of anomalies. Folic acid supplementation has been reported to decrease the incidence of congenital malformations due to anticonvulsant drugs. All anticonvulsants interfere with folic acid metabolism and therefore, patients taking anticonvulsants may develop a folic acid deficiency. Thus, it is recommended that patients taking anticonvulsants take a folic acid supplement both pre and post-conceptually. Neonates of women treated with anticonvulsants, especially barbiturates, should receive vitamin K at birth to reduce the risk of haemorrhage.

Phenytoin

Phenytoin (diphenylhydantoin) is probably the most commonly used anticonvulsant in pregnancy. Phenytoin has been reported to cause a pattern of malformations known as the foetal hydantoin syndrome (FHS).This syndrome includes intrauterine growth retardation (IUGR), distal digital and nail hypoplasia, mental retardation, cleft lip/palate, depressed nasal bridge, low-set ears, ocular hypertelorism, cardiac, and other anomalies.

Carbamazepine

Carbamazepine (Tegeretol) is a commonly prescribed anticonvulsant that was originally thought to be ideal for use in pregnancy as initial reports showed no teratogenic risks above baseline levels. Later, a pattern of malformations similar to those seen in foetal hydantoin syndrome was observed. Similar to phenytoin, carbamezepine is metabolized into oxidative intermediates (epoxides). Clearance of these metabolites relies on epoxide hydroxolase activity. Infants with a decreased enzyme activity would likely be at an increased risk for this pattern of malformations if their mother used carbamezapine during pregnancy.

Valproic acid

Valproic acid, an anticonvulsant is most effective for the treatment of seizures and epilepsy. Valproic acid exposure in the first trimester has been associated with an increased risk of neural tube defects. Valproate has also been associated with increased risks for orofacial clefts and congenital heart defects. It is advisable to evaluate valproate-exposed foetuses for neural tube defects. This should include careful sonographic evaluation and maternal serum alpha foetoprotein with consideration for amniocentesis for acetylcholinesterase and alpha foetoprotein determination.

Antidepressants

Drugs used to treat depression include the tricyclic derivatives, the monoamine oxidase inhibitors (MAOIs), and the selective serotonin reuptake inhibitors (SSRIs). The use of tricyclic antidepressants in pregnancy has not been associated with congenital malformations. MAOIs should be avoided as they have been shown to be teratogenic in animal. Also, there is a risk of severe maternal hypertensive reaction with these medications. The SSRIs are newer to the market and include fluoxetine (Prozac) and sertraline (Zoloft).

Lithium

Lithium, used for the treatment of manic-depressive disorders, has been associated with Ebstein anomaly and other cardiovascular defects. Ebstein anomaly is characterized by a dysplasia of the tricuspid valve with caudal displacement of the septal and posterior leaflets. Other cardiovascular defects associated with lithium ingestion include mitral atresia, patent ductus arteriosus, ventricular septal defects, hypoplasia of the left ventricle, dextrocardia, and anomalies of the great vessels.

Isotretinoin

Isotretinoin is the vitamin A analogue that is singularly effective for the treatment of severe, recalcitrant cystic acne. However, isotretinoin (Accutane) is one of the most potent known human teratogens. Isotretinoin has been associated with an increased rate of spontaneous abortions and up to an 18% incidence of foetal malformations when exposure occurred between 5 and 70 days of conception. The most common abnormalities associated with isotretinoin are craniofacial, followed by cardiac thymus and CNS. Craniofacial abnormalities include: microtic ears, agenesis or stenosis of the external ear canal, micrognathia, malformed calvarium, flattened and depressed nasal bridge, and hypertelorism.

Cardiac malformations include: transposition of the great vessels, tetralogy of Fallot, double-outlet right ventricle, truncus arteriosus communis, ventricular septal defects, aortic arch hypoplasia, and retroesophageal right subclavian artery. Thymic ectopia, hypoplasia, and aplasia occurred most commonly in conjunction with cardiac malformations. Hydrocephalus was the most common central nervous system malformation. Other anomalies included microcephaly, cortical lesions, cerebellar hypoplasia, agenesis, or dysgenesis.

Coumarin derivatives

Coumarin derivatives (warfarin, dicumarol, phenindione) are oral vitamin K antagonists, which are widely used anticoagulants. These agents appear to be capable of inducing foetal malformations in all trimesters. Exposure to these anticoagulants during the first trimester can cause specific anomalies known as foetal warfarin syndrome (FWS). The most consistent features of this syndrome are nasal hypoplasia, depression of the bridge of the nose, and stippled epiphyses. All cases of FWS appear to result from exposure between the 6th and 9th weeks of gestation. CNS defects include hydrocephalus, mental retardation, microcephaly, cerebellar atrophy, meningocele, and others. The use of coumarin derivatives in all trimesters appears to cause significant foetal risk.

Effects of alcohol

Alcohol abuse has been clearly established as a teratogen in humans. The effects of in utero exposure to alcohol include a characteristic collection of anomalies called foetal alcohol syndrome (FAS), which demonstrates clinical features of physical malformations, decreased birth weight, and cognitive anomalies (Figure 2.9).

Spontaneous abortion and stillbirths

Maternal consumption of intoxicating levels of alcohol over prolonged periods is clearly associated with a range of specific adverse foetal outcomes. The risk for spontaneous abortion may be increased two-fold in pregnancies complicated by maternal alcohol abuse.

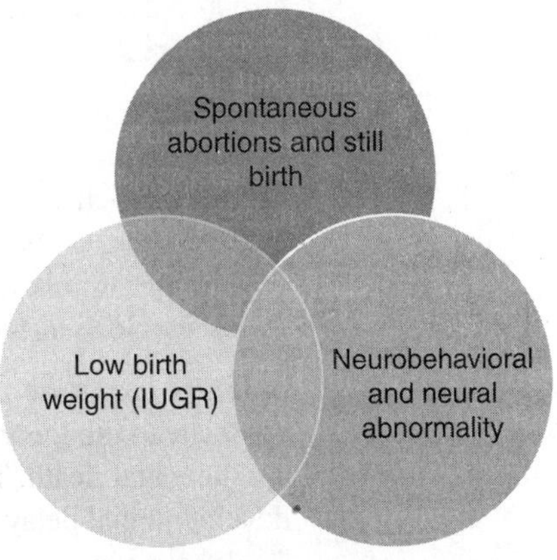

Figure 2.9 Effects of alcohol

Low birth weight

Lowered birth weight is the most reliably documented effect of maternal alcohol abuse.

Alcohol-related pregnancies demonstrate decrease in birth weight, which are primarily due to intrauterine growth retardation (IUGR).

Neurobehavioural and neural abnormality

The adverse effects of alcohol on behavioural development can be detected in the neonatal period. Neonates born to heavy drinkers are more restless during sleep and sleep less than other children. Abnormal electroencephalographic (EEG) activity during sleep has been noted for as long as 6 weeks after birth in some of these children. Children born to alcoholic mothers showed slower mental and motor development and low IQ.

Neural development

Neuroanatomic and biochemical abnormalities undoubtedly underlie the abnormal behavioural development observed in conjunction with foetal alcohol exposure. Microcephaly, a frequent characteristic of FAS, reflects an overall decrease in brain growth.

Prevention

The most conservative advice from a prevention standpoint is abstention from alcohol from the time of conception throughout the entire perinatal period. Such advice has been disseminated through public and professional education efforts.

Effect of chemicals

Many environmental chemicals have a proven track record of teratogenic activity. Exposure to such chemicals through occupation, diet, or accidents results in congenital malformations. Examples of such chemicals include lead, arsenic, mercury, polyaromatic hydrocarbons, ethidium bromide, carbon monoxide, polychlorinated dibenzofurans, etc.

Lead: The human placenta is permeable to lead, and exposure to high environmental levels of lead has been associated with spontaneous abortion, premature rupture of foetal membranes (PROM), and preterm delivery. Research also demonstrates that prenatal lead exposure leads to mental impairment. The levels of lead in breast milk are similar to those in plasma. Mothers with high serum lead levels should avoid breast feeding.

Arsenic: Exposure to arsenic-contaminated drinking water during pregnancy is associated with low birth weight and foetal loss—stillbirth, spontaneous abortion, and neonatal death. There is also concern that arsenic poisoning results in foetal developmental delay.

Mercury: Fish and shellfish have an affinity to accumulate mercury in their bodies, often in the form of methylmercury, a highly toxic organic compound of mercury. When this fish is consumed by an individual, the mercury level is accumulated. Fish-tissue concentrations of mercury increase over time. Thus, species that are high on the food chain collect higher concentrations of mercury that can be many times higher than the species they consume. This process is called biomagnification. Mercury poisoning occurred in Minamata, Japan, and is now referred to as the Minamata disease. Symptoms include ataxia, numbness in the hands and feet, malaise, vision, and speech and hearing defects. In extreme cases, paralysis, coma, and death follow within weeks of the onset of symptoms. A congenital form of the disease affects foetuses in the womb. Figure 2.10 illustrates the transplacental transmission of drugs and chemicals to the foetus.

Effects of radiation

Medical imaging has made rapid and impressive advances in the past two decades. However, prenatal exposure of the foetus to ionizing radiation is an anxiety-provoking issue. Sources of ionizing radiation are high energy X-rays used for diagnosis or for therapy, naturally occurring radioactive materials (for example, radium, radon), nuclear reactors, cyclotrons, and linear accelerators, alternating

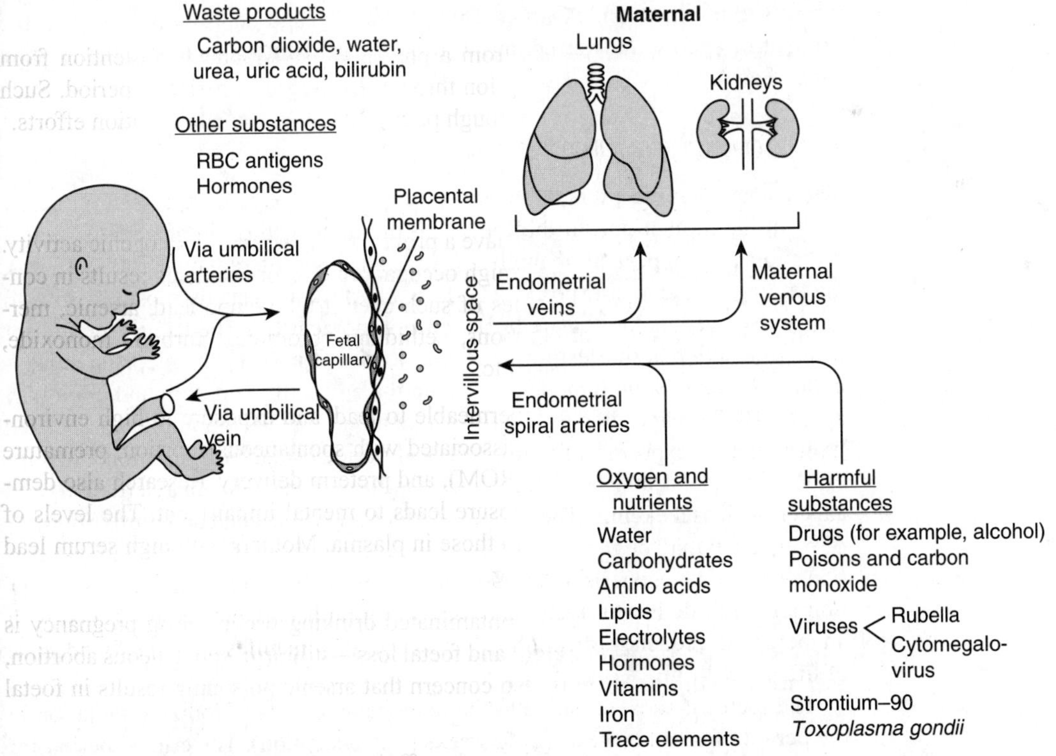

Figure 2.10 Transplacental transmission of molecules to foetus.

gradient synchrotrons, and radioactive materials used in medicine and industry (such as sealed cobalt and caesium). The low levels of background radiation on the earth and in the atmosphere have no detectable effects.

Radiobiology

Ionizing radiation consists of either electromagnetic waves, which are ionizing indirectly (X-rays and gamma rays), or particulates, which are directly ionizing (alpha and beta particles, protons, and neutrons). Because all types of radiation initiate damage by ionization, differences are quantitative rather than qualitative. Ionizing radiation damages tissue either directly or by secondary reaction, as it initiates a chain of chemical reactions that may ultimately result in radiation damage.

These include *physical damage* caused by ionization (takes approximately 10–12 seconds), *physiochemical damage* caused by production of free radicals (takes approximately 10–10 seconds), and *chemical damage* to DNA and RNA structure (takes approximately 10–6 seconds). The *biologic damage* caused from radiation may be expressed minutes to years later and may last a lifetime. Genetic or somatic effects depend on the total dose and dose rate (radiation dose/unit of time), amount of body area exposed, and distribution of the dose within the body.

Linear Energy Transfer (LET) is a measure of the density of ionization along a radiation beam. Higher LET radiation (alpha particles, protons, and neutrons) produces greater damage in a biologic system than lower LET radiation (electrons, gamma rays, and X-rays). Thus, tissue damage depends not only on the amount of energy transferred, but also on the penetrating ability of the specific type of emission.

Effects of ionizing radiation in pregnancy

The damage caused by radiation to cell chromatin may be expressed clinically both in the mother and in the foetus. In the mother, the carcinogenic effect of radiation may appear after moderate to high doses of radiation (50–600 rem), depending on the area exposed. The face and neck are usually most sensitive to damage as well as the female breast during thoracic CT. The latency period for cancer induction is shortest for myeloblastic disorders (for example, leukemia)—about 2–5 years. Solid tumours such as in the breast, thyroid, skin and brain may appear 10–30 years after exposure to radiation. Foetal compromise associated with radiation exposure in utero differs at various stages of gestation. Adverse effects include death, neuropathology, malformations, growth retardation, and cancer, such as leukemia. The developing foetus in the second and third trimesters of pregnancy may be more sensitive to the carcinogenic effect of ionizing radiation. After organogenesis and rapid neuron development (105 days after conception and until delivery), foetal exposure to more than 10 rads is associated with an increased frequency of childhood cancer, usually manifested in the first decade of life.

The foetus is most sensitive to the teratogenic effects of ionizing radiation in the period of organogenesis (2–15 weeks postconception). The critical period for induction of cataracts, microphtalmia, or skeletal defects is at 4–8 weeks of gestation. The CNS remains the most sensitive organ to the effects of ionizing radiation, even at later stages of gestation. Radiation-induced mental and growth retardation and microcephaly may be observed after in utero exposure over 10 rad, between 4–25 weeks of gestation. The risk for childhood cancer may persist until birth. Small head size, seizures, and decline in IQ points were observed with foetal dose over 10 rads in the gestational stage of rapid neuron development and migration (56–105 days after conception).

INFERTILITY

One in six couples experience an unknown delay in conception. Roughly 50% of these couples will conceive either spontaneously or with relatively simple advice and treatment. The other half remain subfertile and need more complex treatment modules such as in vitro fertilization and other assisted conception techniques.

Most couples presenting with fertility problem do not have absolute infertility (i.e. no chance of conception), but rather relative subfertility with reduced chance of conception because of one or more factors in either or both partners. Most couples with subfertility will conceive spontaneously or will be amenable to treatment, so that only 4% remain involuntarily childless.

Therefore, in this chapter the focus is more on subfertility—causes and treatment modules.

Infertility (subfertility): The failure to conceive after one year of unprotected regular sexual intercourse. Subfertility can be primary or secondary.

Primary subfertility: The delay that occurs for couples who have had no previous pregnancies.

Secondary subfertility: The delay that occurs for couples who have conceived previously, although the pregnancy may not have been successful (miscarriage, ectopic pregnancy).

Spontaneous conception: The likelihood of spontaneous conception is affected by age, previous pregnancy, duration of subfertility, timing of intercourse during the natural cycle, extremes of body mass, and pathology present.

FACTORS AFFECTING FERTILITY

Increased chances of conception:

- Woman aged under 30 years
- Previous pregnancy
- Less than three years trying to conceive
- Intercourse occurring during six days before ovulation, particularly two days before ovulation

- Woman's body mass index (BMI) 20–30
- Both partners are non-smokers
- Caffeine intake less than two cups of coffee daily
- No use of recreational drugs

Reduced chances of conception:

- Women aged over 35 years
- No previous pregnancy
- Trying to conceive for over three years
- Intercourse incorrectly timed
- Woman's BMI < 20 or >30
- One or both partners smoke
- High caffeine intake
- Regular use of recreational drugs

CAUSES OF SUBFERTILITY—MALE AND FEMALE SUBFERTILITY

MALE SUBFERTILITY

Abnormal semen quality and sexual dysfunction are contributing factors in 50% of subfertile couples. Subfertility affects one in 20 men. Idiopathic oligoasthenoteratozoospermia is the commonest cause of male subfertility. Less common types of male subfertility are caused by testicular or genital tract infection, disease, or abnormalities. Systemic disease, external factors (drugs, lifestyle), or combinations of these also result in male subfertility.

Semen analysis terminology and seminal fluid analysis parameters are given in Tables 2.8 and 2.9.

Table 2.8 Semen analysis terminology

Normozoospermia – All semen parameters normal
Oligozoospermia – Reduced sperm numbers (Mild to moderate: 5–20 million/ml of semen, Severe: <5 million/ml of semen)
Asthenozoospermia: Reduced sperm motility
Teratozoospermia: Increased abnormal forms of sperm
Oligoasthenoteratozoospermia: Sperm variables all subnormal
Azoospermia: No sperm in semen
Aspermia (anejaculation): No ejaculate (ejaculation failure)
Leucocytospermia: Increased white cells in semen
Necrozoospermia: All sperm are non-viable or non-motile

Table 2.9 Normal seminal fluid analysis (World Health Organization)

Volume > 2 ml

Sperm concentration > 20 million/ml

Sperm motility >50% progressive or >25% rapidly progressive

Morphology >15% normal forms

White blood cells <1 million/ml

Immunobead or mixed antiglobulin reaction test* <50%

*Tests for the presence of antibodies coating the sperm.

Table 2.10 Drugs that impair male fertility

Impaired spermatogenesis: Sulphasalazine, methotrexate

Pituitary suppression: Testosterone injections

Antiandrogenic effects: Cimetidine

Ejaculation failure: α blockers, antidepressants

Erectile dysfunction: β blockers, thiazide

Drugs of misuse: Anabolic steroids, heroin, cocaine

Clinical assessment

History taking should include the frequency of coitus, erectile function, ejaculation, scrotal disorders or surgery, urinary symptoms, past illnesses, lifestyle factors, and any drugs taken. Physical examination should seek signs of hypogonadism (small testes), hypoandrogenism (lack of facial and body hair), systemic disease, and abnormalities of the penis or testicles. Scrotal ultrasound is helpful in confirming a varicocele or testicular tumour. Genetic screening (karyotype or DNA analysis for Y chromosome microdeletions) is indicated for men with severe oligozoospermia and most men with azoospermia.

Treatment options for subfertile men

The treatment options available for subfertile men are:

- Stopping adverse drugs and drug misuse like sulphasalazine and anabolic steroids misused by athletes
- Timing and lifestyle changes
- Treating accessory gland infection

Assisted conception: Intrauterine insemination and intracytoplasmic sperm injection and donor insemination.

Drugs that impair male fertility are given in Table 2.10.

FEMALE SUBFERTILITY

Anovulation, tubal subfertility, endometriosis, and fibroids are major reasons for female subfertility.

Anovulation: Disorders of ovulation account for 30% of infertility and often present with irregular periods (oligomenorrhoea) or an absence of periods (amenorrhoea). Many of the treatments are simple and effective; therefore, couples may need only limited contact with doctors. However, not all causes of anovulation are amenable to treatment by ovulation induction. Anovulation can sometimes be treated with medical or surgical induction, but it is the cause of the anovulation that will determine whether ovulation induction is possible.

Causes of anovulation suitable and not suitable for ovulation induction treatment are given in Tables 2.11 and 2.12.

Chromosomal

Turner's Syndrome (45,X): Underdeveloped streak ovaries resulting in primary ovarian failure (premature menopause).

Table 2.11 Causes of anovulation suitable for ovulation induction treatment

Hypothalamic
Low concentration of gonadotropin releasing hormone
Weight or exercise-related amenorrhoea
Kallman's syndrome
Stress
Idiopathic

Pituitary
Hyperprolactinaemia
Pituitary failure
Sheehan's syndrome
Craniopharyngioma
Cerebral radiotherapy

Ovarian
Polycystic ovaries

Other Endocrine
Hypothyroidism
Congenital adrenal hyperplasia

Table 2.12 Causes of anovulation not suitable for ovulation induction treatment ovarian failure

Idiopathic

Radiotherapy/chemotherapy

Surgical removal

Genetic

Autoimmune

Androgen Insensitivity Syndrome (46,XY): Women have 46,XY karyotype with intra-abdominal gonads that are testes but have developed phenotypically as a female because of the absence of androgen receptors. The vagina ends blindly as there is no uterus and pregnancy is impossible.

Diagnosis of anovulatory subfertility

The concentrations of luteinizing hormone, follicle stimulating hormone, and oestradiol will be low. Some women have polycystic ovarian disease (PCOD), which is detected by ultrasound and higher testosterone concentrations.

Management of anovulation

1. Change of weight: Women with PCOD are overweight and are advised to lose weight. Weight loss with exercise reduces the insulin and free testosterone levels, resulting in improved menstrual regularity, ovulation, and pregnancy rates. Women who are underweight are encouraged to gain weight and improve their BMI to normal values.

2. Appropriate treatment for hyperprolactinaemia and hypothyroidism is advised.

3. Gonadotropin-releasing hormone is started under hospital setting for women who have purely hypothalamic cause for their amenorrhoea.

4. Ovulation induction treatment with clomifene is advised. Clomifene acts by blocking oestrogen receptors in the pituitary leading to increased production of the follicle stimulating hormone, which then stimulates development of one or more dominant follicles. Follicle stimulating hormone injections are used in women who failed to respond to clomifene.

5. Laproscopic ovarian diathermy or drilling has replaced wedge resection of the ovaries in women with PCOD. At laproscopy, five to six diathermy or laser punctures are made in the ovary for ovarian stimulation.

Tubal subfertility

Patent fallopian tubes are a prerequisite for normal human fertility. However, patency alone is not enough—normal function is crucial. Fallopian tubes have a crucial role in picking up the eggs and transporting the eggs, sperm, and embryo. The fallopian tubes are also needed for sperm capacitation and egg fertilization. The fallopian tube is vulnerable to infection and surgical damage, which may impair function by affecting the delicate fimbriae or the highly specialized endosalpinx. A fallopian tube obstruction occurs in 12–33% of infertile couples and hence tubal patency should be investigated early.

Causes of tubal damage

Infection: Pelvic infection is a major cause of tubal subfertility. Infective tubal damage can be caused by sexually transmitted diseases, or can occur after miscarriage, termination of pregnancy, puerperal sepsis, or insertion of an intrauterine contraceptive device. Pelvic infections are most commonly caused by *Chlamydia trachomatis*, *Gonorrhoea*, and genital tuberculosis.

Diagnosis of tubal subfertility

1. Infection screening.
2. Hysterosalpingo contrast sonography—it is a procedure where an echocontrast fluid is introduced into the uterine cavity via a 5 French cervical balloon catheter so that the uterine cavity, ovaries, and fallopian tube patency can be assessed accurately.
3. Transvaginal ultrasonography can be helpful in detecting tubal damages.

Endometriosis

Endometriosis is present in 20–40% of women who complain of subfertility. Endometriosis is characterized by the presence of growth of endometrial tissue outside the uterus and is often associated with symptoms of dysmenorrhoea, dyspareunia, and subfertility.

Pelvic examination may show tenderness, nodules of endometriosis on the uterosacral ligaments or an enlarged ovary, which may be secondary to an ovarian endometrioma. The diagnosis of endometriosis is generally confirmed by laproscopy. Preoperative ultrasonography is helpful to diagnose the likely cause of a tender and enlarged ovary.

Fibroids

Fibroids (leiomyomata) are benign tumours of the myometrium, which occur in 30% of women. Fibroids are more likely to reduce the chances of the embryo implanting if the fibroid is in the intracavity. Fibroids are estimated to have a detrimental effect on fertility in upto 10% cases. They are also associated with an increased risk of miscarriage in women who conceive and half the livebirth in vitro fertilization cycles.

The size of the fibroids can be reduced by the administration of superactive gonadotropin releasing hormone analogues (goserelin, buserelin, nafarelin). If the fibroids are intracavity (submucosal) structures, they can be resected easily hysteroscopically. However, if the fibroids are intramural, an abdominal procedure (laprotomy or laproscopic myomectomy) is needed.

ASSISTED REPRODUCTIVE TECHNIQUES

Many assisted conception modules are offered to subfertile couples based on the etiology of subfertility.

A few important assisted conception techniques are described below:

Intrauterine insemination: For men with ejaculatory dysfunction and difficulty in coitus, semen sample is collected, washed, prepared, and deposited into the uterus at a time when ovulation is likely or assisted. The sample is washed; prepared motile sperm is deposited in the uterus just before the release of the egg in a natural or stimulated cycle. The technique is effective when it is combined with mild superovulation using gonadotropins. It is simpler, cheaper, and less invasive than IVF or ICSI and has fewer complications.

Intracytoplasmic sperm injection (ICSI): A single sperm is injected into the cytoplasm of the egg to attain fertilization. Multiple defects of sperm (concentration, motility, and morphology) show poor success in IVF; hence, ICSI is preferred. ICSI is a specialized variant of IVF treatment in which fertilization is achieved by the injection of a single sperm directly into the cytoplasm of the egg. Only mature eggs are suitable for injection with prepared sperm. A single sperm is carefully examined and selected for normality of its morphology and with a fine glass needle it is inserted directly into the cytoplasm of the egg.

In vitro fertilization (IVF): In IVF, oocytes (obtained surgically from ovarian follicles in superovulated cycles) are prepared and are brought together in a dish in the laboratory. Fertilization takes place outside the body (in vitro = glass). Cleavage stage embryos derived from these fertilized oocytes are placed in the uterus (embryo transfer) for pregnancy to occur.

Donor insemination is advised to couples who suffer from azoospermia or failed ICSI. Donors are hired by sperm banks and are screened for history of medical or genetic disorders and sexually transmitted infections. The women must have atleast one fallopian tube functional and must be ovulatory to achieve success by donor insemination. Counselling must be imparted to both partners to explore all the issues related to the use of donor gametes.

The indications for assisted reproductive techniques are given in Figure 2.11.

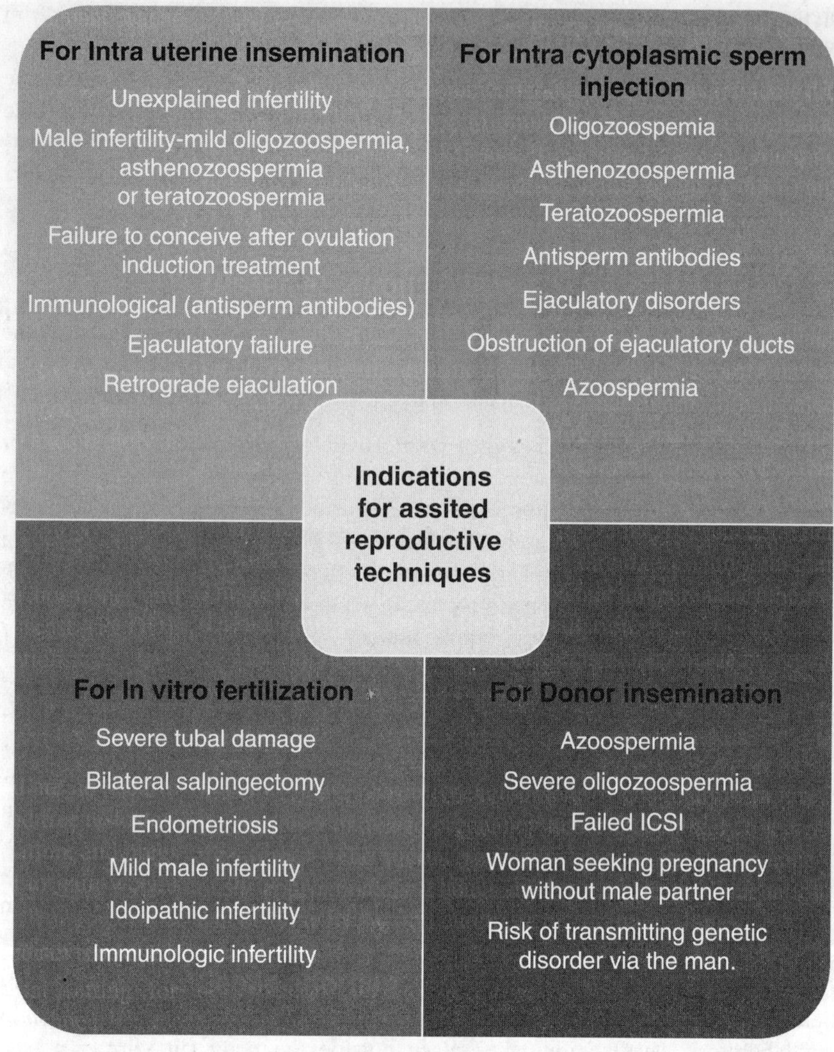

Figure 2.11

SPONTANEOUS ABORTION

The most common complication of pregnancy is spontaneous abortion, which is estimated to occur in 10–15% of pregnancies and about 80% of these abortions occur within 2 to 3 months of gestation. By definition, a complete abortion is the expulsion of all products of conception before the 20th week of gestation.

Spontaneous abortion is one of the least understood pathological processes. The classic definition of RSA (recurrent spontaneous abortion) is the loss of three or more clinically recognized pregnancies spontaneously during early gestation. The modern definition, however, is the spontaneous loss of 2 or more consecutive pregnancies before 20 weeks of gestation, which takes into consideration that a woman over 35 is at greater risk for pregnancy loss than a 25-year-old woman.

The World Health Organization (WHO) has defined miscarriage as the loss of a foetus or embryo weighing ≤ 500 g, which would normally be at 20–22 complete weeks of gestation (WHO 1977).

Recurrent abortion (or as it is sometimes called "habitual abortion") is a form of infertility. Abortion is a common cause of maternal deaths in all countries. The mode of death is by way of haemorrhage, shock, infection, or thromboembolism. These are sometimes associated with the tearing or rupture of the cervix and uterus. They can occur spontaneously or as complications of completing spontaneous abortion.

PATHOPHYSIOLOGY

Potential causes of spontaneous pregnancy loss

It is estimated that foetal viability is achieved only in 30% of all human conceptions, 50% of which are lost prior to the first missed menses (Table 2.13). Patients with a systemic problem will comprise an increasingly larger fraction of all RSA patients with an increased number of previous pregnancy losses.

In the early weeks, death of the foetus often precedes the expulsive action of the uterus and seems to be the precipitating factor for abortion. Later in pregnancy, the foetus is more often born alive and abortion then appears to have been caused by some error in the uterus or in its behaviour. Some of the later abortions begin by rupture of the membranes allowing the liquor amnii to escape. Recognition of these three groups is of practical value in narrowing the search for the cause of abortion. Pathophysiology of a spontaneous abortion may be suggested by the timing of miscarriage.

Chromosomal defects are commonly seen in spontaneous abortions, especially those that occur during 4–8 weeks' gestation. The contribution of chromosomal abnormalities is as high as 70%. Genetic etiologies are common in early

Table 2.13 Potential causes of spontaneous pregnancy loss

Pathologic (blighted) ovum—anembryonic gestation

Embryonic anomalies

Chromosomal anomalies

Increased maternal age

Uterine anomalies

Intra-uterine device

Teratogen

Mutagen

Maternal disease

Placental anomalies

Extensive maternal trauma

first-trimester loss but may be seen throughout gestation. Trisomy chromosomes are the most common chromosomal anomaly.

Insufficient or excessive hormonal levels usually result in spontaneous abortion before 10 weeks' gestation. Infectious, immunologic, and environmental factors generally are seen in first-trimester pregnancy loss. Anatomic factors are usually associated with second-trimester loss. Factor XIII deficiency and a complete or partial deficiency of fibrinogen are associated with recurrent spontaneous abortions.

MECHANISM OF ABORTION

Eighty per cent of diagnosed abortions occur during second and third months of pregnancy. Before the twelfth week, the pregnancy sac tends to be extruded from the uterus in one mass. The membranes rupture at some stage of dilatation of the cervix and the foetus and the placenta are born separately. The process is not likely to be so smooth because the uterus is not properly sensitized and its muscular action is less efficient. Some part of the chorion is often retained and excessive haemorrhage is common.

INCIDENCE

A total of 15–20% of all pregnancies will end in early pregnancy losses. These losses, however, are those recognized pregnancies that are confirmed usually 4–5 weeks after conception. There is now evidence that the pregnancy loss rate before this period, i.e., during the 2–3 weeks following conception, may be as high as 50%.

Habitual abortion is traditionally classified as three or more consecutive abortions. Clinical studies have shown that the risk of pregnancy loss after three previous losses is only 30–40%. A successful outcome after three consequent abortions can be expected to be 55–60%. With a previous live birth, this rate can be as high as 70%.

CLINICAL TYPES OF ABORTION

Table 2.14 Definitions of types of intrauterine pregnancies

Incomplete abortion	Expulsion of some but not all of the products of conception before 20 completed weeks of gestation.
Complete abortion	Spontaneous expulsion of all foetal and placental tissue from the uterine cavity before 20 weeks of gestation.
Inevitable abortion	Uterine bleeding from a gestation of less than 20 weeks, accompanied by cervical dilation but without expulsion of placental or foetal tissue through the cervix.
Anembryonic gestation	An intrauterine sac without foetal tissue present at more than 7.5 weeks of gestation.
First-trimester foetal death	Death of the foetus in the first 12 weeks of gestation.
Second trimester foetal death	Death of the foetus between 13 and 24 weeks of gestation.
Recurrent spontaneous abortion	The loss of more than three pregnancies before 20 weeks of gestation.

Threatened abortion

Threatened abortion is a clinical entity where choriodecidual haemorrhage has begun, but not progressed to the stage of irreversibility. The bleeding is indicative of some degree of separation of the chorion from the deciduas and it varies in amount, duration, and type. It is also accompanied by backache and lower abdominal discomfort due to uterine contractions. This means that the cervix is not open, and the products of conception are not expelled or displaced yet (Figure 2.12).

Treatment

Confinement to bed: Maintained for 2–5 days after all bleeding has ceased.

Sedatives and myometrial inhibitors: Pethidine followed by a sedative to relieve pain and to quell patients' anxiety. They indirectly quieten uterine activity.

Hormones: Endocrine therapy of all types is empirical and of unproven value. Manipulative correction of a retroverted uterus should not be attempted while abortion is threatening. The diagnosis of threatened abortion is so uncertain that it is impossible to state the results accurately. All rhesus factor negative women should be given anti-D immunoglobulin to avoid sensitization.

Inevitable abortion

In this type of abortion the process of abortion has begun and progressed to such an extent that expulsion of the products of conception seems inevitable. With an inevitable abortion, the volume of bleeding is often greater than with other types of abortion. Besides haemorrhage, symptoms like painful uterine contractions, dilatation of the cervix, or extrusion of some part of the conceptus through the os uteri is also seen. Other suggestive signs are ballooning of the upper vagina, tenderness of the uterus, and pyrexia (Figure 2.13).

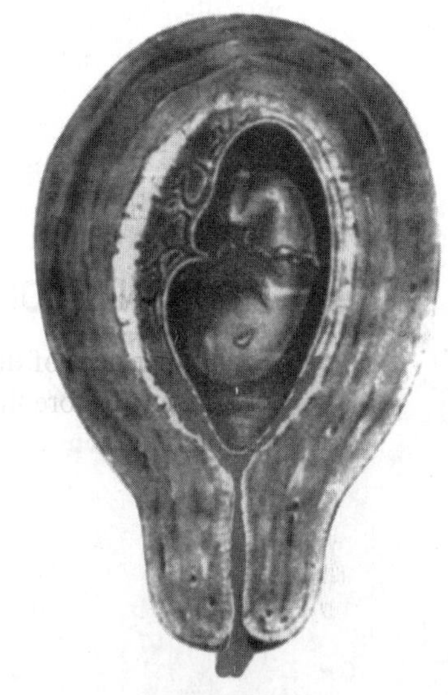

Figure 2.12 Threatened abortion—slight bleeding, membranes intact, and cervical os closed. (See page 246 for the colour image.)

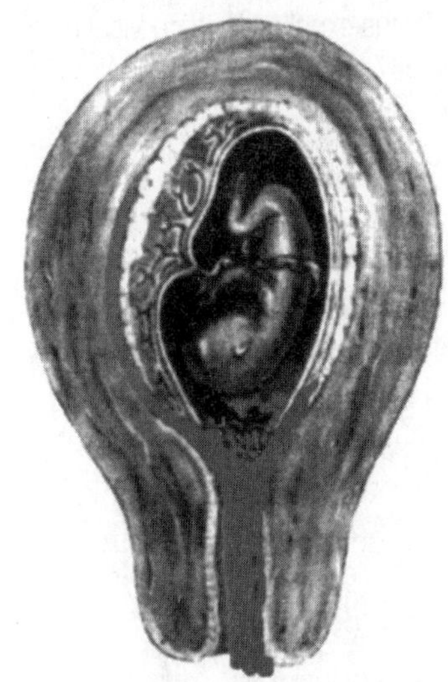

Figure 2.13 Inevitable abortion—moderate bleeding with pain, and cervical os dilated. (See page 246 for the colour image.)

Treatment

The patient is confined to the bed until abortion is complete. Morphine and pethidine can be administered to relieve pain and anxiety. Suction curettage should be performed.

To control profuse bleeding, syntometrine can be administered intramuscularly or intravenously. This treatment can bring about complete evacuation of the uterus and bleeding can be controlled temporarily. Oxytocics can also be administered intravenously to limit bleeding.

Incomplete abortion

In the incomplete variety, the abortion has occurred but the process is incomplete. The cervical os is open and the products of conception are partly expelled. Fragments of chorion often remain in the uterus after apparently complete abortion (Figure 2.14).

When the abortion is incomplete the bleeding does not get progressively less but varies from day to day, becoming heavy from time to time. It continues intermittently for weeks and months and may be accompanied by periodic uterine colic.

Treatment

Dilatation of the cervix and exploration of the uterus under general anaesthesia can be a treatment for incomplete abortion. All rhesus-negative women should be given anti-D immunoglobulin.

Complete abortion

In a case of complete abortion the products of conception are expelled completely from the uterus and the uterine cavity is empty. The entire ovum has been expelled. Once this has occurred, the pain subsides and bleeding decreases. The cervical canal may be closed, as it contracts very rapidly after the complete expulsion of the uterine contents (Figure 2.15).

Treatment

An examination demonstrates that active bleeding has slowed or stopped, there is no tissue visible in the cervix, and the passed tissue appears complete.

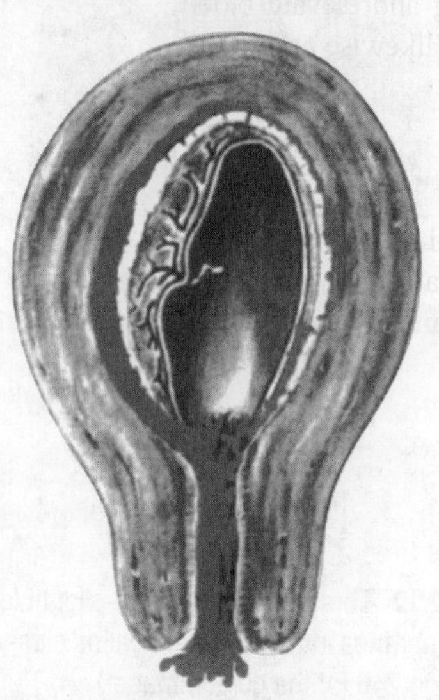

Figure 2.14 Incomplete abortion—free bleeding, foetus expelled, and cervical os dilated. (See page 247 for the colour image.)

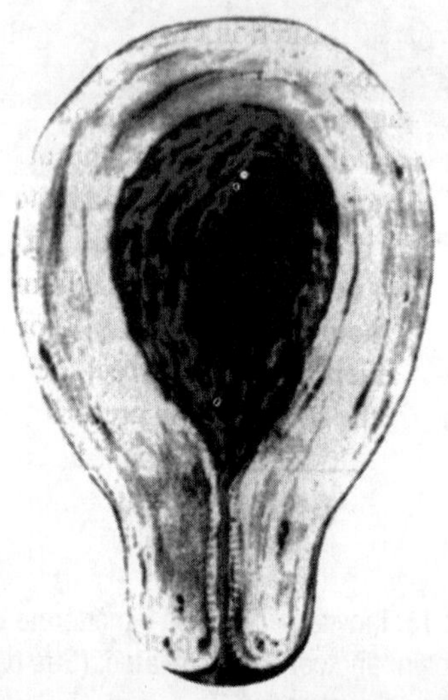

Figure 2.15 Complete abortion—foetus and placenta expelled, bleeding scanty, and cervical os closed. (See page 247 for the colour image.)

Rh-negative women can be given an injection of Rhogam (hyperimmune Rh globulin) within 3 days of the abortion.

Some physicians recommend routinely giving a uterotonic drug (such a Methergine 0.2 mg PO TID × 2 days) to minimize bleeding and to encourage expelling of any remaining fragments of tissue. It also may increase cramping and elevate blood pressure. Antibiotics (such as doxycycline or amoxicillin) are likewise prescribed by some.

Missed abortion

In missed abortion, there is intrauterine death of the foetus and it is then passively retained within the uterine cavity. The foetus becomes macerated or mummified, the liquor amnii is absorbed and the placenta becomes pale and thin. Interesting pathological variant of missed abortion is carneous (blood) mole. Multiple haemorrhages in the choriodecidual space become numerous or extensive that they kill the foetus (Figure 2.16).

In a few cases of missed abortion, products of placental degeneration (probably thromboplastin) enter the maternal circulation and cause intravascular clotting. This results in hypofibrinogenaemia and an increase of the fibrinolysins and fibrin degradation products (FDP) in circulation.

The diagnosis of missed abortion is mostly made by repeated clinical observations, or by the use of ultrasound.

Treatment

Except for the possible development of coagulation failure, the presence of a dead pregnancy in utero is unlikely to harm the women. The uterus generally empties itself spontaneously approximately 21 days after foetal death. Evacuation can be done by suction curettage or curettage alone.

Septic abortion

Septic abortion is a type of abortion associated with sepsis of the products of conception and the uterus. Sepsis is most often caused by a variety of organisms—*E. coli, Enterococcus, Pseudomonas, Streptococcus, Proteus.* According to the severity, septic abortions are graded in to three.

Grade 1: Tenderness confined to the uterus. The infection can be limited to the uterine cavity. Open or closed cervix with a bulky, tender uterus.

Grade 2: The infection will be spread beyond the uterus to the parametrium. The lower abdomen will be slightly rigid and tenderness will be present over the hypogastrium and on either side.

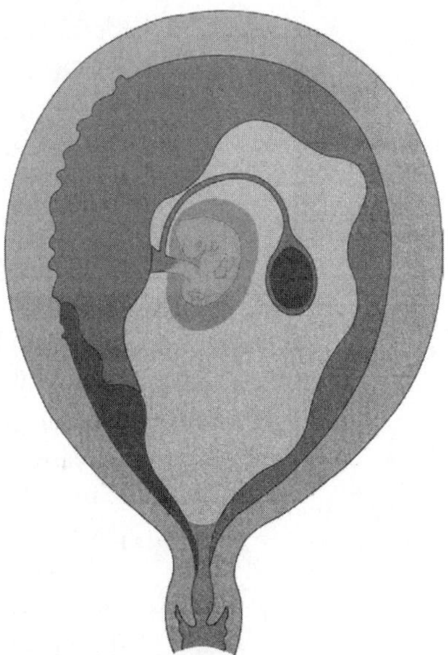

Figure 2.16 Missed abortion—intrauterine death of the foetus. (See page 248 for the colour image.)

Grade 3: Patient will be very ill with signs of peritonitis: fever, dry tongue, rapid pulse, and distended tender abdomen.

Treatment

Patients of all three grades should be hospitalized, and prompt and aggressive therapy should be provided.

The aim of the treatment is to control infection by appropriate antibiotic therapy correction of electrolyte imbalance and blood volume, removal of infected products, and prevention of further bleeding.

Whatever the antibiotic used, it is most important that the initial therapy should always be parenteral, intensive, and in sufficiently high dosage.

RISK OF RECURRENT PREGNANCY LOSS

1. Women who have had at least one liveborn infant:
   (a) With no prior foetal losses—Recurrence risk is 12% for the next pregnancy
   (b) With at least 1 prior foetal loss—Recurrence risk is 24% for the next pregnancy
   (c) With two prior foetal losses—Recurrence risk is 26% for the next pregnancy
   (d) With three prior foetal losses—Recurrence risk is 32% for the next pregnancy
2. Women who have not had at least one liveborn infant with two or more foetal losses:
   (a) Recurrence risk for the next pregnancy is 40–45%.
   (b) Pregnancies involving more than one foetus are at increased risk of miscarriage.
   (c) Uncontrolled diabetes greatly increases the risk of miscarriage.
3. Polycystic ovary syndrome is a risk factor for miscarriage, with 30–50% of pregnancies in women with PCOS being miscarried in the first trimester.
4. High blood pressure and certain illnesses (such as rubella and chlamydia) increase the risk of miscarriage.
5. Tobacco (cigarette) smokers have an increased risk of miscarriage. An increase in miscarriage is also associated with the father being a cigarette smoker. The husband study observed a 4% increased risk for husbands who smoke less than 20 cigarettes/day, and an 81% increased risk for husbands who smoke 20 or more cigarettes/day.
6. Severe cases of hypothyroidism increase the risk of miscarriage. The effect of milder cases of hypothyroidism on miscarriage rates has not been established. Certain immune conditions such as autoimmune diseases greatly increase the risk of miscarriage.
7. Cocaine use increases miscarriage rates.

8. Physical trauma, exposure to environmental toxins, obesity, high caffeine intake (>300 mg/day), high levels of alcohol consumption, high fever (37.8°C = 100°F) or higher), use of an IUD during the time of conception, and use of NSAIDs have also been linked to increased risk of miscarriage.

FACTORS INVOLVED IN RECURRENT EARLY PREGNANCY LOSS

1. Foetal death or disease
2. Genetic factors
3. Endocrine factors
4. Anatomic factors
5. Immunologic factors
6. Infectious factors
7. Environmental factors

Foetal death or disease

The most frequent single cause for abortion is malformation of the foetus and its membranes. This accounts for 50–80% of early (6–8 weeks) abortions. The young pregnancy sac when examined will often be found that the foetus is absent or rudimentary. This condition is called blighted ovum.

Malformations can be caused by defective implantation of a normal trophoblast, by maternal virus infections (especially rubella), and by cytotoxic drugs. Ageing of the ova is a predisposing factor to explain the increased incidence of abortion in older women. Synthesis of nucleic acids in the rapidly dividing cells of the embryo, trophoblast, and decidua plays a part in causing abortion.

Foetal anoxia: Interference with the placental circulation can occur by infarction by placental separation; by faulty placental formation; by hydatidiform mole; and by infection of the placenta as in syphilis.

Foetal anaemia: Incompatibility between the blood groups of the foetus and the mother, resulting in rhesus and other types of isoimmunization, rarely kills the foetus before the 28th week and is an exceptional cause of abortion. Some cases of recurrent abortion may be explained by HLA-incompatible matings.

Poisons and drugs: Chemical poisons that damage the chorion or the foetus are a rare cause of abortion. Cytotoxic agents can certainly cause abortion by killing the foetus.

Pyrexia: Failure of the foetus to withstand very high temperatures can complicate severe maternal infections.

GENETIC FACTORS

Balanced chromosome rearrangements have been found with an increased frequency in couples with recurrent early pregnancy wastage. When balanced rearrangement is present, the chromosomes have difficulty in pairing up and dividing evenly during meiosis. As a result, gametes frequently possess an unbalanced set of chromosomal materials. The clinical consequences of such imbalances are usually lethal to the developing embryo, causing spontaneous abortions.

Major chromosome abnormalities have been found in 4.8–5.5%. Other abnormalities usually encountered include:

1. Sex chromosome mosaicism,
2. Chromosome inversions,
3. Ring chromosomes.

Besides spontaneous abortions, these abnormalities are associated with a high risk of malformations and mental retardation.

Certain chromosomal abnormalities are seen in couples, which are associated with significant cause of RSA (Table 2.15).
It also includes:

Translocation
(a) Robertsonian translocation
(b) Reciprocal translocation
(c) Multiple translocations

Skewed X chromosome inactivation (XCI)

An increase in extremely skewed XCI of 90% has been reported among women who experience RSA. A significant excess of trisomic losses was observed among

Table 2.15 Certain chromosomal abnormalities are seen in couples, which are considered to be a significant cause of RS

Numerical Abnormalities	
45,X/46,XX	45,X/46,XY
46,XX/47,XX	46,XY/47,XY + fragment

Structural Abnormalities	
Variants	
Inversion 9	1 qh +
9 qh +	9 qh + and Y q +
16 qh + inversion 9	14 p +
15 p +	Markers
14 ss	15 ss
22 p +	Y q +
Y q - (pat)	Y q + and 15 ss
Inversion Y	fragile sites 3 p 14 and 6 q

the women who had RSA with skewed XCI versus those without skewed XCI. X-linked mutations (deletions, translocations. etc.) have been clearly associated with skewed XCI and RSA in some families.

Premature centromeric division

At metaphase, the two chromatids of each replicated chromosome are largely held together by a single centromere that also attaches the chromosome to the spindle equator. The centromere then divides and leads the separated chromatids to the spindle poles, ensuring a truly equational division of the chromosome complement.

Rarely, at metaphase, the chromatids of a single chromosome are separated at the centromere. The chromatids of this single chromosome have been interpreted as having separated precociously and the phenomenon has been termed premature centromere division (PCD).

The term premature centromere division (PCD) has been used to describe the premature division of the X chromosome centromere (PCD, X) as compared with the centromeres of other chromosomes in the same metaphase.

Metaphase chromosomes in PCD have separated rod-like straight chromatids and have been described as having a railroad track appearance. The separated centromeres give a localized puffing, which is particularly noticeable in the para-centromeric regions of chromosome 1, chromosome 9, and chromosome 16. This cytogenetic phenomenon is so peculiar to Roberts Syndrome that it is known as the RS effect.

Premature division of the X chromosome centromere (PCD, X) is a relatively common finding in a small proportion of cells in phenotypically normal women. It is positively associated with the age-related X chromosome aneuploidy in lymphocytes.

Mitotic configurations consistent in split centromeres and splayed chromatids in all or most of the chromosomes or PCD have been described in three categories. They are:

1. Low frequency of PCD (up to 3% of the mitosis) observed in colchicines-treated lymphocyte cultures from normal individuals.

2. High frequency of PCD (5% or more) with mosaic aneuploidies involving a variety of chromosomes, called "mosaic variegated aneuploidy", observed in individuals with microcephaly, growth deficiency, severe mental retardation, and risk of malignancy.

3. High frequency of PCD (5% or more) as a sole chromosome abnormality. Individuals with this condition have no recognizable clinical pattern or occur in healthy individuals. Association of this PCD trait with abortions and infertility has been reported.

NON-GENETIC FACTORS

Anatomical factors

The most common malformations associated with RSA are variations of the double uterus (bicornuate, septate, or didelphic (Figures 2.17 and 2.18) with the

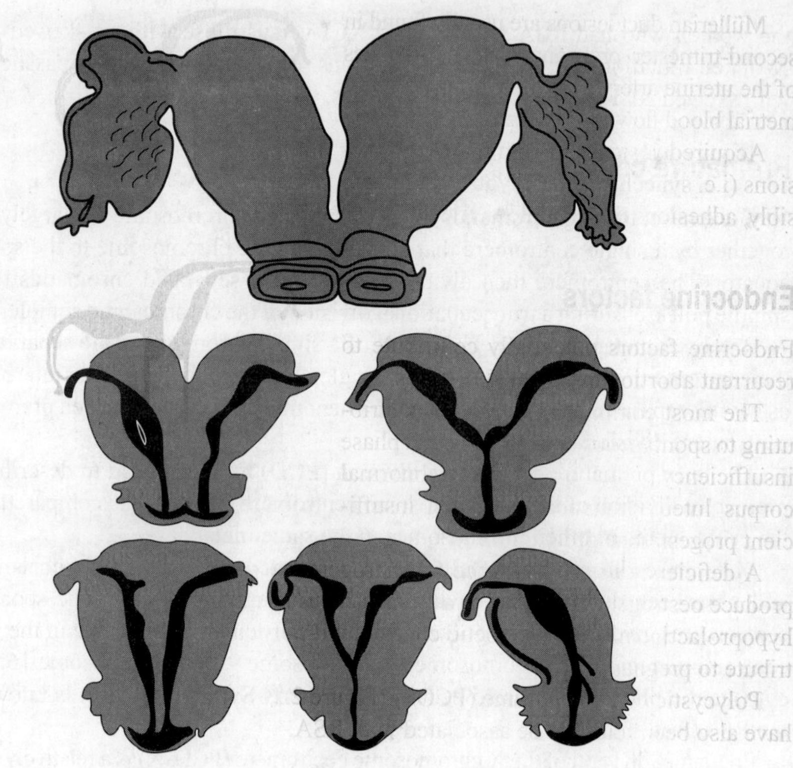

Figure 2.17 Bicornuate uterus.

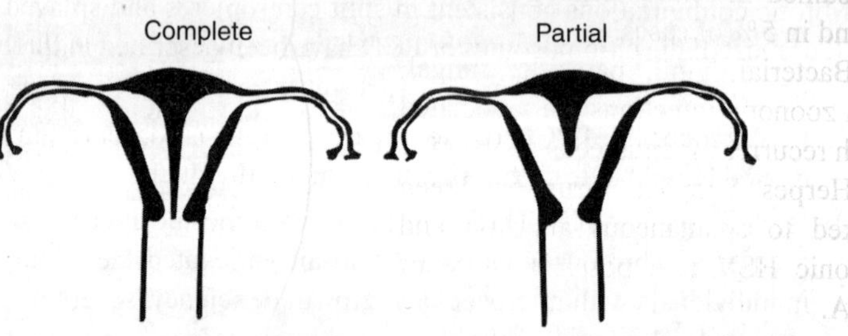

Figure 2.18 Uterine septate. (See page 248 for the colour image.)

septate uterus predominating. Anatomic abnormalities include uterine abnormalities like double uterus, or uterine adhesions as in the case of Asherman's Syndrome; the presence of endometrial polyps, submucous fibroids and, Müllerian duct defect (Figure 2.19).

Congenital or acquired anatomic factors reportedly are present in 10–15% of women who have recurrent spontaneous abortions.

Congenital anatomic lesions include Müllerian duct anomalies (for example, septate uterus, diethylstilbestrol [DES]-related anomalies).

Müllerian duct lesions are usually found in second-trimester pregnancy loss. Anomalies of the uterine artery with compromised endometrial blood flow are congenital.

Acquired lesions are intrauterine adhesions (i.e. synechiae), leiomyomas, and possibly, adhesions due to endometriosis.

Endocrine factors

Endocrine factors potentially contribute to recurrent abortion in 10–20% of cases.

The most common abnormality contributing to spontaneous abortion is luteal phase insufficiency, which occurs when abnormal corpus luteum function results in insufficient progesterone production.

A deficiency or an imbalance of oestrogen and progesterone in circulation to produce oestrogen dominance is a theoretical cause of abortion. Hypothyroidism, hypoprolactinemia, poor diabetic control, and polycystic ovarian syndrome contribute to pregnancy loss.

Polycystic ovary syndrome (PCOS) (Figure 2.20) and Type I diabetes mellitus have also been found to be associated with RSA.

Infectious factors

Presumed infectious etiology may be found in 5% of cases.

Bacterial, viral, parasitic, fungal, and zoonotic infections are associated with recurrent spontaneous abortion.

Herpes Simplex Virus has been linked to spontaneous abortion and chronic HSV is a possible cause of RSA.

Nutritional causes

The deficiency of vitamin A is a cause of increased infant mortality.

A metabolic effect of folate deficiency is an elevation of blood homocysteine. The presence of maternal homocysteine concentrations have been associated both with increased habitual spontaneous abortion and pregnancy complications.

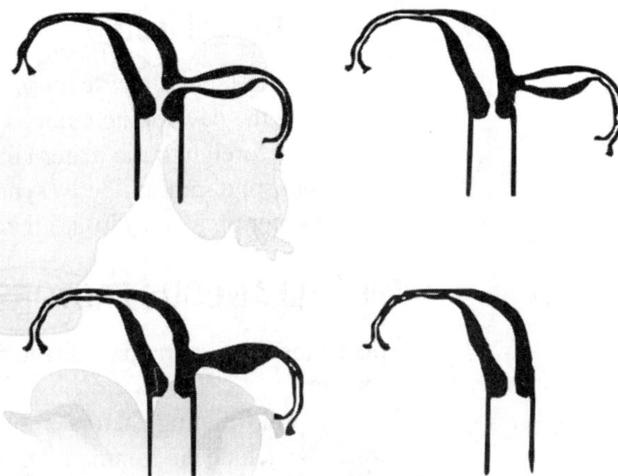

Figure 2.19 Müllerian defect.

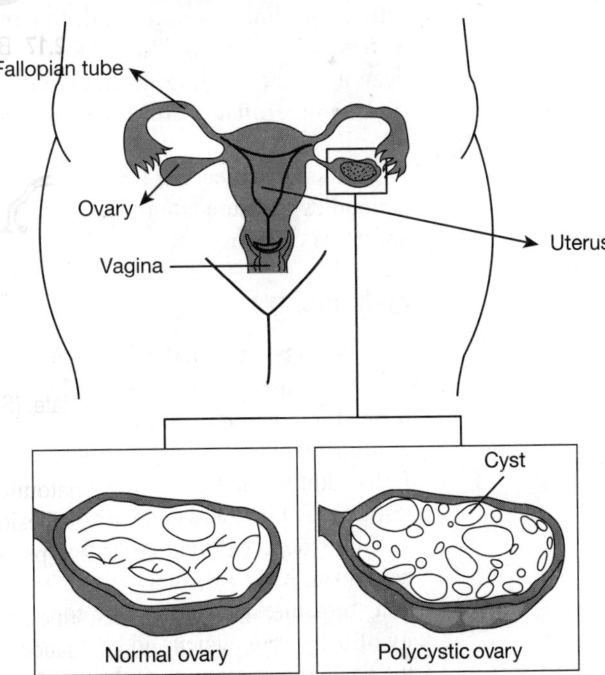

Figure 2.20 Polycystic ovary syndrome (PCOS).

Immunological factors

Immunologic factors may contribute up to 60% of recurrent spontaneous abortions. Both the developing embryo and the trophoblast may be considered immunologically foreign to the maternal immune system.

Antiphospholipid antibody syndrome is generally responsible for more second-trimester pregnancy losses than for first-trimester losses.

MISCELLANEOUS FACTORS

Miscellaneous factors may account for as many as 3% of recurrent spontaneous abortions.

Other contributing factors implicated in sporadic and recurrent spontaneous abortions include environment, drugs, placental abnormalities, medical illnesses, and male-related causes.

Maternal factors

Age and increased parity affect a woman's risk of a miscarriage.

In women younger than 20 years, miscarriage occurs in an estimated 12% of pregnancies; in women older than 20 years, miscarriage occurs in an estimated 26% of pregnancies.

Age primarily affects the oocyte. Women in the advanced reproductive age who have a reduced ovarian reserve are prone to higher risk of repeated miscarriages. Such miscarriages are due to decreased egg quality.

Severe maternal illness (Wilson's disease, maternal phenylketonuria, cyanotic heart disease, hematologic disorders [hemoglobinopathies or aplastic anemia], inflammatory bowel disease, neoplasia) leads to increased risk of abortion.

Women experiencing RSA are more likely to have antisperm antibodies. The antibodies measured were detected in 43.8% of women who had spontaneous abortions compared with 11.8% in women who carried their pregnancy to term.

Male factors

Male fertility may gradually decline with advancing age because morphological changes in the ageing testis, such as an increase of atypical spermatogonia, malformed spermatids, fibrosis of the tubular membrane, and increased desquamation of immature germ cells are observed.

In addition, in ageing men, the weight of the testis, the germinal tissue: total testis tissue ratio, and daily sperm production are significantly reduced.

Oligozoospermia are more frequent in spermatozoa from patients whose partner had an early RSA compared with those who had a late spontaneous abortion or a premature birth. A positive correlation exists between the percentage instability of the sperm nucleus and the percentage of abnormal forms. The alteration in the nuclear chromatin is probably one of the causes of the morphological aberrations in sperm heads.

INDIAN SCENARIO

There is no reliable estimate of the magnitude of abortions that take place in India, but studies suggest that as women in India do not have control on their fertility and have poor health, there are very high chances that they experience abortions (either spontaneous or induced) more than once. It is difficult to attain a reliable estimate on abortion frequencies in the Indian context as the registration of marriages, births, and deaths are usually not complete. Further, studies on spontaneous abortions in India have not been looked upon independently. In most of the studies patients with spontaneous as well as induced abortions have been combined together, and the results therefore do not give a true picture of the causes and their frequency.

Detection of recurrent abortions

The most common symptom of a miscarriage is bleeding. Bleeding during pregnancy may be referred to as threatened abortion. Of women who seek clinical treatment for bleeding during pregnancy, about half will go on to have a miscarriage. Symptoms other than bleeding are not statistically related to miscarriage.

Investigation for recurrent pregnancy loss

Karyotype of the abortus if available.

1. Hysterosalpingiogram: To rule out anatomic causes.
2. Karyotyping of both parents: To rule out genetic factors.
3. Activated partial thrombolastin time (aPPT) and anticardiolipin antibody titer: To rule out immunological factors.
4. T3, T4, and TSH screen for thyroid disease: In suspected cases of hypothyroidism. Thyroid antibodies ATA, AMA in certain cases.
5. Metabolic screening of the mother for certain clinically unrecognized metabolic disorders like:
   (a) Diabetes mellitus
   (b) Phenylketonuria
   (c) Tyrosinemia
   (d) Homocystinuria
   (e) Galactosemia
   (f) Biotinidase deficiency

NEURAL TUBE DEFECTS

Neural tube defect (NTD) is the second most prevalent prenatal anomaly only less frequent than cardiac malformations. Worldwide, there are 400,000 such defects.

NTDs can be separated into two main categories:

1. Abnormalities of the skull and brain, including anencephaly, acrania, or encephalocele

Neural tube defects
Congenital defect caused by incomplete closure of the neural tube during early stages of embryonic development.

2. Malformations of the spine, including meningocele, meningomyelocele, or spina bifida

Anencephaly is defined as a congenital absence of a major portion of the brain, skull, and scalp. The cerebral hemispheres develop without a cranial cover, and the exposure to amniotic fluid damages the brain (Figure 2.21).

Encephalocele refers to the herniation of cranial contents through a defect in the skull. These conditions are usually lethal within the first days of life.

Meningocele is a defect in the vertebrae through which the meningeal sac protrudes. In 90% of cases, neural tissue also protrudes into the meningeal sac, known as meningomyelocele.

Spina bifida refers to both meningocele and meningomyelocele (Figure 2.22). Approximately 90% of these defects are not covered by skin (open neural tube defect) and are associated with spinal nerve damage below the level of the lesion. Disorders in motor, bowel, and bladder function are of various severities depending on the level of the lesion. Intelligence may be normal, but over 50% of affected individuals have a learning disability.

"Closed" spina bifida is a subtle malformation of the caudal neural tube; these defects are difficult to diagnose. They may not be recognized until adult life, basically in the form of cutaneous defects or lipomas in lumbosacral region.

Neural tube defects result from failure of the neural tube to fuse during early embryogenesis, between the third and fifth week of gestation. At 18 days after fertilization, the primitive neural plate forms two lateral neural folds with a central neural groove. The lateral edges of these folds fuse in the mid-portion of the embryo, forming the neural tube. The fusion of the neural tube goes from the cranial to the caudal portion finishing by 26 days of development.

The aetiology of NTD is not clear. Mostly the disorder emerges as a multifactorial trait. Both genetic background and nutritional status influence the incidence. Chromosomal abnormalities (Trisomy 18, triploidy), single gene mutations (Meckel–Gruber Syndrome), maternal disease (diabetes mellitus, hyperthermia), or maternal exposure to teratogens (alcohol, valproic acid) are seen to be observed with NTDs.

Anencephaly
The absence of all or a major part of the brain.

Meningocele
A protrusion of the meninges through an opening in the skull or spinal column forming a sac filled with cerebrospinal fluid.

Spina bifida
A neural tube defect in which a part of the spinal cord protrudes through the spinal column resulting in neurological impairment.

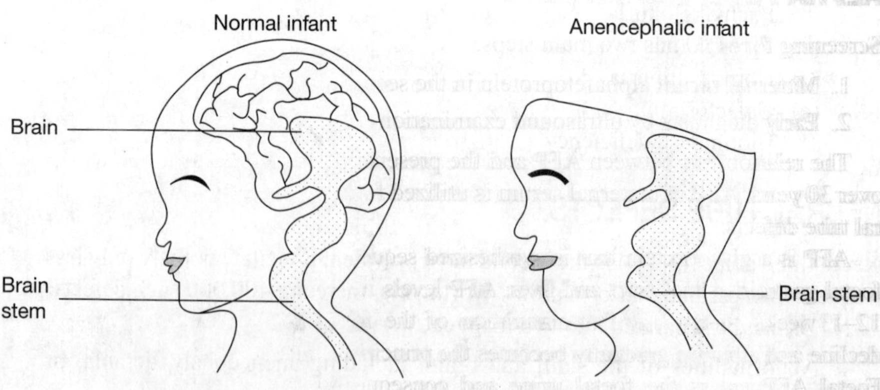

Figure 2.21 Anencephaly. (See page 250 for the colour image.)

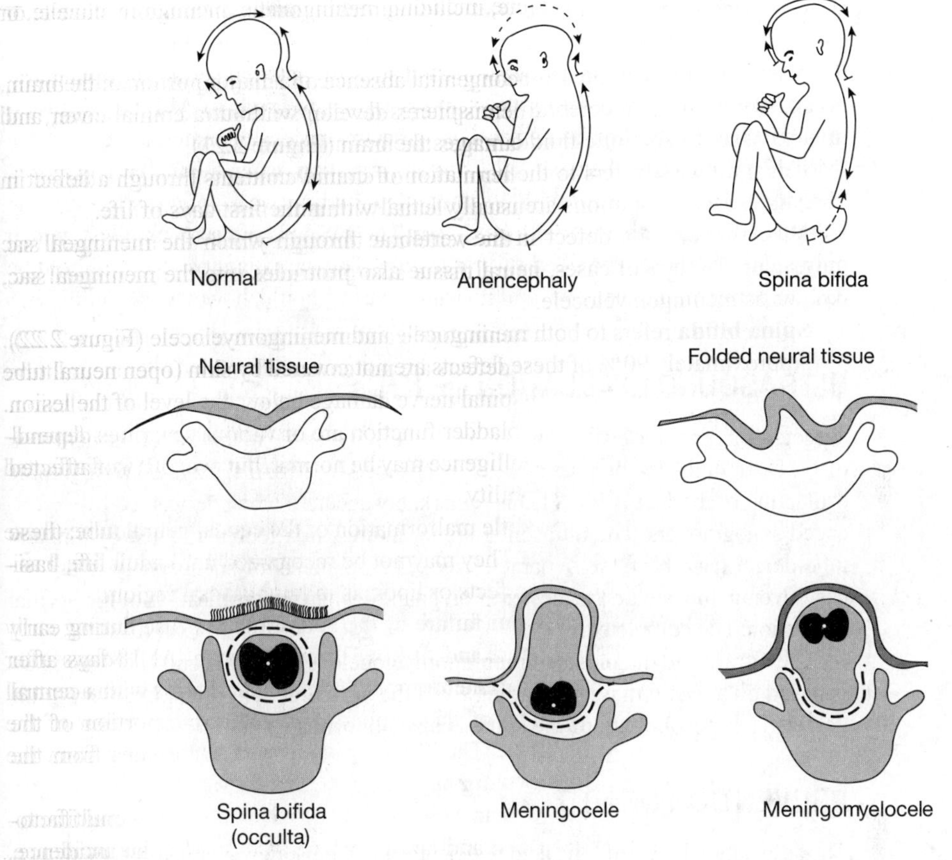

Figure 2.22 Spina bifida, meningocele, and meningomyocele. (See page 250 for the colour image.)

SCREENING OF NTD WITH MATERNAL SERUM ALPHA-FETOPROTEIN (AFP)

Screening for NTD has two main steps:

1. Maternal serum alphafetoprotein in the second trimester of pregnancy
2. Early diagnosis by ultrasound examination

The relationship between AFP and the presence of NTD has been known for over 30 years. AFP in maternal serum is utilized for the prenatal diagnosis of neural tube defects.

AFP is a glycoprotein that is synthesized sequentially by the yolk sac and the foetal gastrointestinal tract and liver. AFP levels in foetal plasma are maximal at 12–13 weeks gestation. After maturation of the foetal liver, plasma AFP levels decline and albumin gradually becomes the principal plasma protein of the foetus. Foetal AFP enters the foetal urine and consequently the amniotic fluid. Peak concentrations of amniotic fluid AFP are reached at 12–14 weeks gestation and steadily decline parallel to the foetal serum concentration. Amniotic fluid AFP passes into maternal circulation, probably by diffusion through the membranes or the placenta. AFP appears in low concentrations in maternal serum; its concentration peaks at 28–32 weeks' gestation. Maternal serum levels of AFP can be measured as early as the first trimester. For screening purposes, maternal serum AFP (MSAFP) is measured between 15–20 weeks gestation, when the increase is linear.

Only 5–10% of women with elevated MSAFP have been found to be carrying a foetus affected with a neural tube defect. The MSAFP is a screening test, which only identifies those who need further testing. The next diagnostic step should be easy to perform, inexpensive, and non-invasive. It should, however, be definitive.

ULTRASOUND EVALUATION OF NTDs

Targeted sonographic evaluation is currently offered as the main test for the detection of NTD. In high-risk pregnancies, as determined by MSAFP, targeted sonographic evaluation of the foetus for NTD is remarkably accurate when performed by experienced sonographers. The ultrasonographic findings in a foetus affected by a neural tube defect have been well characterized. The diagnosis of anencephaly is usually easy, even in the late first trimester of pregnancy, when the ossification of the normal skull should be completed.

The ultrasound diagnosis of meningomyelocele is more difficult. The diagnosis is based on a cystic mass protruding from the vertebrae without skin covering the defect. The morphology of the spine is also abnormal.

PREVENTION OF NTD

Folic acid
It is called Vitamin B. It helps the foetus during neural tube closure. Its deficiency leads to neural tube defects.

The association between folic acid deficiency and the incidence of neural tube defects has long been appreciated. Epidemiological observations have explored differences in socioeconomic status, seasonal variation, prevalence in different countries, and the association between poor diets and the incidence of NTDs. These variations are a function of both genetic background and nutritional status. The general conclusion has been that NTDs are partially precipitated by functional folic acid deficiencies.

GENETIC SUSCEPTIBILITY FOR NTD AND FOLIC ACID INTAKE

Despite the known evidence relating folic acid intake to prevention of NTDs, the underlying pathophysiologic mechanism is unknown.

1. Folate plays an important role in serving as a methyl donor in DNA synthesis, purine–pyrimidine metabolism, and protein synthesis. The reduced folate coenzyme 5, 10- methylene tetrahydrofolate catalyses the main rate-limiting step during the DNA synthesis.
2. Reduced folate is also a cofactor in the synthesis of homocysteine to methionine, an important factor for protein synthesis. These activities help cell proliferation and gene expression.

Possible influences include insufficient diet, the haemodilution of pregnancy, increased plasma clearance, and genetic disorders that might affect production, transport, and metabolism. Genetic background, either of the mother or the foetus, may play an important role in the development of NTDs. In dichorionic pregnancies, one of the foetuses could be affected by the defect, while the other could be completely normal, despite the fact that each foetus is exposed to the same folate status from their mother.

FORTIFICATION DURING PREGNANCY

Numerous epidemiological and clinical studies have demonstrated that folic acid intake has health implications in addition to NTD prevention. Folic acid interventions may also decrease the incidence of other birth defects, epithelial cancers, neurological problems, and cardiovascular disease.

Observational studies have also demonstrated a reduction in the incidence in other birth defects, in addition to NTDs. There seems to be a lower rate of cleft palate and cardiac defects among pregnant women who have taken folic acid supplementation in the pre-conceptional months and during the first trimester of pregnancy.

DOWN SYNDROME (TRISOMY 21)

- Down syndrome is the most common chromosomal condition affecting newborn babies.
- Characteristics may include intellectual delay, distinct facial features, problems with the heart, and digestive tract.
- Down syndrome is due to one of the following:
  - An additional copy of chromosome 21 (*trisomy 21*) in all of the cells of the body (about 95% of cases).
  - An additional copy of chromosome 21 in some of the cells of the body (*mosaic trisomy 21*—about 1% of cases).
  - A chromosomal *translocation* involving chromosome 21 (about 4% of cases).
- The chance for having a child with Down syndrome due to *trisomy 21* increases with advanced maternal age.
- Screening and diagnostic testing (where indicated) for Down syndrome is available in pregnancy.

Trisomy 21/Down syndrome is one of the most common and best-known chromosomal disorders and is the single most cause of moderate mental retardation. The incidence rate is 1 in 800 and for foetuses of mothers who are 35 years or older, the incidence rate is higher (Figure 2.23).

The syndrome was first described clinically by Langdon Down in 1866.

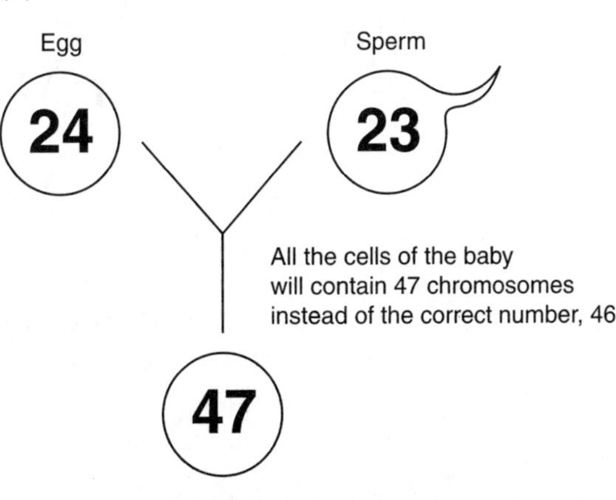

Figure 2.23 (A) Free trisomy 21,

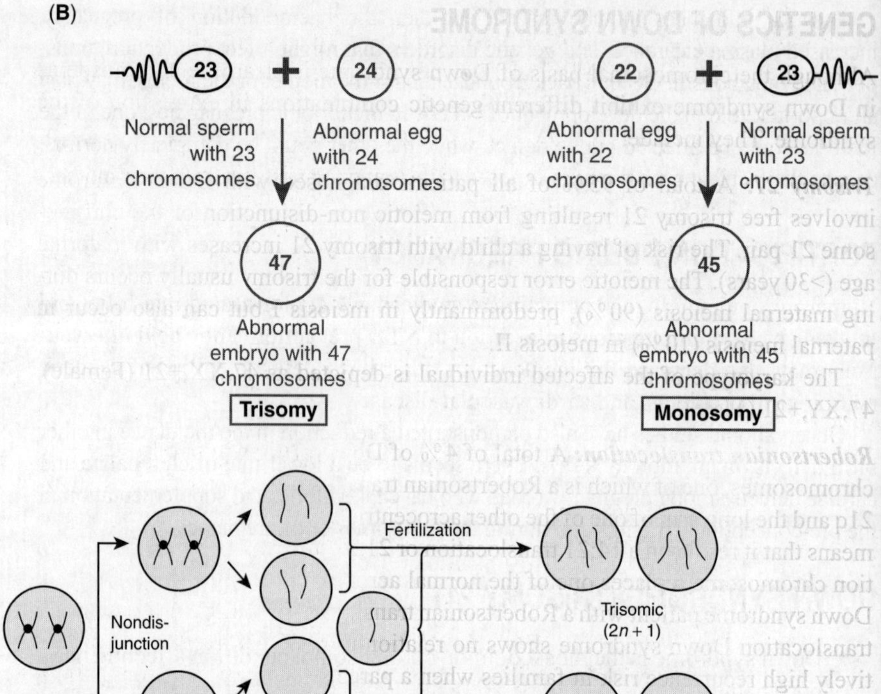

Figure 2.23 (B) Non-disjunction (See page 243 for the colour image.) **(C)** Mechanism of non-disjunction. (See page 244 for the colour image.)

GENETICS OF DOWN SYNDROME

Although the chromosomal basis of Down syndrome is clear, the chromosomes in Down syndrome exhibit different genetic combinations in expression of the syndrome. They include:

Trisomy 21: A total of 95% of all patients diagnosed with Down syndrome involves free trisomy 21 resulting from meiotic non-disjunction of the chromosome 21 pair. The risk of having a child with trisomy 21 increases with maternal age (>30 years). The meiotic error responsible for the trisomy usually occurs during maternal meiosis (90%), predominantly in meiosis I but can also occur in paternal meiosis (10%) in meiosis II.

The karyotype of the affected individual is depicted as 47,XX,+21 (Female), 47,XY,+21 (Male).

Robertsonian translocation: A total of 4% of Down syndrome patients have 46 chromosomes, one of which is a Robertsonian translocation between chromosome 21q and the long arm of one of the other acrocentric chromosomes (14 or 21). This means that it results in a 14;21 translocation or 21;21 translocation. The translocation chromosome replaces one of the normal acrocentrics and the karyotype of a Down syndrome patient with a Robertsonian translocation. Unlike free trisomy 21, translocation Down syndrome shows no relation to maternal age but has a relatively high recurrence risk in families when a parent is a carrier of the translocation. For this reason, parental karyotyping and genetic counselling can be advised.

Mosaic Down syndrome: A small percentage of Down syndrome patients are referred to as mosaics. When a person has a chromosome abnormality, the abnormality is usually present in all of his/her cells. Sometimes, however, two or more different chromosome complements are present in an individual. This condition is referred to as **Mosaicism**. A common cause of mosaicism is non-disjunction in an early postzygotic mitotic division. The effects of mosaicism on development vary with the timing of non-disjunctional event, the nature of the chromosomal abnormality, the proportions of the different chromosome complement present and the tissues affected.

The phenotype of a mosaic Down syndrome patient may be milder than free trisomy 21, but there is variability in phenotypes among mosaic patients, possibly reflecting the variable proportion of trisomy 21 cells in the embryo during early development.

ADVANCED MATERNAL AGE IN DOWN SYNDROME

Down syndrome, one of the most common congenital anomalies, affects 1 of every 1,000 newborns. It is the most intensively studied human chromosome abnormality, yet little is known about its cause, and only advanced maternal age has been confirmed as a risk factor. *Refer to the chapter on Advanced Maternal Age.*

CHARACTERISTIC FEATURES/PHENOTYPE OF DOWN SYNDROME

- Hypotonia.
- Dysmorphic facial features that include: flat nasal bridge, small mouth, protruding tongue, small low set ears, and upward slanting eyes with epicanthal fold. The eyes have Brushfield spots around the margin of the iris.
- Short in stature and have brachycephaly with a flat occiput. The neck is short with loose skin on the nape.
- The hands are short and broad with short fingers, and may have a single transverse palmar crease (Simian Crease) and clinodactyly (incurved fifth digits).
- The dermatoglyphics (patterns of ridged skin) are highly characteristic.
- The feet show a wide gap between the first and second toes with a furrow extending proximally on the plantar surface.
- Developmental delay and mental retardation: Normal growth and development is usually delayed and individuals with Down syndrome do not reach the developmental milestones of unaffected individuals. Developmental delay is obvious by the end of one year and the IQ is usually 30–60 when the child is old enough to be tested. However, many children in spite of these limitations grow to be happy, responsive and self-reliant persons.
- Congenital heart diseases, duodenal atresia, and tracheoesophageal fistula are more common in Down syndrome.
- There is a 15-fold increase in the risk of developing leukemia.

Figure 2.24 depicts clinical features of Down syndrome.

MEDICAL CONDITIONS ASSOCIATED WITH DOWN SYNDROME

- ***Heart defects:*** A total of 50% of children born with Down syndrome are affected with ventricular septal defects. Other related heart defects that are usually observed in affected children are atrio-ventricular septal defects, teralogy of Fallot, and patent ductus arteriosus. Neonatal surgical correction is a good treatment module available.
- ***Gastrointestinal abnormalities:*** These are also frequently observed in children with Down syndrome. Oesophageal atresia, tracheoesophageal fistula, duodenal atresia, or stenosis, Hirschsprung's disease, and imperforate anus are some of the more common conditions. Celiac disease progresses in 5–15% of children with Down syndrome. Surgical intervention may be of help for some of these gastrointestinal conditions.
- ***Leukemia:*** Children with Down syndrome are also at an increased risk of developing acute lymphoblastic leukemia, myeloid leukemia, and testicular cancer.

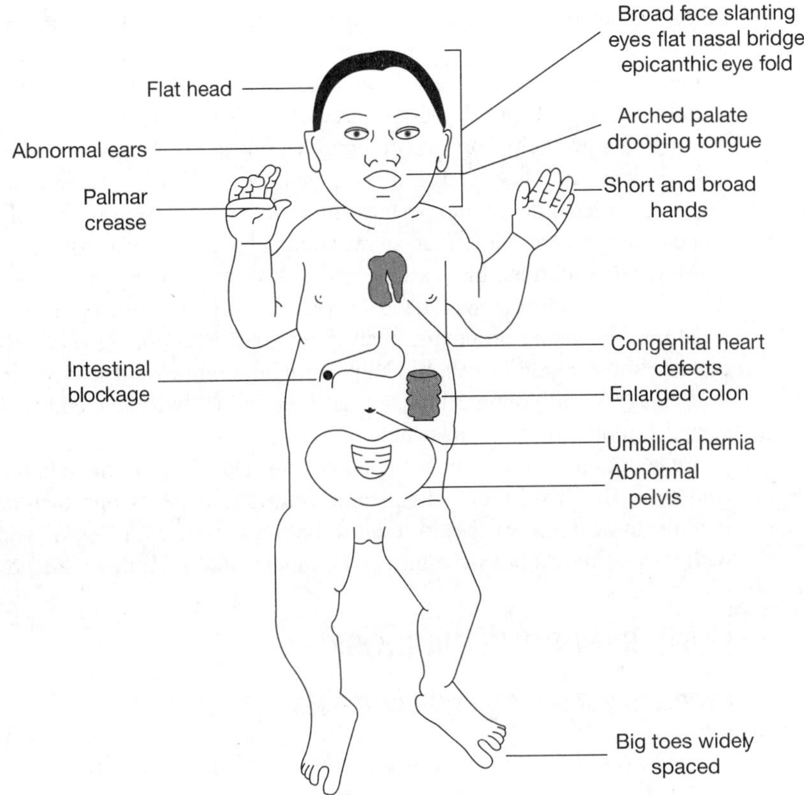

Figure 2.24 Clinical features of Down syndrome. (See page 245 for the colour image.)

- ***Other frequently related medical conditions observed with Down syndrome:*** These include attention deficit hyperactivity disorder (ADHD), autism, obsessive compulsive disorder (OCD), depression infantile spasms, frequent ear infections (otitis media), hearing loss, visual impairment, sleep apnea, underactive thyroid (hypothyroidism), cervical spine instability, constipation, obesity, seizures, dementia, and early-onset Alzheimer's disease.

DOWN SYNDROME MANAGEMENT

As in most genetic syndromes, although the genetic cause of Down syndrome is known, currently there are no treatment modules available for aneuploidies/Down syndrome. Scientists are exploring the role of the extra 21st chromosome and the additional genes responsible for the disorder. The syndrome is characterized by cognitive malfunction and much of the research focuses on understanding and improving cognitive skills.

Many children with Down syndrome despite their limitations are able to perform better and show good improvement in cognitive skills and have shown signs of self-reliance under appropriate special education systems. Special education and training for children with intellectual and developmental disabilities is offered in most countries. Early intervention programs, such as physical therapy, occupational therapy, and speech therapy, are helpful. Audiology, speech, language, and hearing therapy help improve communication skills. Physical therapy helps in independent mobility and improves self-dependence. Occupational therapy improves independence and performing tasks. Mental health care helps the child and parents combat with mood swings and behavioural disturbances.

Medical conditions like cardiac and gastrointestinal anomalies in individuals with Down syndrome will need corrective surgery soon after birth. Regular screening for vision problems, hearing loss, ear infections, hypothyroidism, and other medical conditions should be performed to improve their survival.

Teenagers and younger adults must be provided with sex education to avoid sexual exploitation and harassment.

Behavioural training can help people with Down syndrome and their families deal with the frustration, anger, and compulsive behaviour that often occur. Parents and caregivers should learn to help a person with Down syndrome deal with frustration. At the same time, it is important to encourage independence.

DOWN SYNDROME DIAGNOSIS

Prenatal screening and diagnosis

- **Maternal Serum Screening (MSS)/AFP assay at 16 weeks:** MSS also known as triple screen measures three blood markers and is made available to most pregnant women at 15 to 20 weeks of gestation to identify those at increased risk for Trisomy 21, Trisomy 18, and Neural Tube defects (NTDs). The three serum components measured in this screening test include Alpha Feto protein (AFP), human chorionic gonadotropin (HCG) and unconjugated oestriol (uE3). In pregnancies with Down syndrome, the levels of AFP and uE3 are reduced in maternal serum. HCG in maternal serum is significantly higher than normal when the foetus has Down syndrome.

- **NTD test by MSS and ultrasound:** When the foetus has an open NTD, the concentration of AFP is likely to be higher than normal in maternal serum as well as in amniotic fluid. A number of foetal abnormalities can be detected by ultrasound. An example of useful ultrasound marker for evaluating the risk of foetal aneuploidy is the measurement of foetal nuchal translucency (NT), which quantifies ultrasonographic translucency between the skin and soft tissue overlying the cervical spine. NT can be increased because of an abnormal accumulation of fluid between the foetal neck in the first trimester (10 to 14 weeks). The risk of aneuploidy, which varies with maternal age and gestational age, is also dependent on the degree of NT. Increased NT can also be indicative of underlying cardiac defect or genetic syndrome.

Cardiac defects, absence of nasal foetal bone, and short humerus and femur observed in Down syndrome can also be detected by ultrasound.

Several invasive diagnostic tests reliably detect Down syndrome. Most of these procedures carry a small risk of pregnancy loss.

- **Amniocentesis** refers to the procedure of removing a sample of amniotic fluid transabdominally by syringe. The amniotic fluid contains cells of foetal origin that can be cultured for diagnostic tests. Amniocentesis is typically performed between 16 and 20 weeks of pregnancy.

- **Chorionic villus sampling (CVS)** involves the biopsy of tissue from the villous area of the chorion transcervically or transabdominally generally between the 10th and 12th week of pregnancy. The major advantage of CVS over amniocentesis is that CVS allows the results to be available at an early stage of pregnancy, thus reducing the period of uncertainty and allowing termination, if elected to be performed in the first trimester.

- **Cordocentesis** is a procedure used to obtain a sample of foetal blood directly from the umbilical cord with ultrasonographic guidance. Cordocentesis is usually performed at 19 to 21 weeks of pregnancy.

- **Fluorescent in situ hybridization** (FISH) is a quick tool to detect chromosomal abnormalities using fluorescent probes. This can be done on blood, foetal cells from amniotic fluid, and embryos used in IVF. However, the technique is expensive.

REVIEW QUESTIONS

Essay Questions

1. Explain the common bacterial infections affecting pregnant women with examples.

2. Explain the common viral infections affecting pregnant women in detail.

3. Explain with examples the teratogenic effects of drugs, chemicals, and radiation in detail.

4. Explain the inheritance of genetic disease conditions in consanguineous marriage with an example (pedigree).

5. Explain the physiological changes and nutritional requirements during pregnancy in detail.

6. Explain the common food allergies in detail. Add a note on the symptoms of food allergy.

7. Explain the concept of advanced maternal age and aneuploidies with three examples.

8. Explain with examples the different prenatal diagnostic tools available for genetic testing in detail.

9. Explain amniocentesis as a diagnostic tool for prenatal diagnosis in detail. Add a note on its advantages/disadvantages over CVS.

10. Explain the non-invasive testing methods employed in prenatal diagnosis with examples in detail.

11. Explain the causes and management options of male and female subfertility in detail.

12. Explain the different assisted reproductive techniques available for subfertility management in detail.

13. Explain the different clinical types of abortion with treatment options in detail.

14. Explain the different factors involved in recurrent pregnancy loss in detail.

15. Explain the investigation options available for recurrent pregnancy loss.

16. Define neural tube defects. Add a note on the types, screening methods available to detect NTDS, and the role of folic acid in lowering the risk of NTDs.

17. Explain in detail the genetics and clinical features of Down syndrome. Add a note on its diagnosis and management

Short Notes

1. Write short notes on the following:
   (a) *E. coli* and *H. influenza* infections during pregnancy
   (b) Rubella infection during pregnancy
   (c) CMV and HSV infection during pregnancy
   (d) Foetal Alcohol Syndrome
   (e) Effects of radiation on human pregnancy
   (f) Mechanism of teratogenesis
   (g) Teratogenic effect of chemicals
   (h) Anticonvulsants and antidepressants—teratogenic action

2. Write short notes on the following:
   (a) Consanguinity
   (b) Haemophilia and consanguinity

3. Prenatal nutrition

4. Physiological changes during pregnancy

5. Nutritional requirements during pregnancy

6. Symptoms of food allergy

7. Common food allergies

8. Write short notes on the following:
   (a) Older egg model
   (b) Advanced maternal age
   (c) Advanced maternal age in Down syndrome
   (d) Sex chromosomal aneuploidies
   (e) Aneuploidy

9. Write short notes on the following:
   (a) Invasive testing
   (b) Non-invasive testing
   (c) Indications for prenatal diagnosis
   (d) Goals of prenatal diagnosis
   (e) Amniocentesis
   (f) Chorionic villus sampling
   (g) Preimplantation genetic diagnosis
   (h) Foetal cell sorting
   (i) Ultrasound
   (j) Maternal serum screening

11. Write short notes on the following:
   (a) Subfertility
   (b) Male subfertility
   (c) Female subfertility
   (d) Anovulation
   (e) Endometriosis
   (f) Tubal damage
   (g) Factors affecting fertility
   (h) IVF
   (i) ICSI
   (j) Drugs that impair male fertility

12. Write short notes on the following:
   (a) Pregnancy
   (b) Spontaneous abortion
   (c) Risk of pregnancy loss
   (d) Premature centromeric division
   (e) Genetic factors involved in recurrent pregnancy loss
   (f) Maternal factors involved in recurrent pregnancy loss
   (g) Anatomical factors involved in recurrent pregnancy loss

13. Write short notes on the following:
   (a) Anencephaly
   (b) Spina bifida
   (c) Maternal serum screening for detection of NTDs
   (d) Ultrasound evaluation of NTDs
   (e) Folic acid fortification

14. Genetics of Down syndrome

15. Advanced maternal age in Down syndrome

16. Clinical features of Down syndrome

17. Diagnosis of Down syndrome

Explain the Screening Methods for Genetic Defects and Diseases in Neonates and Children

3

CHAPTER OBJECTIVES

Newborn Screening
Heterozygote Screening
Presymptomatic Testing
Congenital Abnormalities (Birth Defects) and Dysmorphology
Clinical Dysmorphology—Classification of Foetal and Birth Defects

Diagnostic Approach to the Dysmorphic Foetus
Teratology
Basic Principles of Teratology
Developmental Milestones

Improvements in our understanding of human heredity and the identification of numerous disease-causing genes have led to the progress of many tests for genetic conditions. The ultimate goal of genetic testing is to recognize the potential for a genetic condition at an early stage. In some cases, genetic testing allows early intervention that may lessen or even prevent the development of the condition. In other cases, genetic testing allows people to make informed choices about reproduction. For those who know that they are at risk for a genetic condition, genetic testing may help lessen anxiety associated with the uncertainty of their situation.

Generally, genetic testing in adults, neonates and the foetus includes newborn screening, heterozygote screening, presymptomatic diagnosis, and prenatal testing.

NEWBORN SCREENING

Testing for genetic disorders in newborn infants is called **newborn screening**. Most states in the United States and many other countries screen newborn infants for phenylketonuria and galactosemia. These biochemical disorders are also known as metabolic disorders and follow autosomal recessive inheritance. Early detection and intervention can prevent mental retardation to a large extent. In most countries, a heel prick is done on the newborn to collect a drop of blood, and the screening test is performed. Because of widespread screening, the frequency of mental retardation due to these genetic conditions has dropped tremendously. Screening newborns for additional genetic diseases such as sickle-cell anemia and hypothyroidism is also common.

HETEROZYGOTE SCREENING

Testing members of a population to identify heterozygous carriers of recessive disease-causing alleles, who are healthy but have the potential to produce children with the particular disease, is termed **heterozygote screening**. Testing for Tay–Sachs disease is a successful example of heterozygote screening.

PRESYMPTOMATIC TESTING

Evaluating healthy people to determine whether they have inherited a disease-causing allele gene is known as **presymptomatic genetic testing**. For example, presymptomatic testing is available for members of families that have an autosomal dominant form of breast cancer. In this case, early identification of the disease-causing allele allows for closer surveillance and the early detection of tumors. Presymptomatic testing is also available for some genetic diseases for which no treatment is available, such as Huntington disease, an autosomal dominant disease that leads to slow physical and mental deterioration in middle age.

CONGENITAL ABNORMALITIES (BIRTH DEFECTS) AND DYSMORPHOLOGY

In many developed countries, congenital malformations represent the most frequent cause of mortality during the first year of life; for example, they account for more than 20% of all infant deaths. At birth, about 2–3% of infants are found to have major structural defects and this frequency increases to 3–4% by the age of 1 year. Additionally, birth defects contribute substantially to childhood morbidity and long-term disability. Many of the birth defects are now detected by ultrasound prior to birth.

Clinical investigation of the causes and consequences of birth defects is called **Dysmorphology**.

CLINICAL DYSMORPHOLOGY—CLASSIFICATION OF FOETAL AND BIRTH DEFECTS

Congenital defects can be classified in different ways. The most common classification is based on organ systems or body regions.

The following five major causes of malformations are generally recognized:

1. Chromosome abnormalities including microdeletion/microduplication syndromes
2. Single gene defects
3. Multifactorial disorders (involving both genetic and environmental factors)
4. Teratogenic exposition (environmental factors)
5. Unknown

The increasing knowledge of the pathogenesis of human congenital defects has led to a better understanding of the developmental relationship of the defects in malformation syndromes. Birth defects can be categorized into the four main types of pathogenic processes:

1. Malformation
2. Deformation
3. Disruption
4. Dysplasia

The categories of structural defects are illustrated in Figure 3.1.

Malformation

This term is reserved for intrinsic abnormalities caused by an abnormal completion of one or more of the embryonic processes. Thus, such anomalies may be limited to a single anatomic region, involve an entire organ, or produce a

Deformation
An alteration in shape/structure.

Dysplasia
Abnormal growth or development of cells, organs, or tissues.

Syndrome
A group of symptoms that occur together and characterize a particular abnormality.

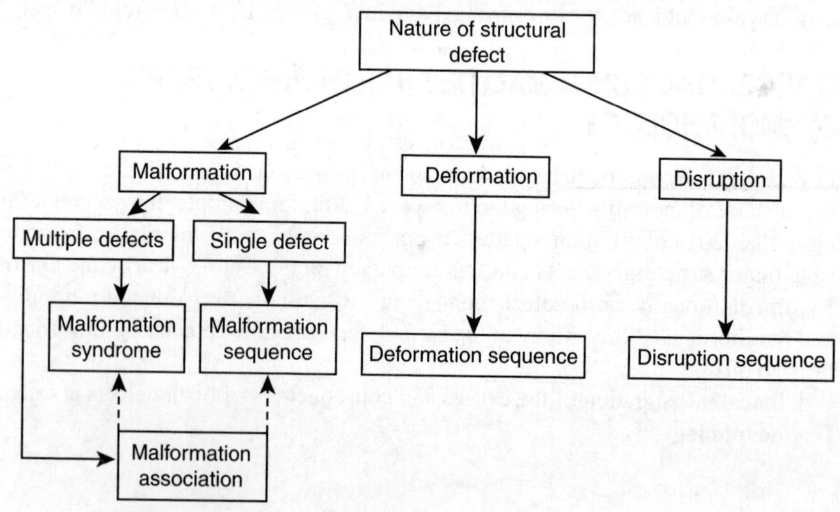

Figure 3.1 Categories of structural defects

malformation syndrome affecting a number of different body systems. The early development of a particular tissue or organ system may be arrested, delayed, or misdirected, resulting in persistent structural abnormalities. Although defining an anomaly as a malformation does not imply any specific etiology, it strongly suggests that the developmental error occurred early in gestation, either during tissue differentiation or during organogenesis.

Deformation

Deformations are secondary events that may be extrinsic or intrinsic to the foetus (Table 3.1) Mechanical forces that alter the shape or position of normally formed body structures can produce them. Although deformations can result in severe changes in the configuration of various body parts, they occur usually in the foetal period and not during embryogenesis. Most deformational abnormalities induced by mechanical forces involve cartilage, bone, and joints, probably because these tissues yield to intrauterine pressure; however, they often tend to resolve spontaneously toward their original forms once the abnormal mechanical stresses are

Table 3.1 Causes of deformations

Extrinsic

Mechanical Forces

Small maternal stature

Premature rupture of membrane

Unusual implantation site

Large uterine leiomyomas

Uterine malformations

Multifoetal pregnancy

Breech presentation

Intrinsic

Malformations

Spina bifida

CNS malformations

Bilateral renal agenesis

Severe hypoplastic kidneys

Severe polycystic kidneys

Urethral atresia

Dysfunctions

Neuromuscular disorders

Connective tissue defects

removed. Abnormal foetal presentation, severe and long-standing oligohydramnios of any cause, or even a pre-existing malformation or disruption that limits foetal mobility can produce a deformation. Other causes include maternal factors such as intrauterine constraint due to primigravidity, a small pelvic outlet, or structural abnormalities of the uterus. Crowding can be produced by multifoetal pregnancies. Examples of congenital deformations comprise talipes equinovarus (clubfoot), congenital hip dislocation, congenital postural scoliosis, positional plagiocephaly (flat head), torticollis, and mandibular asymmetry.

Deformations can be intrinsic and secondary to malformations or neuromuscular disorders. In such cases the deformity can be progressive after birth.

Disruption

Structural defect of an organ, part of an organ, or a larger region of the body may be caused also by an interference with, or an actual destruction of a previously normal organ or tissue. In contrast to deformities, disruptions may result from mechanical forces as well as by events such as ischemia, haemorrhage, or adhesion of denuded tissues. These secondary abnormalities do not conform to the boundaries normally imposed by the embryonic development, and they commonly affect several different tissue types in a delimited anatomic region. For example, in the amnion band sequence, an amniotic band may result in amputation of a limb, or damage the foetal face, penetrating skin, muscle, bone, and soft tissue without regard to their embryonic relationships. Disruptions usually affect structures that had previously developed normally, and their presence does not imply intrinsic abnormality of the tissue involved. There is seldom a need for concern about mental deficit or other hidden problems. The recurrence risk is low unless uterine malformation is found in the mother.

Dysplasia

The last major category of pathogenic processes that leads to birth defects is dysplasia. The structural changes are caused by a primary defect involving abnormal cellular organization or function within a specific tissue type throughout the body. For an increasing number of these disorders, a specific biochemical deficiency has been defined, often involving abnormalities of enzyme production or synthesis of structural protein. Major mutant genes that may be diagnosed by DNA analysis cause almost all dysplasias. These abnormal mixtures of tissue types often produce discrete tumours such as haemangiomas. An important feature of most dysplastic conditions is their progressive course. Since the tissue itself is intrinsically abnormal, clinical effects tend to persist or worsen as long as the tissue continues to grow or function.

DIAGNOSTIC APPROACH TO THE DYSMORPHIC FOETUS

Pregnancy history is important because a specific non-genetic cause for the structural defect may be revealed such as a teratogenic exposure (infection, drug) or a uterine factor resulting in a deformity or disruption. Other features such as oligohydramnios and lack of foetal movements may provide a clue to the cause of the defect. Information on the family history and a full pedigree is often needed as in any situation where genetic counselling will be provided. An examination of both parents is sometimes needed to arrive at a correct diagnosis. The foetal scan should be conducted to a high standard using a systematic approach and can be helped by a checklist. When examining the foetus, careful measurement is essential especially when a skeletal dysplasia is suspected. Precise measurements allow serial evaluations to be made and compared.

Chromosome analysis should be undertaken in all foetuses with multiple defects and, often also, when the defect appears to be isolated given the limitations of foetal evaluation by ultrasound for minor signs and the possibility of hidden problems. Biochemical studies are currently helpful in only a limited number of dysmorphic foetuses; for example, peroxisomal disorders such as Zellweger Syndrome and some lysosomal storage diseases. Molecular analysis is becoming increasingly important in the diagnosis of malformation syndromes and its application will be essential in the future.

The evaluation of a dysmorphic infant involves taking the medical history, physical examination (Figure 3.2), imaging and laboratory studies, and perinatal autopsy (when the infant dies).

Single-system defect

Malformations that involve only a single organ system of the body make up the largest proportion of birth defects. Such abnormalities include the most common birth defects: cleft lip and palate, clubfoot, pyloric stenosis, congenital hip dislocation, and congenital heart disease. These anomalies occur with increased frequency in some families and ethnic groups but do not follow the classic Mendelian patterns of inheritance expected for disorders caused by major mutant genes. The concordance rate in identical twins for these defects is low, providing strong evidence for the influence of environmental factors in their causation. Most of the disorders in this group are therefore thought to be of multifactorial etiology, implying the additive effects of multiple genes, each contributing a small effect, and presumably an environmental "trigger" of unknown nature.

Syndrome

When a particular set of primary anomalies thought to originate from a single etiology (for example, trisomy 18 syndrome) repeatedly occurs in a consistent pattern, it is called a syndrome (from the Greek "running together").

Prenatal syndrome diagnosis still relies heavily on the ability of the ultrasonographer to detect and correctly interpret morphological and developmental findings, and to recognize a pattern in them. Discussion with a clinical geneticist is therefore often rewarding. In many cases a final syndrome diagnosis can only be reached or confirmed after birth, when additional evaluation can be performed, or following termination of pregnancy after the post-mortem examination.

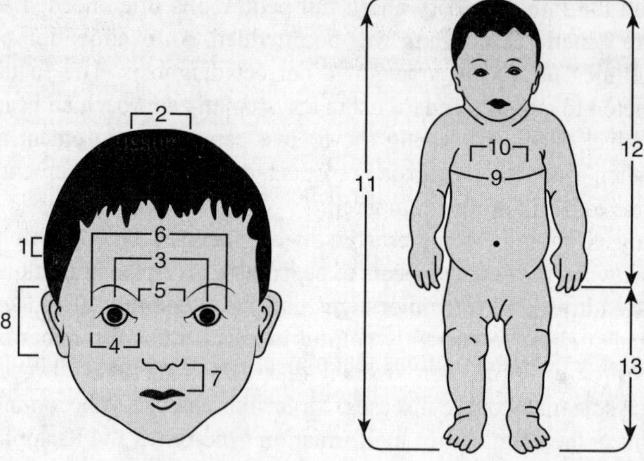

Measurement	Range (cm)	
	Term (38–40 wk)	Preterm (38–40 wk)
1 Head circumference	32–37	27–32
2 Anterior tontanelle $\left(\dfrac{L-W}{2}\right)$	0.7–3.7	…
3 Interpupillary distance	3.3–4.5	3.1–3.9
4 Palpebral fissure	1.5–2.1	1.3–1.6
5 Inner canthal distance	1.5–2.5	1.4–2.1
6 Outer canthal distance	5.3–7.3	3.9–5.1
7 Philtrum	0.6–1.2	0.5–0.9
8 Ear length	3–4.3	2.4–3.5
9 Chest circumference	28–38	23–29
10 Internipple distance*	6.5–10	5–6.5
11 Height	47–55	39–47
12 Hand (palm to middle finger)	5.3–7.8	4.1–5.5
13 Ratio of middle finger to hand	0.38–0.48	0.38–0.5
14 penis (pubic bone to tip of glans)	2.7–4.3	1.8–3.2

* Internipple distance should not exceed 25 % of chest circumference.

Figure 3.2 Physical evaluation of dysmorphic infant. (See page 249 for the colour image.)

Diagnoses based on clinical observation show a wide range of latitude, and thus there may be no gold standard. No single congenital malformation is pathognomonic for a specific syndrome. Furthermore, there is inherent variability in the manifestations of most dysmorphic disorders, both in type and in severity of the various structural abnormalities.

Sequence/cascade

Some patterns of multiple malformations appear to be the result of a cascade of related consequences, proceeding often from one primary single-system malformation or event. During intrauterine life, this primary abnormality interferes with normal embryologic and foetal developmental processes resulting at birth in seemingly separate and distinct abnormalities that may involve different body areas and organ systems. The etiology of most sequences is unknown, but some have features compatible with multifactorial inheritance, as might be expected by their derivation from often a single underlying malformation.

The clinical value of recognizing malformation sequences lies in the differentiation from other multiple defect conditions that may have different implications in terms of prognosis and recurrence risk. The oligohydramnios sequence is the most illustrative example (Figure 3.3).

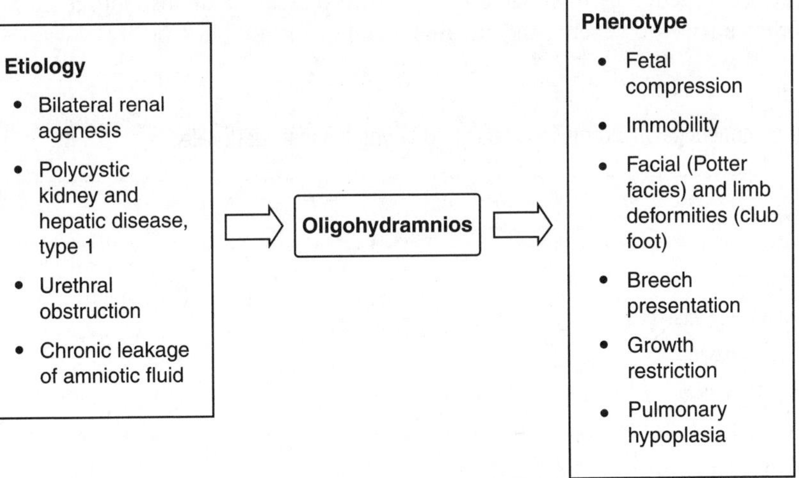

Figure 3.3 Oligohydramnios cascade

Genetic testing in neonates and children for congenital abnormalities/developmental delay include:

1. New born screening—Heel prick; for example, Phenylketonuria.
2. Chromosomal analysis of blood to look for structural or numerical chromosomal abnormality—Small amount of blood is collected from the patient. The lymphocytes in blood are stimulated to divide "in vitro" by adding a mitogen called phytohaemagglutinin. Cells are allowed to grow and divide and are arrested at metaphase of cell division using a spindle block called colchicine. Cells at metaphase are harvested by subjecting them to hypotonic treatment and fixed using Carnoy's fixative (methanol:acetic acid; 3:1). The fixed sample is casted on glass slides and stained with giemsa to look for chromosome morphology, for example, aneuploidies, deletions, etc.

3. Molecular testing—DNA analysis that detects mutations in genes. A small amount of blood is collected from the patient. Whole genomic DNA is isolated from whole blood using standard protocols. The quality of the DNA is checked and the exon of interest is amplified using polymerase chain reaction and RFLP (Restriction Fragment Length Polymorphism) methods are used to detect mutations, for example, Cystic fibrosis, Duchene muscular dystrophy.

4. Biochemical genetic testing for inborn errors of metabolism—Blood (serum) or urine sample is subjected to Enzyme Linked Immunosorbent Assay (ELISA) to test for the presence of specific biochemical markers.

5. Genetic counselling offered before and after a genetic test. *Refer the chapter on Genetic Counselling.*

TERATOLOGY

There have been dramatic advances in understanding the causes of human birth defects. The aetiology of congenital malformations can be divided into three categories: unknown, genetic, and environmental factors (Table 3.2).

Table 3.2 Etiology of human congenital malformations observed during the first year of life

Suspected Cause
Unknown
Polygenic
Multifactorial (gene–environment interactions)
Spontaneous errors of development
Synergistic interactions of teratogens
Genetic
Autosomal and sex-linked inherited genetic disease
Cytogenetic (chromosomal abnormalities)
• *Trisomy 21, Trisomy 13, Turner Syndrome, Wolf Hirschhorn Syndrome*
New mutations
Environmental
Maternal conditions: Alcoholism, Diabetes, Endocrinopathies; Phenylketonuria; Smoking and Nicotine; Starvation; Nutritional deficits
Infectious agents: Rubella, Toxoplasmosis, Syphilis, Herpes simplex, Cytomegalovirus, Varicella-zoster, Venezuelan equine encephalitis, Parvovirus B19
Mechanical problems (deformations): Amniotic band constrictions; Umbilical cord constraint; disparity in uterine size and uterine contents
Chemicals, drugs, high dose ionizing radiation, hyperthermia

The aetiology of the majority of human malformations, approximately 65–75 %, is still unknown. However, a significant proportion of congenital malformations of unknown aetiology is likely to be polygenic (i.e. due to two or more genetic loci) or at least to have an important genetic component. Malformations with an increased recurrent risk, such as cleft lip and palate, anencephaly, spina bifida, certain congenital heart diseases, pyloric stenosis, hypospadias, inguinal hernia, talipes equinovarus, and congenital dislocation of the hip, can fit the category of multifactorial disease, as well as the category of polygenic inherited disease. The multifactorial threshold hypothesis involves the modulation of a continuum of genetic characteristics by intrinsic and extrinsic (environmental) factors.

Although the modulating factors are not known, they probably include placental blood flow, placental transport, site of implantation, maternal disease states, infections, drugs, chemicals, and spontaneous errors of development. Spontaneous errors of development may account for malformations that occur without apparent involvement of genetic abnormalities or environmental influences; most often referred to as unknown causes.

Understanding the pathogenesis for the large group of malformations with unknown aetiology will depend on identifying the genes involved in polygenic or pleurogenic processes, the interacting genetic and environmental determinants of multifactorial traits, and the statistical risks for error during embryonic development.

The known aetiologies of teratogenesis include genetic and environmental factors that affect the embryo during development (for example, drugs, chemicals, radiation, hyperthermia, infections, abnormal maternal metabolic states, or mechanical factors). Environmental and genetic causes of malformations have different pathologic processes that result in abnormal development. Congenital malformations due to genetic reasons have a cascade of pathologic processes that are a direct consequence of gene deficiency, a gene abnormality, chromosome deletion, or chromosome excess. The pathologic nature of this process is determined before conception, or at least before differentiation, because of inherited or newly acquired genetic abnormalities present in all or most of the cells of the embryo. Although environmental factors may modify the development of the genetically abnormal embryo, the genetic abnormality is usually the predominant contributor to the pathologic process.

Environmental risk parameters or modifiers

1. ***The importance of the stage of exposure:*** The susceptibility of an embryo or foetus to teratogenic influences is related to the stage of development at which the exposure occurs. The explanation for this phenomenon is that the foetus is constantly changing during its development with respect to tissue receptors, metabolism, drug distribution, and cell proliferation. Thus, tissue response to an exposure and the ability of the foetus to recuperate from the insult vary with the gestational stage. Although detrimental effects can be induced at any time during pregnancy, most major malformations result from exposures during days 18–40 of postconception in the human.

However, the palate, central nervous system, and genital structures can be affected at later stages of development. Our knowledge of the time of resistance or susceptibility of the embryo to various environmental influences has expanded over the past three decades. This information is vital in evaluating the significance of individual exposures or epidemiologic studies.

2. ***The threshold concept and the importance of the magnitude of exposure (dose and dose rate):*** Every teratogenic agent that has been tested in mammals has exhibited a dose–response relationship and a threshold dose response—that is, a dose below which there is no difference between the exposed and non-exposed in the incidence of malformations. The dose to which the foetus is exposed is determined by maternal pharmacokinetics, placental exchange, foetal, and placental metabolism of the substance (and the teratogenic activity of the metabolites), the foetal distribution of the substance, and the presence of tissue-specific receptors. Factors that influence the response include maternal toxicity and drug–drug interactions.

   The most significant mistake by scientists or lay individuals uneducated in the fields of general and radiation toxicology is to ignore the importance of the dose or the exposure of the environmental agent. Environmental chemicals and physical agents (such as radiation) have deleterious effects at high exposures and represent no measurable risk at low exposures. This includes all environmental agents, even water.

3. ***Maternal disease states:*** Maternal disease states may produce deleterious effects on the foetus that are difficult to separate from a possible teratogenic effect of a therapeutic agent. This is an especially relevant consideration for long-standing conditions such as diabetes or the autoimmune diseases.

BASIC PRINCIPLES OF TERATOLOGY

The principles are as follows:

1. Exposure to teratogens follows a toxicological dose response curve. There is a threshold below which no effect will be observed and as the dose of the teratogen is increased both the severity and frequency of reproductive effects will increase.

2. The period of exposure is critical in determining what effects will be produced and whether any effects can be produced by a known teratogen. Some teratogenic effects have a broad, and others, a very narrow period of sensitivity.

3. Even the most potent teratogenic agent cannot produce every malformation.

4. Most teratogens have a confined group of congenital malformations that result after exposure during a critical period of embryonic development. This confined group of malformations is referred to as the syndrome that describes the agent's teratogenic effect.

The various teratogenic agents and their action have been described in chapter 9. Table 3.3 lists the factors that influence susceptibility to developmental toxicants.

Table 3.3 Factors that influence susceptibility to developmental toxicants

1. **Stage of development:** The developmental period at which an exposure occurs will determine which structures are most susceptible to the adverse effects of chemicals and drugs and to what extent the embryo can repair the damage.

2. **Magnitude of the exposure:** Both the severity and incidence of toxic effects increase with dose.

3. **Threshold phenomena:** The threshold dose is the dose below which the incidence of death, malformation, growth retardation, or functional deficit is not statistically greater than that of non-exposed subjects.

4. **Pharmacokinetics and metabolism:** The physiologic changes in the pregnant woman and during foetal development and the bioconversion of compounds can significantly influence the developmental toxicity of drugs and chemicals by affecting absorption, body distribution, active metabolites, and excretion.

5. **Maternal diseases:** A maternal disease may increase the risk of foetal anomalies or abortion with or without exposure to a chemical or drug.

6. **Placental transport:** Most drugs and chemicals cross the placenta. The rate and extent to which a drug or chemical crosses the placenta are influenced by molecular weight, lipid solubility, polarity or degree of ionization, plasma protein binding, receptor mediation, placental blood flow, pH gradient between the maternal and foetal serum and tissues, and placental metabolism of the chemical or drug.

7. **Genotype:** The maternal and foetal genotypes may result in differences in cell sensitivity, placental transport, absorption, metabolism, receptor binding, and distribution of an agent, and account for some variations in toxic effects among individual subjects and species.

Growth and development are important aspects of childhood. Growth refers only to physical development, whereas development refers to the way in which children attain the ability to perform complex tasks as they grow. Physical development follows a regular pattern; however, cognitive (mental process of knowing, reasoning, perception, and judgment) and behavioural development is variable, and its measurement is quite complex and subjective.

Cognition
The process of knowing/understanding.

DEVELOPMENTAL MILESTONES

Child development refers to the process by which children undergo changes in skill development during defined time periods called developmental milestones.

A number of factors influence the development of a child. These consist of genetic and environmental factors that include rearing pattern, socioeconomic status of the parents, cultural practices, and temperament of the child.

Developmental milestones
A skill that a child acquires within a specific time frame, for example, taking the first step.

Developmental domains: The development of a child can be evaluated and understood by classifying it into several domains:

1. Motor development
2. Cognitive development
3. Emotional and social development

4. Hearing and speech development
5. Bowel and bladder function development

Normal development

Development is continuous from conception to maturity. The progression of development through different milestones is the same in all children but the rate of development varies. Development is intimately related to the maturation of the central nervous system. Normal development in children includes the following skills:

1. Gross motor skills—Sit, stand, walk, run, etc.
2. Fine motor skills—Using hands to eat, draw, dress, play, write, etc.
3. Language skills—Speaking, using body language and actions to communicate.
4. Social skills—Interacting with others, developing relationships with family and friends, responding to feelings of others.

Motor skills
Ability to perform complex muscle and nerve acts to produce movement.

Developmental delay

It occurs when children have not reached the developmental milestones by the expected time period. For example, if the normal range for talking is 15 months to two years, and a 2.5-year old has still not begun speaking words, this would be considered a developmental delay. However, most pediatric neurologists do not make a diagnosis of mental retardation in children until after 4 years of age, unless the delay is severe. This is because the rate of development in every child is different and should not be mistaken for mental retardation.

The causes of developmental delay are listed in Table 3.4.

Table 3.4 Causes of developmental delay

Time of Occurrence	Cause	Examples
Prenatal	Genetic	Trisomy 21, Fragile X Syndrome
	Infections	Congenital infections
Perinatal	Intrauterine or neonatal	Low birth weight, prematurity, hypoxia, seizures
Postnatal	Brain injury from multiple causes	Malnutrition, infection (meningitis)
	Environmental factors	Child neglect, abuse

Diagnosis

A complete medical and physical examination is an important tool in evaluation. The history includes pedigree analysis, pregnancy and perinatal history, development and medical history of the child, parents, and affected members of family.

A complete analysis of the clinical and genetic data will help the pediatrician formulate a diagnosis.

Identification

Developmental delay is identified through two types of assessments:

- Developmental screening
- Developmental evaluation

A developmental screening test is a quick and general measurement of skills. Its purpose is to identify children who require further evaluation. A screening test is done giving the parent a questionnaire that queries the developmental milestones or a simple test is given to the child by a health professional.

An evaluation of a child for development involves in depth assessment of the child's skills, and this is performed by highly trained child psychologists. The evaluation test report details on the child's strengths and weaknesses in all areas of development (known as development profile) and this is used to determine if the child is in need of any intervention or treatment plan.

Developmental disorders

Learning disability (LD)

It is a neurological disorder that affects the brain's ability to receive, transmit, store, or respond to information. The term learning disability is used to describe the seemingly unexplained difficulty of a person in acquiring basic academic skills.

Types: LD can affect a person's ability in the areas of listening, speaking, reading, writing, and mathematics.

Causes: Heredity, problems during pregnancy and birth (maternal exposure to alcohol/drugs, low birth weight, premature or prolonged labour), and physical injuries (head injury) after birth or nutritional deprivation.

The treatment plan is individualized depending upon the type and severity of LD.

Attention deficit hyperactivity disorder (ADHD)—Behavioural disorder

ADHD is characterized by inappropriate levels of inattention, impulsivity, and hyperactivity. Early identification and treatment is extremely important because ADHD may have serious consequences including failure in school, family stress, depression, delinquency, and risk of accidental injuries.

Symptoms:

Fails to pay attention to fine details

Has difficulty in sustaining attention

Struggles to follow instructions

Easily distracted

Loses things easily and is forgetful in nature
Talks, climbs, or runs excessively

Causes: Research clearly demonstrates that ADHD runs in families, and the patterns of transmission are to a large extent genetic.

Diagnosis: There is no single test to diagnose ADHD. Therefore, a comprehensive evaluation is required to establish diagnosis. Such an evaluation should include careful history and clinical assessment of the individuals' academic, social and emotional functioning, and developmental level.

Treatment is a multimodal comprehensive approach, which includes:

- Parental and child education about diagnosis and treatment
- Specific behaviour management techniques
- Medication

REVIEW QUESTION

Essay Questions

1. Explain in detail the causes of congenital abnormalities and diagnostic tools available to screen/detect them.
2. Define teratology. Explain the principles of teratology; add a note on environmental risk parameters/modifiers.

Short Notes

1. Write short notes on the following:
   (a) Congenital abnormalities
   (b) Birth defects
   (c) Dysmorphology
   (d) Malformation
   (e) Dysplasia
   (f) Deformation
   (g) Disruption
   (h) Genetic causes of congenital abnormalities
   (i) Teratology
   (j) Principles of teratology
   (k) Factors that influence susceptibility to developmental toxicants

4

Identify Genetic Disorders in Adolescents and Adults

CHAPTER OBJECTIVES

Cancer as a Genetic Disease
DNA Repair Genes
Chromosome Mutations and Cancer
The Molecular Genetics of Colorectal Cancer
Inborn Errors of Metabolism
Classification of inherited metabolic diseases
Enzyme Defects (Aminoacidopathies)
Defects in Purine Metabolism
(Lesch Nyhan Syndrome)

Lysosomal storage diseases
Genetic Haemochromatosis (GH)
Huntington's Disease
Deregulation in Protein pathways
NRSE Mediated Pathway
Therapeutic Modalities for Management of HD
Mental Health

Normal cells grow, divide, mature, and die in response to a complex set of internal and external signals. A normal cell receives both stimulatory and inhibitory signals, and its growth and division are regulated by a balance between these opposing forces. In a cancer cell, one or more of the signals has been disrupted, which causes the cell to proliferate at an abnormally high rate. As they lose their response to the normal controls, cancer cells gradually lose their regular shape and boundaries, eventually forming a distinct mass of abnormal cells—a tumour. If the cells of the tumour remain localized, the tumour is said to be **benign**; if the cells invade other tissues, the tumour is said to be **malignant**. Cells that travel to other sites in the body, where they establish secondary tumours, have undergone **metastasis**.

CANCER AS A GENETIC DISEASE

Cancer arises as a result of fundamental defects in the regulation of cell division, and its study therefore has significance for our basic understanding of cell biology.

Early observations suggested that cancer might result from genetic damage:

1. It was recognized that many agents such as ionizing radiation and chemicals that cause mutations also cause cancer (are carcinogens).

Benign
A benign tumour is a tumour that is non invasive, non progressive and lacks the ability to metastasize. Example: Uterine Fibroid.

Malignant
Malignancy is a medical condition characterized by anaplasia, invasiveness, and metastasis. It is progressive in nature and is capable of spreading to distant tissues (metastasizing property).

Metastasis
Spreading of a disease (cancer) from one part of the body to another.

2. Some cancers are consistently associated with particular chromosome abnormalities. About 90% of people with chronic myeloid leukaemia, for example, have a reciprocal translocation between chromosome 22 and chromosome 9.

3. Some specific types of cancers tend to be familial (run in families). Retinoblastoma, a rare childhood cancer of the retina, appears with high frequency in a few families and is inherited as an autosomal dominant trait.

The clonal evolution of tumours

Cancer begins when a single cell undergoes a mutation that causes the cell to divide at an abnormally rapid rate. The cell proliferates, giving rise to a clone of cells, each of which carries the same mutation. Because the cells of the clone divide more rapidly than normal, they soon outgrow other cells. Additional mutations that arise in the clone may further enhance the ability of those cells to proliferate, and cells carrying both mutations soon become dominant in the clone. In this process, called **clonal evolution**, the tumour cells acquire more mutations that allow them to become increasingly more aggressive in their proliferative properties (Figure 4.1). The rate of clonal evolution depends on the frequency with which new mutations arise. Any genetic defect that allows more mutations to arise will accelerate cancer progression.

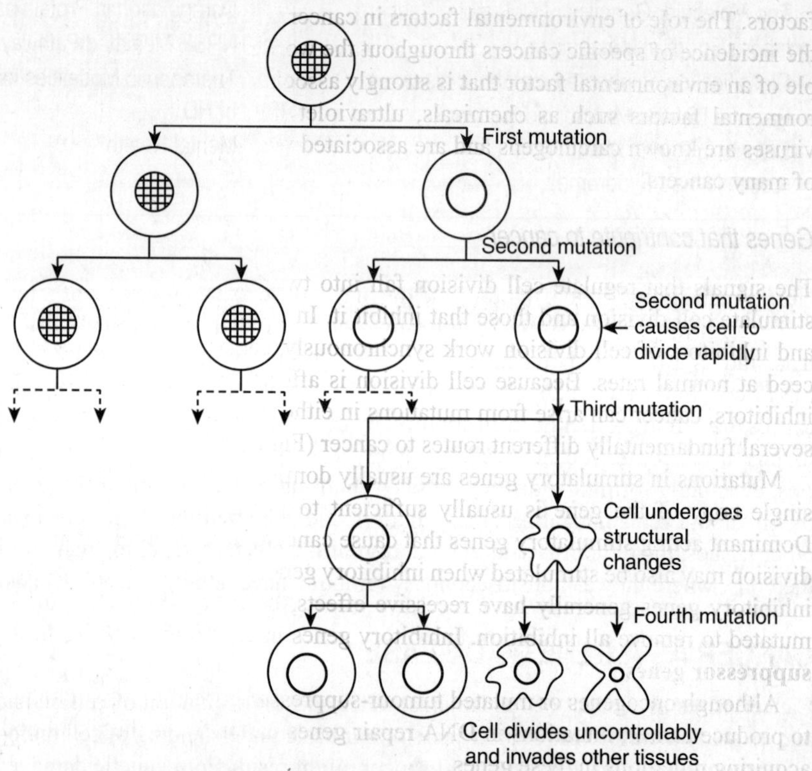

Figure 4.1 Clonal evolution of tumours

Genes that regulate DNA repair are often found to have been mutated in the cells of advanced cancers, and inherited disorders of DNA repair are usually characterized by increased incidences of cancer. Because DNA repair mechanisms normally eliminate many of the mutations that arise, without DNA repair, mutations are more likely to persist in all genes, including those that regulate cell division. Xeroderma pigmentosum, for example, is a rare disorder caused by a defect in DNA repair. People with this condition have elevated rates of skin cancer when exposed to sunlight (which induces mutation). Mutations in genes that affect chromosome segregation also may contribute to the clonal evolution of tumours. Many cancer cells are aneuploid, and it is clear that chromosome mutations contribute to cancer progression by duplicating some genes (those on extra chromosomes) and eliminating others (those on deleted chromosomes). Cellular defects that interfere with chromosome separation increase aneuploidy and therefore may accelerate cancer progression.

The role of environment in cancer

Although cancer is fundamentally a genetic disease, most cancers are not inherited, and there is little doubt that many cancers are influenced by environmental factors. The role of environmental factors in cancer is suggested by differences in the incidence of specific cancers throughout the world. Smoking is a good example of an environmental factor that is strongly associated with cancer. Other environmental factors such as chemicals, ultraviolet light, ionizing radiation, and viruses are known carcinogens and are associated with variation in the incidence of many cancers.

Genes that contribute to cancer

The signals that regulate cell division fall into two basic types: molecules that stimulate cell division and those that inhibit it. In normal cells, both stimulators and inhibitors of cell division work synchronously, causing cell division to proceed at normal rates. Because cell division is affected by both stimulators and inhibitors, cancer can arise from mutations in either type of signal, and there are several fundamentally different routes to cancer (Figure 4.2).

Mutations in stimulatory genes are usually dominant, because a mutation in a single copy of the gene is usually sufficient to produce a stimulatory effect. Dominant acting stimulatory genes that cause cancer are termed **oncogenes**. Cell division may also be stimulated when inhibitory genes are made *inactive*. Mutated inhibitory genes generally have recessive effects, because both copies must be mutated to remove all inhibition. Inhibitory genes in cancer are termed **tumour-suppressor genes**.

Although oncogenes or mutated tumour-suppressor genes or both are required to produce cancer, mutations in DNA repair genes can increase the likelihood of acquiring mutations in these genes.

Oncogene
Tumour/cancer-causing gene.

Tumour suppressor gene
A gene that suppresses cellular proliferation.

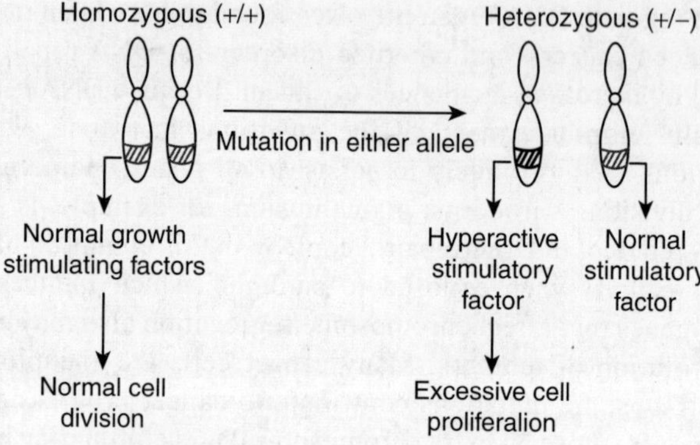

(a) Oncogenes–Dominant acting mechanism

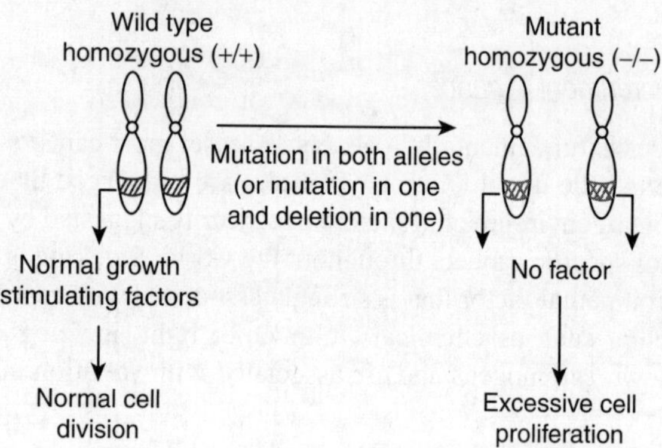

(b) Tumour suppressor genes–Recessive acting mechanism

Figure 4.2 Action of oncogenes and tumour-suppressor genes in cancer

DNA REPAIR GENES

Cancer arises from the accumulation of multiple mutations in a single cell. Some cancer cells have normal rates of mutation, and multiple mutations accumulate because each mutation gives the cell a replicative advantage over cells without the mutations. Other cancer cells may have higher-than-normal rates of mutation in all of their genes, which leads to more frequent mutation of oncogenes and tumour-suppressor genes.

Two processes control the rate at which mutations arise within a cell: (1) the rate at which errors arise during and after replication and (2) the efficiency with which these errors are corrected. The error rate during replication is controlled by the fidelity of DNA polymerases and other proteins in the replication process. However, defects in genes encoding replication proteins have not been strongly linked to cancer.

The mutation rate is also strongly affected by whether errors are corrected by DNA repair systems. Defects in genes that encode components of these repair systems have been consistently associated with a number of cancers. People with xeroderma pigmentosum, for example, are defective in nucleotide-excision repair, an important cellular repair system that normally corrects DNA damage caused by a number of mutagens, including ultraviolet light. Likewise, about 13 % of colorectal, endometrial, and stomach cancers have cells that are defective in mismatch repair, another major repair system in the cell.

Genes affecting chromosome segregation

Most advanced tumours contain cells that exhibit a variety of chromosome anomalies, including extra chromosomes, missing chromosomes, and chromosome rearrangements. Aneuploidy in somatic cells usually arises when chromosomes do not segregate properly in mitosis. Normal cells have a checkpoint that monitors the proper assembly of the mitotic spindle; if chromosomes are not properly attached to the microtubules at metaphase; the onset of anaphase is blocked. Some aneuploid cancer cells contain mutant alleles for genes that encode proteins having roles in this checkpoint; in these cells, anaphase is entered into despite the improper or lack of assembly of the spindle, and chromosome abnormalities result.

The tumour-suppressor gene *p53*, in addition to controlling apoptosis, plays a role in the duplication of the centrosome, which is required for proper formation of the spindle and for chromosome segregation. Normally, the centrosome duplicates once per cell cycle. If *p53* is mutated or missing, however, the centrosome may undergo extra duplications, resulting in the unequal segregation of chromosomes. In this way, mutation of the *p53* gene may generate chromosome mutations that contribute to cancer. The *p53* gene is also a tumour-suppressor gene that prevents cell division when the DNA is damaged.

p53 gene
A gene that regulates cell death/apoptosis, suppresses tumour, regulates cell cycle, and stops the cells from dividing when the DNA is damaged.

Sequences that regulate telomerase

Another factor that may contribute to the progression of cancer is the inappropriate activation of an enzyme called telomerase. Telomeres are special sequences at the ends of eukaryotic chromosomes. In DNA replication in somatic cells, DNA polymerases require a 3-OH group to add new nucleotides. For this reason, the ends of chromosomes cannot be replicated, and telomeres become shorter with each cell division. This shortening eventually leads to the destruction of the chromosome and cell death; so somatic cells are capable of a limited number of cell divisions. In germ cells, telomerase replicates the chromosome ends, thereby maintaining the telomeres, but this enzyme is not normally expressed in somatic cells. In many tumour cells, however, sequences that regulate the expression of the telomerase gene are mutated so that the enzyme is expressed, and the cell is capable of unlimited cell division. Although the expression of telomerase appears to contribute to the development of many cancers, its precise role in tumour progression is still being investigated.

Telomerase
An enzyme involved in the formation and repair of telomeres, so that the chromosomes are not shortened during cell division.

Genes that promote vascularization and the spread of tumours

A final set of factors that contribute to the progression of cancer includes genes that affect the growth and spread of tumours. Oxygen and nutrients, which are essential to the survival and growth of tumours, are supplied by blood vessels, and the growth of new blood vessels (angiogenesis) is important to tumour progression. Angiogenesis is stimulated by growth factors and others proteins encoded by genes whose expression is carefully regulated in normal cells. In tumour cells, genes encoding these proteins are often overexpressed compared with normal cells, and inhibitors of angiogenesis-promoting factors may be inactivated or underexpressed. At least one inherited cancer syndrome—Van Hippel–Lindau disease, in which people develop multiple types of tumours—is caused by the mutation of a gene that affects angiogenesis.

In the development of many cancers, the primary tumour gives rise to cells that spread to distant sites, producing secondary tumours. This process of metastasis is the cause of death in 90% of human cancer cases; it is influenced by cellular changes induced by somatic mutation. By using microarrays to measure levels of gene expression researchers have identified several genes that are transcribed at a significantly higher rate in metastatic cells compared with non-metastatic cells. These genes encode components of the extracellular matrix and the cytoskeleton, which are thought to affect the migration of cells. Other genes that affect metastasis include adhesion proteins that help hold cells together.

Oncogenes are dominant in their action and stimulate cell proliferation. Tumour-suppressor genes are recessive in their action and inhibit cell proliferation. Defects in DNA repair genes allow a higher-than-normal rate of mutation in oncogenes and tumour-suppressor genes. Mutations in genes that control chromosome segregation allow chromosome mutations to accumulate, which may then contribute to cancer progression. Mutations that allow telomerase to be expressed in somatic cells and that affect vascularization and metastasis also may contribute to cancer progression.

CHROMOSOME MUTATIONS AND CANCER

Most tumours contain cells with chromosome mutations. Some types of tumours are consistently associated with *specific* chromosome mutations, suggesting that in these cases the specific chromosome mutation played a pivotal role in the development of the cancer. However, many cancers are not associated with specific types of chromosome abnormalities, and individual *gene* mutations are now known to contribute to many types of cancer. Nevertheless, chromosome instability is a general feature of cancer cells, causing them to accumulate chromosome mutations, which then affect individual genes that contribute to the cancer process. Thus, chromosome mutations appear to both *cause* and *be a result* of cancer.

At least three types of chromosome rearrangements—deletions, inversions, and translocations—are associated with certain types of cancer. Deletions may result in the loss of one or more genes that normally hold cell division in check. When these so-called tumour-suppressor genes are lost, cell division is not regulated and cancer may result. Inversions and translocations contribute to cancer in several ways. First, the chromosomal breakpoints that accompany these mutations may lie within tumour-suppressor genes, disrupting their function and leading to cell proliferation. Second, translocations and inversions may bring together sequences from two different genes, generating a fused protein that stimulates some aspect of the cancer process. Such fusions are seen in most cases of chronic myeloid leukaemia, a fatal form of leukemia affecting bone marrow cells. About 90% of patients with chronic myeloid leukemia have a reciprocal translocation between the long arm of chromosome 22 and the tip of the long arm of chromosome 9 (Figure 4.3). This translocation produces a shortened chromosome 22, called the Philadelphia chromosome because it was first discovered in Philadelphia. At the end of a normal chromosome 9 is a potential cancer-causing gene called *c-ABL*. As a result of the translocation, part of the *c-ABL* gene is fused with the *BCR* gene from chromosome 22. The protein produced by this *BCR–c-ABL* fusion gene is much more active than the protein produced by the normal *c-ABL* gene; the fusion protein stimulates increased, unregulated cell division and eventually leads to leukaemia.

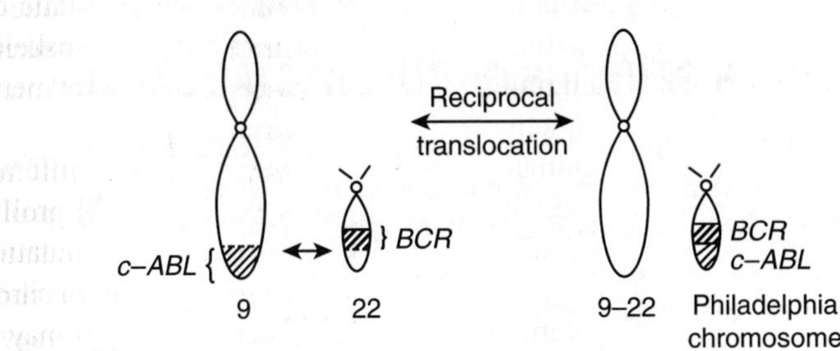

Figure 4.3 Reciprocal translocation between chromosomes 9 and 22-chronic myeloid leukemia (CML)

A third mechanism by which chromosome rearrangements may produce cancer is by the transfer of a potential cancer-causing gene to a new location, where it is activated by different regulatory sequences. Burkitt lymphoma is a cancer of the B cells, the lymphocytes that produce antibodies. Many people having Burkitt lymphoma possess a reciprocal translocation between chromosome 8 and chromosome 2, 14, or 22, each of which carries genes for immunological proteins (Figure 4.4). This translocation relocates a gene called *c-MYC* from the tip of chromosome 8 to a position in one of the above mentioned chromosomes that is next to a gene for one of the immunoglobulin proteins. At this new location, *c-MYC* comes under the control of regulatory sequences that normally activate the production of immunoglobulins, and *c-MYC* is expressed in B cells. The *c-MYC* protein stimulates the division of the B cells and leads to Burkitt lymphoma.

Most tumours contain a variety of types of chromosome mutations. Some tumours are associated with specific deletions, inversions, and translocations. Deletions can eliminate or inactivate genes that control the cell cycle; inversions

Burkitt lymphoma
A type of lymphoma of B-cell origin that occurs especially in children of Central Africa and is associated with Epstein–Barr virus.

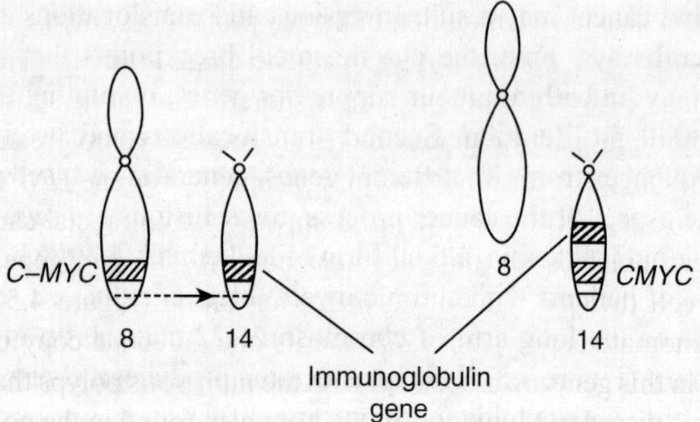

Figure 4.4 Reciprocal translocation between chromosomes 8 and 14—Burkitt Lymphoma

and translocations can cause breaks in genes that suppress tumours, fuse genes to produce cancer-causing proteins, or move genes to new locations, where they are under the influence of different regulatory sequences.

THE MOLECULAR GENETICS OF COLORECTAL CANCER

Mutations that contribute to colorectal cancer have received extensive study, and this cancer is an excellent example of how cancer often arises through the accumulation of successive genetic defects. Colorectal cancers arise in the cells lining the colon and rectum. More than 135,000 new cases of colorectal cancer are diagnosed in the United States each year, where this cancer is responsible for more than 56,000 deaths annually. If detected early, colorectal cancer can be treated successfully; consequently, there has been much interest in identifying the molecular events responsible for the initial stages of colorectal cancer.

Colorectal cancer is thought to originate as benign tumours called adenomatous polyps. Initially, these polyps are microscopic, but in time they enlarge, and the cells of the polyp acquire the abnormal characteristics of cancer cells. In the later stages of the disease, the tumour may invade the mus cle layer surrounding the gut and metastasize. The progression of the disease is slow; from 10 to 35 years may be required for a benign tumour to develop into a malignant tumour. Most cases of colorectal cancer are sporadic, developing in people with no family history of the disease, but a few families display a clear genetic predisposition to this disease. In one form of hereditary colon cancer, known as familial adenomatous polyposis coli, hundreds or thousands of polyps develop in the colon and rectum; if these polyps are not removed, one or more almost invariably becomes malignant.

Because polyps and tumours of the colon and rectum can be easily observed and removed with a colonoscope (a fiber optic instrument that is used to view the interior of the rectum and colon), much is known about the progression of colorectal cancer, and some of the genes responsible for its clonal evolution have been identified. About 75% of colorectal cancers have mutations in tumour-suppressor gene *p53,* and many also have a mutation in the *ras* protooncogene. Families with adenomatous polyposis coli carry a defect in a gene called *APC,* and mutations in *APC,* are found in the cells of tumours that arise sporadically (in persons without a family history). Additional genes that are frequently mutated in colorectal cancer include the oncogenes *myc* and *neu* and the tumour-suppressor gene *HNPCC.* Mutations in these genes are responsible for the different steps of colorectal cancer progression. One of the earliest steps is a mutation that inactivates the *APC* gene, which increases the rate of cell division, leading to polyp formation (Figure 4.5). A person with familial adenomatous polyposis coli inherits one defective copy of the *APC* gene, and defects in this gene are associated with the numerous polyps that appear in those who have this disorder. Mutations in *APC* are also found in the polyps that develop in people who do not have adenomatous polyposis coli.

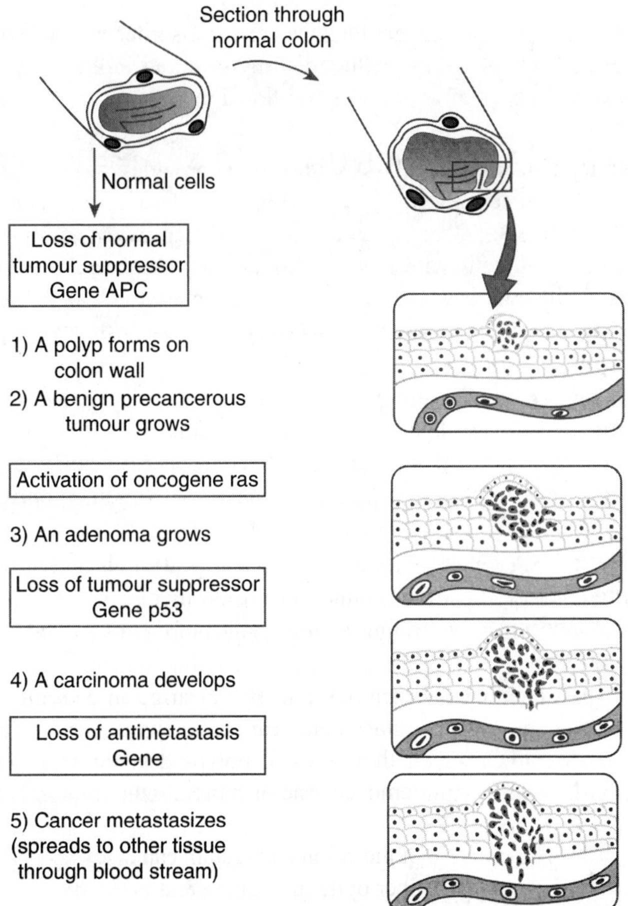

Figure 4.5 Mutations in multiple genes contribute to progression of colorectal cancer (See page 251 for the colour image.)

Mutations of the *ras* oncogene usually occur later, in larger polyps comprising cells that have acquired some genetic mutations. The protein produced by the normal *ras* proto-oncogene sits inside the cell membrane. From there it relays signals from growth factors that stimulate cell division. When *ras* is mutated, the protein that it encodes continually relays a stimulatory signal for cell division, even when growth factor is absent. Mutations in *p53* and other genes appear still later in tumour progression; these mutations are rare in polyps but common in malignant cells. Because *p53* prevents the replication of cells with genetic damage and controls proper chromosome segregation, mutations in *p53* may allow a cell to rapidly acquire further gene and chromosome mutations, which then contribute to further proliferation and invasion into surrounding tissues. The sequence of steps just outlined is not the only route to colorectal cancer, and the mutations need not occur in the order presented here, but this sequence is a common pathway by which colon and rectal cells become cancerous.

To summarize, cancer is fundamentally a genetic disorder, arising from somatic mutations in multiple genes that affect cell division and proliferation. If one or more mutations is inherited, then fewer additional mutations are required for cancer to develop.

- A mutation that allows a cell to divide rapidly provides the cell with a growth advantage; this cell gives rise to a clone of cells with the same mutation. Within this clone, other mutations occur that provide additional growth advantages, and cells with these additional mutations become dominant in the clone. In this way, the clone evolves. Environmental factors play an important role in the development of many cancers by increasing the rate of somatic mutations.

- Several types of genes contribute to cancer progression. Oncogenes are dominant mutated copies of genes that normally stimulate cell division. Tumour-suppressor genes normally inhibit cell division; recessive mutations in these genes may contribute to cancer. Oncogenes and tumour-suppressor genes often control the cell cycle or regulate apoptosis.

- Defects in DNA repair genes and genes that control chromosome segregation often increase the overall mutation rate of other genes, leading to defects in proto-oncogenes and tumour-suppressor genes that may contribute to cancer progression.

- Mutations in sequences that regulate telomerase, an enzyme that replicates the ends of chromosomes, are often associated with cancer. Telomerase allows cells to divide indefinitely but is not usually expressed in somatic cells. Mutations in tumour cells allow telomerase to be expressed.

- Tumour progression is also affected by mutations in genes that promote vascularization and the spread of tumours.

INBORN ERRORS OF METABOLISM

The term inborn errors of metabolism was coined by Archibald Garrod who proposed the "one gene, one enzyme" hypothesis based on his research on the nature and inheritance of alkaptonuria. Most biochemical genetic disorders are in born errors of metabolism which occur due to defects in single genes that code for specific enzymes that catalyze the conversion of various biochemical substrates into products. In most of these biochemical disorders, problems arise due to accumulation of substrates due to lack of enzyme expression. This accumulation results in toxic effects which interfere with normal function.

Metabolism
The chemical processes by which cells produce the substances and energy needed to sustain life.

Enzymes
A group of proteins produced in living cells that catalyze the metabolic processes of an organism.

CLASSIFICATION OF INHERITED METABOLIC DISEASES

S No	Metabolism Involved	Examples
1	Disorders of carbohydrate metabolism	Mucopolysaccharidoses
2	Disorders of aminoacid metabolism	Phenylketonuria, Maple syrup urine disease
3	Disorders of purine metabolism	Lesch Nyhan syndrome
4	Lysosomal storage disorders	Tay Sach's disease

Proteins carry out an astounding number of different functions. Proteins are coded by genes. Mutations in virtually every functional class of protein can lead to a genetic disorder. The recognition that a disease results from abnormality in a protein of a particular class is often useful in understanding its pathogenesis and inheritance, and in devising therapy.

ENZYME DEFECTS (AMINOACIDOPATHIES)

Enzymes are the biological catalysts that mediate, with great efficiency, the conversion of a substrate to a product. Apart from the few catalytic ribonucleic acids (RNAs) involved in RNA processing, enzymes are proteins. One of the best known groups of inborn errors of metabolism, the hyperphenylalaninemias arise from deficient activity of phenylalanine hydroxylase. *Refer the case study on phenylketonuria.*

DEFECTS IN PURINE METABOLISM (LESCH NYHAN SYNDROME)

A good example of a genotype phenotype relationship due to allelic heterogeneity is provided by mutations at the Hprt locus encoding the X linked enzyme hypoxanthine guanine phosphoribosyltransferase (Hprt). Patients with no residual Hprt

Purine
A base that is a constituent of DNA or RNA.

activity have a remarkable phenotype called the Lesch Nyhan syndrome, characterized by choreoathetosis (a movement disorder), spasticity, variable mental retardation, uric acid overproduction that causes gout and renal stones. The neurological manifestations may result from changes in brain purine levels produced by the disease. Finally, patients with Hprt deficiency also illustrate how loss of normal feedback inhibition on the regulation of a metabolic pathway can have pathophysiological consequences, an important principle of biochemical genetic disease.

LYSOSOMAL STORAGE DISEASES

Lysosomes are membrane bound organelles containing an array of hydrolytic enzymes involved in the degradation of variety of biological macromolecules. Genetic defects of these hydrolases lead to the accumulation of their substrates inside the lysosome, resulting in cellular dysfunction and eventually, cell death.

Tay Sach's disease

Tay Sach's disease is one of a group of heterogenous lysosomal storage diseases, the G_{M2} gangliosides that result from the inability to degrade a sphingolipid, G_{M2} ganglioside. The biochemical lesion is a marked deficiency of hexosaminidase A (hex A). Although the enzyme is ubiquitous, the disease has its impact almost solely on the brain, the predominant site of G_{M2} synthesis. The clinical course of Tay Sachs disease is particularly tragic. Affected infants appear normal until about 3 to 6 months of age but then gradually undergo progressive neurological deterioration until death at 2 to 4 years. The effects of neuronal cell death can be seen directly in the form of the so called cherry red spot in the retina, which is surrounded by a pale macula. In the chronic form of adult onset, the manifestations include lower motor neuron dysfunction and ataxia due to spinocerebellar degeneration, nut in contrast to infantile disease, vision and intelligence usually remain normal, although psychosis develops in one thirds of these patients.

Mucopolysaccharidoses

Mucopolysaccharides
A group of polysaccharides with high molecular weight which contain amino sugars and often form complexes with proteins.

Mucoploysaccharides or glycosaminoglycans (GAGs) are polysaccharide chains synthesized by connective tissue cells as normal constituents of many tissues. They are made up of long disaccharide repeating units; the nature of the sugar molecules is the distinguishing feature of a specific GAG. The degradation of these molecules occurs in the lysosome and requires the stepwise removal of the monosaccharide unit by an enzyme. A series of enzymes is thus required for the degradation of any one GAG, and a single enzyme often participates in the catabolism of more than one GAG.

The mucopolysaccharidoses are a heterogeneous group of storage diseases in which mucoploysaccharides accumulate in lysosomes as a result of a deficiency of one of the enzymes required for their degradation. Examples of mucopolysaccharidoses are given in Table 4.1.

Table 4.1 Examples of mucopolysaccharidoses

Syndrome	Clinical Feature	Enzyme Defect	Genetics
Hurler	Diagnosed at 6–18 months, corneal clouding, skeletal changes on radiograph, hepatospleno-megaly, coarse facies, nasal discharge, hydro-cephalus, death <10 years	α L Iduronidase	Autosomal recessive
Hunter	Similar to Hurler syndrome, but with slower pro-gression, no corneal clouding and a uniquely pebbly skin lesion	Iduronate sulphatase	X-linked recessive
Sanfilippo A	Hyperactivity and retardation, progressive neu-rodegeneration	Heparan N sulphatase	Autosomal recessive
Sanfilippo B	Similar to Sanfilippo A syndrome	α N acetylglucosaminidase	Autosomal recessive

Haemoglobinopathies

A molecular disease is one in which primary disease causing event is a mutation, either inherited or acquired. This chapter outlines basic genetic and biochemical mechanisms underlying genetic disease, using disorders of haemoglobin—Haemoglobinopathies as examples.

Disorders of human haemoglobins, called haemoglobinopathies occupy a unique position in medical genetics for several reasons. They are easily the most common single gene diseases in the world and they cause substantial morbidity. Haemoglobin is the oxygen carrier in vertebrate red blood cells. The molecule contains four subu-nits: two α and two β chains. Each subunit is composed of a polypeptide chain, globin and a prosthetic group, heme, which is an iron containing pigment that com-bines with oxygen to give the molecule its oxygen transporting ability.

The study of the structure of haemoglobin allows one to predict which types of mutations are likely to be pathogenic. Thus, a mutation alters globin conforma-tion, substitutes highly conserved amino acids or disrupts the hydrophobic shell—that excludes water from the interior of the molecule—by replacing one of the non polar residues, is likely to cause a haemoglobiopathy.

Haemoglobin
An oxygen-carrying pigment of the red blood cells which gives them the red colour and transports oxygen from lungs to tissues.

Haemolytic anemias—Sickle cell disease

Sickle cell haemoglobin (Hb S) was the first abnormal haemoglobin to be detected and is of great clinical importance. It is due to a single nucleotide substitution that changes the codon of the sixth amino acid of β globin from glutamic acid to valine (GAG to GTG: Glu6Val). Homozygosity for this mutation is the cause of sickle cell disease, a serious disorder that is common in characteristic geographic distri-bution—equatorial Africa, Mediterranean area and India).

Sickle cell disease is a severe autosomal recessive haemolytic condition characterized by a tendency of the red blood cells to become grossly abnormal in shape (i.e. sickled) under conditions of low oxygen tension. Heterozygotes,

Glutamic acid
An amino acid obtained by hydrolysis from wheat gluten and sugar-beet residues.

Valine
An essential amino acid present in most plant and animal proteins, required for growth.

who are said to have sickle cell trait, are clinically normal, but their red blood cells sickle when subjected to very low oxygen pressure in vitro. Under conditions of low oxygen tension, the sickle haemoglobin molecules aggregate in the form of rod shaped polymers of fibers, which distort the shape of the erythrocyte to a sickle shape. These misshapen erythrocytes are less deformable than normal and unlike normal red blood cells cannot squeeze in single file through capillaries, thereby blocking blood flow and causing local ischemia.

Thalassemia

Haemoglobin E (Hb E) is a β globin structural variant (Glu26Lys) that causes thalassemia because it is synthesized at a reduced rate.It is probably the most common structural abnormal haemoglobin in the world occurring at high frequency in South East Asia.

The thalassemias, collectively the most common human single gene disorders are a heterogenous group of diseases of haemoglobin synthesis in which mutations reduce the synthesis or stability of either the α or β globin chain, to cause α and β thalassemia respectively.

Alpha thalassemias

The name "thalassemia" is derived from the Greek word for sea, *thalassa*, and signifies that the disease was first discovered in persons of Mediterranean origin. Both α and β thalassemia have a high frequency in many populations, although α thalassemia is more prevalent and widely distributed.

Genetic disorders of the α globin production affect the formation of both fetal and adult haemoglobins and therefore cause intrauterine and postnatal disease. In the absence of α globin chains with which to associate, the chains of β globin cluster are free to forma homotetrameric haemoglobin. Haemoglobin with γ_4 composition is known as Hb Bart's and the β_4 tetramer is called Hb H. Because neither of these haemoglobins is capable of releasing oxygen to tissues in normal conditions, they are completely ineffective oxygen carriers. Consequently infants with severe α thalassemia and high levels of Hb Bart's suffer severe intrauterine hypoxia and are born with massive generalized fluid accumulation, a condition called hydrops foetalis. In milder α thalassemias, an anemia develops because of the gradual precipitation of the Hb H in the erythrocyte. This leads to the formation of inclusions in the mature red blood cell, and the removal of these inclusions by the spleen damages the cells, leading to their premature destruction.

Hydrops foetalis
Serious and extensive oedema of the foetus.

Beta thalassemias

The β thalassemias share many features with α thalassemia. Decreased β globin production causes a hypochromic, microcytic anemia and the imbalance in globin synthesis leads to precipitation of the excess α chains, which in turn leads to damage of the red cell membrane. In contrast to α globin, however the β chain is important only in the postnatal period. The onset of β thalassemia is not apparent until a few months after birth, when β globin normally replaces γ globin as the major non- α chain and only the synthesis of the major adult haemoglobin Hb, A is reduced. The excess α chains are insoluble, so that they precipitate in red cell precursors are destroyed in the bone marrow; this process causes ineffective erythropoiesis.

Most individuals with two β thalassemia alleles have **thalassemia major**, a condition characterized by severe anemia and the need for lifelong medical management. Carriers of one β thalassemia allele are clinically well and are said to have **thalassemia minor**. Such individuals have hypochromic, microcytic red blood cells and may have a slight anaemia.

GENETIC HAEMOCHROMATOSIS (GH)

Haemochromatosis is a clinical condition characterized by classic triad of hepatomegaly, diabetes and bronzing of the skin. The disease was thought to be caused by a 'chromogenic' substance carried in the heme, hence its name. GH may be defined based on genetic, biochemical or clinical criteria or a combination of them. Genetically, GH is a recessively inherited clinical syndrome of iron overload due to mutations in the HFE gene. These mutations may lead to iron loading and subsequently to organ damage.

The cause of the iron overload is a malregulation of dietary iron absorption in the duodenum. At comparable levels of body iron stores, GH patients fail to down regulate intestinal iron absorption compared to normal subjects. This causes accumulation of iron with no compensatory mechanism of elimination. Over time, excess iron accumulates in vulnerable tissues like liver causing cirrhosis and eventually hepatocellular carcinoma; in the heart causing congestive failure and dysrhythmias; in the pancreas causing diabetes; in the skin causing melanoderma; in organs of the endocrine system causing amenorrhea or loss of libido.

Symptoms due to the tissue iron overload of GH depend on degree of overload, age of presentation and sex.

The diagnosis is made by a combination of clinical suspicion and biochemical and genetic testing. Serum ferritin measurements are a good reflection of body iron stores. Liver biopsy with Prussian blue stain classically shows accumulation of iron in parenchymal cells. Advanced disease condition will show nodular cirrhosis.

Phlebotomy is the treatment of choice but must be started before irreversible damage has occurred. Early diagnosis and intervention with phlebotomy prevents cardiomyopathy, cirrhosis and cancer associated with tissue iron overlaod. Phlebotomy therapy is inexpensive and widely available.

Anaemia
A deficiency in the number of red blood cells or in the haemoglobin content.

Hepatomegaly
Enlargement of the liver (due to infection or trauma).

Chromogenic
A substance capable of generating a colour in combination with other chemical compounds.

Cardiomyopathy
A disease condition where the myocardium (heart muscle) is affected resulting in heart failure.

Phlebotomy
Technique employed to collect blood (for diagnostic tests) by venipuncture.

HUNTINGTON'S DISEASE

Huntington's disease (HD) formerly referred as Huntington's chorea, is a rare progressive neurodegenerative disorder that primarily affects the functions of the central nervous system. Individuals affected with HD are typically presented with dual involuntary (choreiform and hypokinetic) movements along with psychiatric disturbances and dementia. Of all signs and symptoms, the disease is readily recognised and identified by its classic sign – chorea, which spreads progressively to all the muscles of the human body. Such choreatic movements are irregular in nature and are well observed affecting the trunk, upper and lower limbs as well as the respiratory and buccolingual muscles. Owing to this condition, HD affected patients have uncontrolled body movements and also have difficulties performing basic activities such as swallowing – dysphagia. In addition, debilitating features such as unintended weight loss, autonomic nervous system dysfunction and sleep-and circadian rhythm disturbances, are quite less common in those suffering from this disease. Eventually, as the disease becomes severe, individuals acquire the ability to develop aspiration pneumonia which is the most common cause of death. Studies have highlighted that dysphagia caused during advanced stages of the disease, can cause aspiration complications with the likelihood of developing fatal aspiration pneumonia. Cardiorespiratory complications and subdural hematoma are other common causes of death in the diseased population. Moreover, depression caused in HD patients is associated with higher suicidal rates which are several folds higher than that of the general population.

The prevalence of Huntington's disease is approximately 5-10 per 100,000 persons belonging to the Caucasian population. On the contrary, Japan has much lower prevalence which is about one-tenth of that of the Caucasian descent. HD's age of onset is usually between 30 and 50 years of age, with a range of 2 to 85 years. Post age of disease onset, individuals will have a survival period of 17-20 years on an average.

Genetic background

Genetics has a strong impact in influencing the course of HD pathogenesis and the type of genetic mutation determines the clinical phenotype of the affected individual. This means that the genetic variations that are caused in the disease specific gene has the tendency to influence the age of onset of developing the disease, the severity of disease symptoms, the ability of juvenile (early onset) disease to develop and get inherited from the father to the progeny and sporadic appearance of developing new mutations to HD. From the above fact, it is clearly evident that understanding genetic background and the genetic susceptibility of Huntington's disease is crucial in establishing a confirmed diagnosis of the disease as well as in deciding the therapeutic strategy for HD affected individuals.

Huntington's disease is caused because of the mutations in the gene named as Huntingtin (HTT) which is located on chromosome 4 and its cytogenetic location is 4p16.3. Mutations in the HTT gene lead to repeat expansion of three main nucleotides namely: cytosine (C), adenine (A) and guanine (G). Three bases together make up a genetic codon and they have the ability to code for an amino acid that leads to synthesis of polypeptides (functional protein molecule). Therefore, mutations in the HTT gene leads to repeat expansion of these three nitrogenous bases and is scientifically termed as trinucleotide repeat expansion. In simple terms, Huntington's disease is a trinucleotide repeat expansion of the codon CAG. This CAG codon is located on the 5' end of exon 1 of the HTT gene and they code for the amino acid – glutamine. The HTT gene has 67 exons. Mutations in the HTT gene lead to formation of a mutant huntingtin protein (mHTT) which consists of abnormally long repeats of polyglutamine protein sequences.

Under normal circumstances, the CAG triplet is usually repeated about 20 times. However, in the case of Huntington's disease this CAG triplet is repeated more than 20 times and the number of times these repeats are expanded varies from person-to-person. Also, the affected individuals will have mild to moderate and/or moderate to severe symptoms of HD, which is based on the increased number of triplet expansion. This in turn influences and affects the penetrance and variable expressivity of the disease. The normal population will have CAG repeats generally in the range of 10-27. Individuals who have CAG repeat expansion in the range 27-35 are unaffected (do not have any symptoms) however, they have the ability to transmit the CAG repeat expansions to their offspring and that number could be higher than that of the parental generation. For example, a father who has repeats in the range of 27-35 will transmit the abnormal repeat expansion to his son and the son will have a repeat of 40 times. This condition is termed as anticipation – a genetic terminology that refers to passing of genes from the parental generation to their offspring and each time the genes get passed down the generation, the disease expression and its symptoms get more severe. The offspring will tend to develop the disease at an early age and the symptoms will be severe. Another important factor that needs to be understood is that, HD follows Mendelian pattern of inheritance and it is inherited in autosomal dominant fashion. With reference to the repeat expansion factor, individuals who have CAG repeats in the range 36-39 will have late onset of the disease development. However, in this category there is an interesting observation. There are individuals who have repeats within the range 36-39, but do not develop the disease phenotypically and are not presented with any obvious signs and symptoms. This attribute is known as reduced (or incomplete penetrance). They are however, capable of passing on the genetic mutations to their progeny(s). Individuals who have CAG repeats in the range 40-50 will have the typical adult onset disease symptoms, whereas those who have the longest repeats will develop severe forms of infantile and juvenile cases of HD. Such juvenile cases of HD are possible because of high allele instability that happens during parental transmission.

Therefore, the number of CAG triplet repeats is the primary determinant of disease severity that accounts for nearly 30-60% of variance in the age of onset of developing the disease's initial symptoms. The remaining factors for variance are assigned with other genetic as well as environmental factors. From a clinical perspective, it was found that there is a positive correlation between the number of CAG repeats and Vonsattel grades of neuropathological severity. This means that higher the CAG repeat length, higher will be the degree of cell death in the striatal region of the brain and hence higher Vonsattel grades.

Molecular mechanisms underlying disease pathogenesis

Being a rare molecular and hereditary neurodegenerative disease, HD is no exception. There are a myriad of complex dynamic pathways and activities that are involved behind the series of neurodegeneration in the striatum (caudate nucleus and putamen) of the brain. Starting from DNA to cellular level, the molecular pathogenesis of HD is complex and involves a few protein pathways that are responsible for altering the cellular dynamics. As a result of genetic variations, the otherwise normal wild type protein gets transcribed into a mutant form, which in turn undergoes aggregation by forming protein oligomers. These oligomer aggregates tend to disrupt many of the vital cellular functions by altering key organelles function. Despite a well-defined genetic architecture behind the disease progression, the exact molecular underpinning behind these mechanisms still remains as an unresolved puzzle. This section will highlight some of the molecular pathways that get disorganised during the course of disease pathogenesis. Figure 4.6 represents a schematic illustration of the prime major steps that are involved in the disease pathogenesis.

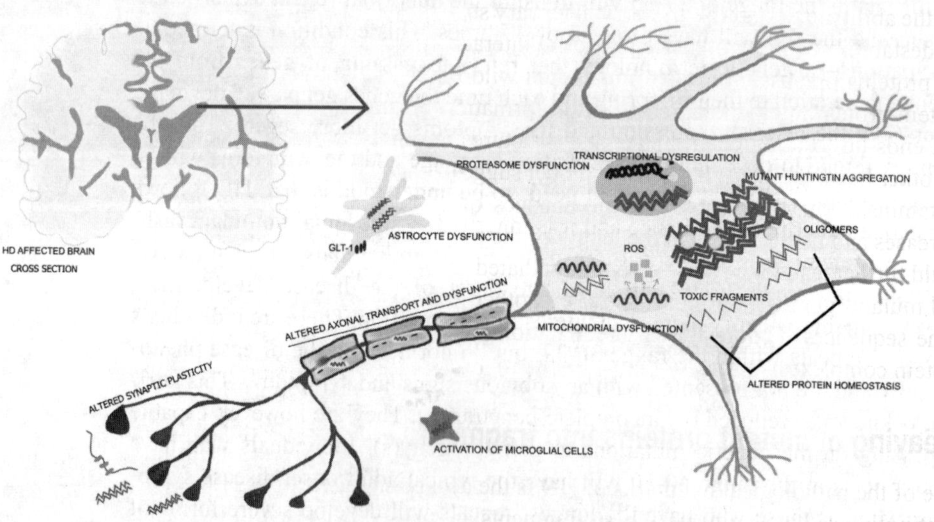

Figure 4.6 Schematic illustration of the major steps that are involved in the initiation and progression of HD pathogenesis. Starting from transcriptional dysregulation till alteration of synaptic plasticity, the continued process results in progressive neurodegeneration of striatal neurons that are predominantly located in the basal ganglia region of the brain, during the course of disease progression. Abbreviation: ROS: reactive oxygen species, GLT-1: glutamine transporter, HD: Huntington's disease.

The disease pathogenesis includes the following steps:

a) Protein aggregate formation
b) Transcriptional dysregulation
c) Altered protein homeostasis
d) Mitochondrial dysfunction
e) Altered synaptic plasticity and axonal transport defect
f) Neuroglia dysfunction

Protein aggregate formation

Huntingtin protein is composed of >3100 amino acids by having a molecular mass of 349 KDa, depending upon the total number of glutamine residues. The protein consists of polyglutamine sequences coined at the NH_2 terminal and has multiple consensus repeat sequences called HEAT (huntingtin, elongation factor 3, protein phosphatase 2A, and TOR1 [target of rapamycin 1]) that are inevitable for protein-protein interactions. Mutations in the HTT gene results in the formation of mHTT protein - a ubiquitously expressed protein and has CAG repeats more than 36 in number. mHTT protein has the ability to induce nerve cell dysfunction and death through varied mechanisms. Before inducing cellular dysfunction as such the mutated protein first undergoes aggregation. There are two proposed models that help in understanding the probable mechanisms of mHTT aggregation namely polar zip model and the transglutaminase model.

According to polar zip model, the presence of polyglutamine tract in the protein has the ability to destabilise the normal tertiary structure of the protein. As a result, the destabilised huntingtin protein tends to interact with other polyglutamine bearing proteins (inclusive of other mutant and wild-type huntingtin proteins). These protein-protein interactions result in the formation of insoluble β-pleated sheets that ends up forming polar zipper like structures through hydrogen bonding. On the other hand, the transglutaminase model suggests that huntingtin being a transglutaminase enzyme's substrate, the chances of enzyme-mediated crosslinking increases and that is based on the length of the polyglutamine stretch. This in turn could further lead to the same enzyme-mediated crosslinking with other wild-type and mutant-huntingtin proteins as well as other proteins consisting of polyglutamine sequences. This results in precipitation and accumulation of intraneuronal protein complexes.

Cleaving of mutant proteins into fragments

One of the pathological hallmarks of HD is the accumulation of toxic N-terminal huntingtin protein fragments. These fragments are caused because of proteolysis initiated by caspases and other protease enzymes. Additionally, mechanisms such as aberrant splicing at exon 1 of the protein can also contribute to its fragmentation. Thus, both wild type and mutant forms of huntingtin protein gets fragmented during the disease progression, wherein presence of mHTT fragments correlates with increased toxicity because of its propensity to form more nuclear and less-cytoplasmic aggregates.

Transcriptional dysregulation

DNA microarray based studies have evidenced the fact that mHTT has the propensity to interfere and imped transcription. This particular mutant protein interferes with some of the key regulators that are involved in cell function and survival such as p53, cAMP response element-binding (CREB) protein, CREB–binding protein (CBP), PGC-1a (peroxisome proliferator-activating receptor-g coactivator-1 a), Sp1 along with its cofactor TAFII130 and cystathionine γ-lyase.

DEREGULATION IN PROTEIN PATHWAYS

There are two key pathways namely CREB and neuron restrictive silencer elements (NRSE) pathway whose transcription process gets deregulated during HD pathogenesis.

CREB pathway

Under normal physiological conditions, CREB transcription factor binds to CRE promoter region on the DNA sequences and aids in the transcription process that is necessary for neuronal survival. However, during HD progression, mHTT interrupts CRE-mediated transcriptional regulation. This deregulation is initiated by the direct interaction of mHTT with CBP which results in sequestration of CBP as well as TAFII130 in the nucleus. Owing to this condition, the duo loses its ability to get attached to CRE sites in the cellular DNA promoters. In addition to this, RNA Pol II enzyme does not get positioned properly to initiate the overall process. Thus, mHTT results in impeding transcription.

NRSE MEDIATED PATHWAY

In this pathway, the wild-type HTT regulates the action of genes that consists of NRSE binding sites e.g. Brain-derived neurotropic factor (BDNF). REST-NRSF (repressor-element-1 transcription factor-neuron restrictive silencer factor) attaches to the NRSE regions that lie on BDNF promoter sequences. Wild-type HTT interacts with REST-NRSF and decreases its availability in the nucleus and thus restricts the binding of the same with BDNF promoter region. In the case of HD, the mHTT fails to interact with REST-NRSF because of which their levels tend to increase in the nucleus. REST-NRSF, as a result binds to the NRSE in the BDNF gene promoter region, thereby enhancing the incorporation of a molecule named Sin3A-histone-deacetylase complex (HDACs). Owing to this association, the expression of NRSE, NRSF, REST and BDNF are suppressed and thus transcription of BDNF gene and BDNF synthesis is deranged.

Altered protein homeostasis

There are two main protein degradation systems - the ubiquitin– proteasome system (UPS), and autophagy–lysosome system. The former helps in cleaving and degradation of the wild-type HTT protein while the latter helps in cleaving of expanded mHTT forms of protein. The UPS gets impaired during the pathogenesis of HD because of the accumulation of mHTT in the nucleus. In normal conditions, Hsp70 and Hsp40 aids in regulating transcription, however in HD the mutated forms of HTT protein induces misfolding of protein aggregates including the chaperons. This in turn disrupts the entire protein clearance pathway eventually leading to mitochondrial dysfunction. With regard to autophagy and lysosomal systems' functions during HD, differing observations were raised across several experimental studies. Certain *in vivo* studies using HD animal models have revealed that the formation of autophagosome complexes are not affected either by the wild-type or mHTT forms of protein. Although this mechanism is not disrupted, studies elucidated the fact that these autophagosomes are not efficient enough to sequestrate and degrade any unwanted harmful proteins. Nevertheless, it was proposed that autophagosome's impaired axonal transport in HD eventually leads to incapable autophagosome - lysosome fusion along with decreased degradation of these contents.

Mitochondrial dysfunction

The mitochondrial organelle gets disrupted during the disease pathogenesis which in turn affects several cellular dynamics such as defects in ATP synthesis, reduced mitochondrial oxygen consumption, reduced glucose metabolism and cAMP levels, and depressed Ca^{++} buffering capacity. Eventually, there will be an elevation in the formation of reactive oxygen species and consequently the neuronal cells will have increased oxidative stress and thus the neurons undergo apoptotic cell death. mHTT, in addition, interferes with organellar axonal transport and can reduce the transport of the mitochondria to synapse junctions, as well as in ATP synthesis.

Altered synaptic plasticity and axonal transport defect

Decreased transcription of significant genes that are involved in signaling and neurotransmission tend to disrupt the neuronal homeostasis. These alterations have further implications on synaptic plasticity and therefore there are defects caused along the axonal length. Such defects could impair the transport and delivery of proteins and other organelles along the neuronal axons, which is further exacerbated by increased mHTT levels. Abnormalities that are caused in neurons and synaptic terminals are the earliest molecular derangements in HD pathogenesis. Studies have demonstrated that mutations in the HD gene also affect the trafficking of NMDAR in striatal neuron, which is because of alteration in balance between the synaptic and extrasynaptic NMDAR activity in HD.

HD is characterised by a failure of either GABAA (gamma-aminobutyric acid type A) or AMPA (amino-3-hydroxy-5-methyl-4-isoxazole propionic acid) receptor delivery, which inhibits synaptic excitability. mHTT impairs the contact where HAP1 binds these receptors to the kinesin motor factor KIF5. Moreover, mHTT inhibits the release of BDNF, cortical transport, and the retrograde trafficking of its receptor TrkB in the striatum, all of which are necessary to initiate survival signals in the cell body. All these factors eventually end up in causing defects along the neuronal axons.

Neuroglia dysfunction

Astrocytes and microglial neuronal cells are most predominantly affected during the course of HD. Astrocytes are glial cells that provide support to neurons by enabling uptake of extracellular glutamate, thereby preventing excitotoxicity. During the disease progression, HD animal model based studies that elucidated that astrocytes contribute to neurological dysfunction reduced levels of GLT-1 glutamate transporter. This is because of the expression of N-terminal huntingtin with 160Q in astrocytes. Additional defects that were induced because of HD in astrocytes include reduced BDNF discharge or impaired secretion of the chemokine CCL5. Although the huntingtin protein aggregates are more common in neuronal than non-neuronal glial cells, these glial cells contribute to disease progression which is probably because of lack of cell division in neurons or a less efficient protein regulation system. ROS and neurotoxic chemicals (quinolinic acid) that can trigger molecular pathways resulting in neuronal death, are further produced by reactive astrocytes and activated microglial cells.

Diagnostic methods used for HD

Diagnosis of HD involves several procedures and is complete only when the suspected/affected individuals' medical history, family history background, clinical examinations including neuroimaging studies and genetic diagnostic testing is performed. HD diagnostic evaluation should be performed by taking certain factors into consideration, especially before one decides to perform genetic testing for a suspected individual. This is because there are certain other genetic disorders that mimic symptoms of HD.

Before the concerned group of medical specialists could decide to proceed with any other confirmed diagnostic testing, the suspected individual should be screened for the following

- Progressive motor disability – involuntary chorea movements. Sometimes voluntary movements may also be affected.
- Mental disturbances that includes decline in cognitive functions, behavioral changes and/or signs of depression.
- Family history having strong background of persistent autosomal dominance inheritance patterns.

Gathering a thorough family history of the suspected individual is crucial in establishing the initial investigation of the suspected individual. As an alternate for HD diagnosis, performing neurodiagnostic imaging studies could also provide an indication of HD pathogenesis. A CT or an MRI scan, can diagnose and look for symptoms of cerebral atrophy or atrophy in the caudate nucleus region. In addition to this, positron emission topography (PET) can also help in revealing signs of diminution in metabolic rate of the brain's striatal region. Genetic testing on the other hand helps in establishing a confirmatory diagnosis. Interestingly, HD has the reputation of being the first genetic anomaly mapped to a distinct chromosome using a restriction fragment length polymorphism (RFLP) marker in the year 1983.

Genetic diagnosis for HD can be performed in three ways namely predictive testing, diagnostic genetic testing and prenatal and pre-implantation genetic diagnosis. Predictive genetic testing, otherwise known as pre-symptomatic testing, can be performed for individuals who are at risk of developing the disease in the near future, but do not have any symptoms of HD at the current moment. Importantly, predictive testing is not suggested for asymptomatic at-risk individuals who are less than 18 years of age.

Predictive testing is generally conducted by a team of genetic counselors, neurologists and other healthcare related professionals who can help in providing support to such concerned individuals, particularly with the intention of helping them to educate themselves about the disease outcomes and prognosis. It is important to ensure that the individual should not be forced to undergo complete predictive testing by any of their family members including the concerned medical team at any point of time. Obtaining a signed informed-consent and complete willingness from the patient is recommended before engaging in any sort of genetic evaluation and/or genetic counseling. Adapting the ethics and principles of an ideal genetic counseling session is necessary and has to be followed at all costs from the beginning till the end of their testing sessions.

For patients who have already displayed signs and symptoms of HD, confirmatory diagnostic genetic testing can be performed. There are few scenarios where diagnostic genetic testing is highly recommended for the following group of individuals. They are:

- The patient (proband) with a positive family history and has specific motor symptoms.
- The patient with a positive family history and has prodromal symptoms (suggesting the impending likelihood of developing HD).
- The patient has no family history, but has specific symptoms that are likely to be associated with HD.
- Child with a family history of HD and has features of juvenile HD.

Regardless of the above criteria for enabling a patient to undergo diagnostic genetic testing, there are certain pre-requisites that need to be met before initiating genetic testing. First, the concerned clinician or neurologist should recommend and approve the need for following up with a diagnostic genetic testing, the patient should be well educated about the pros and cons of undergoing genetic testing. Next, the option for referral of a genetic counseling session should also be put forward to the patients. This is necessary because these counseling sessions can help in educating the patient about the disease's genetic background as well as the risk of transmission of the disease to the next generation. It also helps predict risk assessment for close relatives to develop HD. Pedigree analysis and information collection can help in establishing appropriate genetic testing for confirmatory diagnosis, since HD is a trinucleotide repeat expansion disease with variable penetrance and expressivity. However, educating the patients is essential and genetic counseling sessions are indeed put into practice with the scope of providing psychological support to patients in addition to establishing genetic diagnosis and performing appropriate diagnostic testing.

Currently, molecular testing of the HTT gene for establishing HD diagnosis is performed by using targeted analysis for CAG trinucleotide expansions. Conventional polymerase chain reaction (PCR), triplet-primed PCR (TP-PCR), and expanded repeat analysis techniques are used to detect the number of CAG repeats in the HTT gene. Normally, PCR based methods can help in the detection of alleles up to about 115 CAG repeats (e.g. Long-range PCR, PCR- RFLP). PCR assays used for detecting CAG repeats involve amplification using primers flanking CAG repeat region, followed by the usage of capillary electrophoresis. Sometimes, polymorphisms in the flanking sequence region may contribute to allele-specific PCR failure and might cause misdiagnosis of HD. On the other hand, TP-PCR aids in detection of an expanded allele that has >200 CAG repeats and helps in the expansion of alleles that have a characteristic CE pattern, thereby distinguishing patterns from non-expanded alleles. Unlike long-range PCR that requires the usage of Southern blotting techniques, TP-PCR doesn't require Southern blotting.

Prenatal testing is essential and required for pre- conceptional planning when either one of the parent is affected or at risk of developing HD. Under such circumstances, either chorionic villus sampling (CVS) at 10-12 weeks of pregnancy or by performing amniocentesis at 14-20 weeks is recommended. In special cases, when the couple plan for opting *in vitro* fertilisation technique (IVF) for conception, pre-implantation genetic diagnosis (PGD) can be employed. PGD test is performed on a single cell that is obtained from the eight-cell stage embryo (post IVF). The HD genetic mutation analysis is then performed on this single cell which allows for detection of HTT gene repeat sizes for that embryo. After analysis, only embryos that are tested negative for HD gene mutation, is selected and then implanted into the posterior wall of the uterus (as part of IVF related pregnancy procedures).

THERAPEUTIC MODALITIES FOR MANAGEMENT OF HD

HD being a monogenic autosomal dominant disorder in addition to progressive neurodegenerative changes in the brain and altered abnormal body movements poses challenges for defining standard care of treatment for HD affected patients. At the most there is no definite or complete curative therapy owing to its complex functionalities. The current treatment strategies are primarily involved in alleviating pain and symptoms with the help of pharmacological and non-pharmacological maneuvers. In the recent times, revolution in the field of molecular biology has pioneered Huntington's disease research that aims in probing and solving underlying defects at the molecular level. These trials are conducted at the preliminary and preclinical studies with a few that have reached the clinical trials stage. Despite, the limited reach in bringing up these innovative therapeutic trials from bench-to-bedside, understanding and validating such strategies through extensive clinical trials could pave a way in the long run in further enhancing treatment options for affected individuals.

Currently, the point of care for HD patients is through administration of drugs for improving motor dysfunction symptoms and the usage of surgical ailments. Chorea medication, antipsychotic medication, mood stabilising medicines, and antidepressants are used in treating HD based on the kind of motor dysfunction and movement disorders the patients are affected with. Mostly patients are treated with medications that enable to reduce chorea. This is because one of the major pathological hallmarks of HD is the degeneration of neurons in the basal ganglia (particularly the striatum) which leads to development of chorea movements. To treat and reduce these involuntary chorea movements, Tetrabenazine (TBZ) was the first drug to be invented and implemented for the same. TBZ's mechanism of action has been proposed to selectively result in depletion of central monoamines at the nerve terminal by the reversible inhibition of human vesicular monoamine transporter 2 (VMAT2). Deutetrabenazine (DBZ) is another drug similar to that of TBZ in reducing chorea, except that it is an isotopic isomer of TBZ and has six deuterium atoms have been substituted in the place of hydrogen. Dopamine antagonists, also known as antipsychotics or neuroleptics are the second line of choice of drugs for treating chorea. Since nearly 40% of HD patients experience either partial or HD associated depression, antidepressants are used to treat depressive symptoms. However, these medications are not useful for treating other psychotic symptoms or HD associated chorea. Selective serotonin reuptake inhibitors (SSRIs) are the most commonly used antidepressants to treating HD patients. Citalopram is the most commonly used SSRI antidepressant in HD treatment strategy.

Surgical treatment as an alternate therapy can be used in improving chorea symptoms. For example, deep brain stimulation therapy is highly effective in alleviating chorea symptoms in HD patients who are resistant to pharmacological therapy. Nevertheless, this surgical therapy is rarely used in management of Huntington's chorea since patients who are resistant to pharmacological therapy in HD is quite rare.

In the past decade, pioneering research in genetics and neurosciences have embarked the potential application of using molecular i.e. root cause therapy for management of HD. These therapies particularly aim at restoring the effects of wild type HTT protein or in other words they help in lowering the levels of mHTT. Antisense oligonucleotide (ASO), RNA interference (RNAi), zinc-finger protein (ZFP), transcription activator-like effector nuclease (TALEN),clustered regularly interspaced short palindromic repeats (CRISPR)/CRISPR-associated System (Cas) therapies, stem cell and antibody therapies are some of the major innovations that have been bought forth into pre-clinical and clinical trials for testing their efficacy in targeting HD at the molecular level. ASOs are single stranded analogues to oligonucleotides and at present three ASOs have been tested for their potential therapeutic efficiency for HD in clinical trials: Tominersen, WVE-120101 and WVE-120102. ASOs can be either allele specific (target mHTT) or non-allele specific i.e. they can target both wild-type as well as the mutant HTT protein. RNAi therapies make use of transgenes that helps in expression of molecules such as microRNA (miRNA), short hair pin RNA (shRNA), short interfering RNA (siRNA). These varied RNAi molecules inhibits the action of messenger RNA (mRNA) thereby halting protein translation process and thus results in protein degradation (mHTT). RNAi therapies require the usage of viral vectors for its delivery and have its own limitations despite its beneficial action. Currently, AMT-130 (UniQure Biopharma B.V) is the only RNAi-based gene therapy that is tested for its utility in clinical trial studies. With regard to stem cell therapy, more emphasis is placed on utilising them as potential future therapeutic agents owing to its ability to help in regeneration of depleted neurons that are lost during the course of HD. Currently, Cellavita HD is the most progressed stem cell therapy for HD that utilises mesenchymal stem cells (MSCs) and is administered through intravenous injection.

Overall, there is continuing progress in the areas of diagnostic and therapeutic maneuvers for management of Huntington's disease with the aim of restoring motor dysfunction symptoms and also by improving overall psychological and physical well-being of affected individuals. Life style modifications, physiotherapy, and occupational therapy when offered to HD patients could further enable them in carrying their day-to-day activities on a regular basis. With careful monitoring and regular follow up, the concerned medical team could very well contribute their level best in assessing HD affected as well as at risk individuals.

The simplest way to conceptualize a psychiatric disorder is a disturbance of cognition (thought), conation (action) or affect (feeling) or any disequilibrium between these three domains.

MENTAL HEALTH

According to the world Health Organization (WHO), health is a state of complete physical, mental and social well being and not mere absence of disease or infirmity. Normal mental health is rather difficult to define and some of the following traits demonstrate normal mental health:

1. Reality orientation
2. Self-awareness and self-knowledge
3. Self-esteem and self-acceptance
4. Ability to exercise voluntary control over their behaviour
5. Ability to form affectionate relationships
6. Pursuance of productive and goal directive activities

Schizophrenia
Mental illness characterized by disruption of thinking ability and emotional sensitivity.

Table 4.2 gives details on parameters involved in mental status examination. Mental disorders may be broadly classified as follows:

→ Organic mental disorders
→ Schizophrenia

Table 4.2 Parameters involved in mental status examination

1. General appearance and behaviour
   General appearance
   Attitude
   Comprehension
   Gait and posture
   Motor activity
   Rapport
2. Speech
   Rate and quantity
   Volume and tone
   Flow and rhythm
3. Thought
   Stream and form
   Content
4. Mood and affect
5. Perception
6. Cognition (Higher mental functions)
   Consciousness
   Orientation
   Attention
   Concentration
   Memory
   Intelligence
   Abstract thinking
7. Insight
8. Judgement

→ Mood disorders

→ Psychotic disorders

→ Stress-related disorders

→ Disorders of adult personality and behaviour

→ Sexual disorders

→ Sleep disorders

Causes of mental disorders include the following:

- Metabolic causes—hypoxia, hypoglycaemia
- Endocrine causes—hormonal imbalances

Psychosis
Psychosis is the disorder/phenomenon describing psychotic action/behavior characterized by hallucinations, delusions and abnormal condition of the mind.

- Drugs—sedatives, alcohol, hypnotics, antipsychotics, anticonvulsants
- Nutritional deficiencies—thiamine, niacin, protein, Vitamin B12, folic acid
- Intracranial causes—epilepsy, head injury, intracranial infections, migraine, stroke
- Environmental—abuse, failure in life, career, stress, sleep deprivation
- Genetic—chromosomal and gene defects

Genetics in mental retardation is detailed in Table 4.3. Mental retardation is observed in the following genetic disorders:

Table 4.3 Genetic disorders associated with mental disorders

1. Chromosomal abnormalities—Down Syndrome, Fragile X Syndrome, Turner Syndrome, Klinefilter's Syndrome

2. Inborn errors of metabolism—Phenylketonuria, Homocystinuria, Tay Sach's disease, Gaucher's disease, Galactosemia, Glycogen storage disorders, Lesch Nyhan Syndrome, Hurler's Syndrome, Hunter's Syndrome

3. Single gene disorders—Neurofibromatosis

4. Cranial anomalies—Microcephaly

Diagnosis

1. Family history
2. General physical examination
3. Detailed neurological examination
4. Mental status examination
5. Investigations

    Routine—urine and blood (inborn errors of metabolism)

    EEG

    Chromosome studies (Down Syndrome)

    CT and MRI of brain

    Thyroid function test
6. Psychological tests

Management options

1. Improvement of socio-economic condition
2. Medical measure
3. Adequate treatment for psychological and behavioural problems
4. Genetic and parent counselling
5. Rehabilitation

SUGGESTED READING

1. Jimenez-Sanchez M, Licitra F, Underwood BR, Rubinsztein DC. Huntington's disease: mechanisms of pathogenesis and therapeutic strategies. Cold Spring Harbor perspectives in medicine. 2017 Jul 1;7(7):a024240.
2. Ferguson MW, Kennedy CJ, Palpagama TH, Waldvogel HJ, Faull RL, Kwakowsky A. Current and possible future therapeutic options for Huntington's disease. Journal of Central Nervous System Disease. 2022 Apr 7;14:11795735221092517.
3. Gil JM, Rego AC. Mechanisms of neurodegeneration in Huntington's disease. European Journal of Neuroscience. 2008 Jun;27(11):2803-20.

REVIEW QUESTION

Essay Questions

1. Explain the various genetic mechanisms involved in the expression of cancer with diagrams in detail.
2. Explain in detail various haemoglobinopathies. Add a note on their genetics.
3. Explain the causes, diagnosis and treatment options of mental disorders in detail. Add a note on the role of genetic disorders in mental illness.
4. Explain in detail about the genetics and pathophysiology of Huntington's disease.

Short Notes

1. Write short notes on the following:
   (a) Cancer genetics
   (b) Oncogenes
   (c) Tumour-suppressor genes
   (d) Chromosomal abnormalities in cancer
   (e) Molecular genetics of colorectal cancer
   (f) Genes that promote vascularization and spread of tumours
   (g) DNA repair genes and cancer
   (h) Telomerase activity and cancer

2. Write short notes on the following:
   (a) Genetic haemochromatosis
   (b) Sickle cell anemia
   (c) Thalassemia
   (d) Molecular mechanisms of Huntington's Disease

3. Write short notes on the following:

   (a) Causes of mental disorders
   (b) Diagnosis and management of mental disorders
   (c) Genetics in mental illness
   (d) Parameters involved in mental status examination

Describe the Role of Nurse in Genetic Services and Counselling

5

CHAPTER OBJECTIVES

Types of Gene Therapy
Classification Based on Type of Therapy
Classification Based on the Method of Therapy
Vectors Used
Non-viral Vector Systems
Special Gene Therapy Strategies
Impact of Genetic Condition on Families
Genetic Counselling

Legal and Ethical Issues
Ethical Issues in Prenatal Diagnosis (Adapted from WHO Guidelines on Ethical Issues in Medical Genetics)
Ethical Issues in Genetic Testing of Children
Privacy of Genetic Information and Its Misuse
Role of a Nurse

Gene therapy
A technique for the treatment of genetic disease in which a gene that is absent or defective is replaced by a functional gene.

TYPES OF GENE THERAPY

There are various types of gene therapy that can be done. This is based on either:

- the type of therapy that is done or
- the mode of therapy (how it is done)

CLASSIFICATION BASED ON TYPE OF THERAPY

There are 2 types of gene therapy done in this case. It includes:

- gene augmentation and
- gene inhibition

Gene augmentation

This technique is usually performed if the diseased gene is recessive. Thus, adding a normal functional gene will cause the expression of only the dominant gene (normal functional) and thus prevents the diseased recessive gene's expression.

Gene inhibition

This technique is usually carried out if the diseased gene is dominant. Therefore adding a normal functional gene will have no counteracting effect. Therefore the diseased gene must be inhibited.

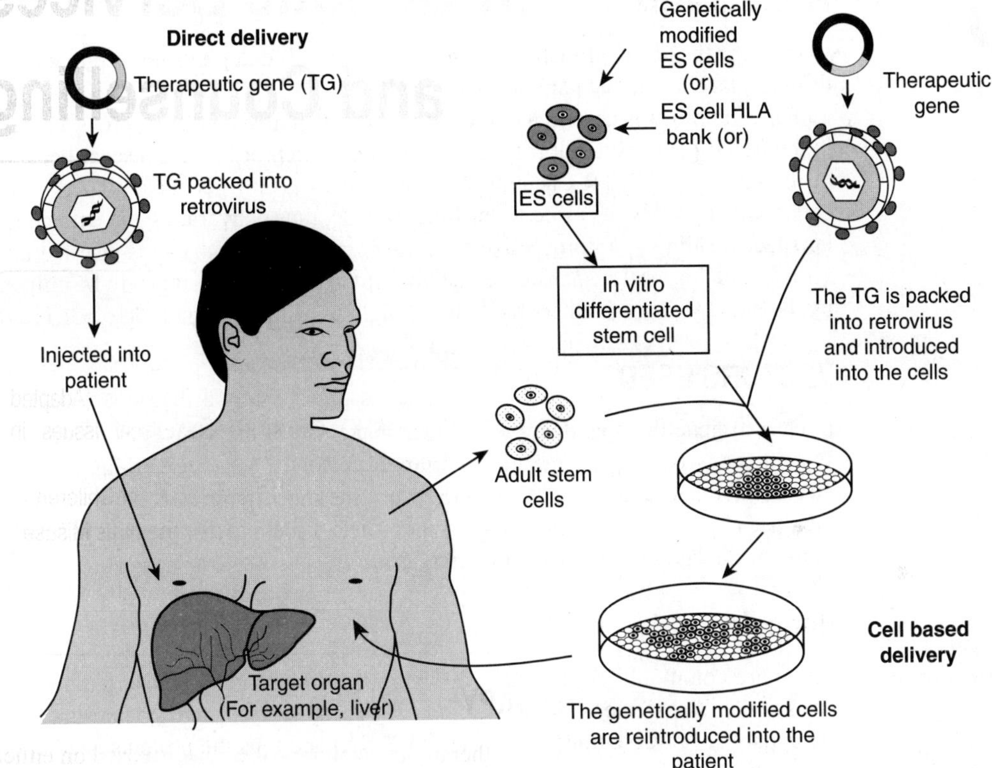

Figure 5.1 Modes of gene therapy. (See page 252 for the colour image.)

CLASSIFICATION BASED ON THE METHOD OF THERAPY

There are 2 types of gene therapy done in this case (Figure 5.1). It includes:

- Ex vivo therapy
- In vivo therapy

Ex vivo therapy

In this case, the target cell (with the diseased gene) is taken outside the body, the desired therapy is carried out and then it is cultured and then inserted back into the body.

Ex vivo
Artificial environment outside the living organism.

For example, it is used in the treatment of familial hypercholesterolemia, where there is accumulation of cholesterol in the body. Hepatocytes that metabolize LDL do not have genes coding for LDL and thus there is no LDL binding because the liver cells do not recognize LDL and so no LDL metabolism occurs. The treatment strategy is to isolate liver cells and insert the gene coding for LDL into these cells by using viruses, culture them and then insert them back into the body so that normal LDL functioning proceeds.

In vivo therapy

In vivo
Occurring within a living organism.

In this case the normal functional gene (for the diseased target gene) is put into the desired place inside the patient's body itself.

For example, it is used in the treatment of cystic fibrosis, where there is a defect in the CFTR gene (cystic fibrosis transmembrane receptor). In this disease because of the absence of CFTR Cl- transport is affected, i.e. they get accumulated in the cell, so the cell absorbs more water from outside, thus dehydrating the extracellular space, leading to a fibrosis like appearance. So the CFTR gene is inserted into viruses and this viral suspension is usually kept in a nasal spray that will be utilized by the patients. Thus it enters the lungs straight and aids in formation of CFTR.

VECTORS USED

In case of gene therapy, many techniques make use of the viruses as a transport system. Thus viruses are the most common vectors. There are various kinds of viruses that can be used in gene therapy, but the most important fact underlying their use is governed by the fact they do not cause disease inside the patient's body. Some of the common viral vectors used are:

Retrovirus

Retrovirus
Group of RNA viruses whose RNA is used as a template inside a host cell for the formation of DNA by means of the enzyme reverse transcriptase.

These are commonly used viruses in which the desired gene is inserted and the virus is then transfected into the desired cell. These viruses are used because they are capable of reverse transcription (RNA DNA) and thus the proteins needed by the host are synthesized by the virus as it synthesizes proteins necessary for its survival and function.

Disadvantage: It has propensity for causing viral infections. To prevent this, the envelope gene has to be removed, the virus must now be cultured in vitro in large amounts after inserting gene of interest and then transfection must be carried out. It is however not 100% effective. Yet another disadvantage of these retroviruses is that they act only on cells that are dividing.

Transfection
Transfer of genetic material isolated from a cell or virus into another cell.

Adenovirus

To overcome the problems faced by using retroviruses, adenoviruses came in to play. The same procedure as above is used. One advantage of adenoviral vectors over retroviral ones is that they act on all cells (dividing or non-dividing).

Disadvantage: They do not integrate with the host genome and thus are lost in the successive generations of cells. Thus recurrent therapy must be given to overcome this. These viruses are not specific to a particular cell type.

Adeno-associated virus

These viruses came into play to overcome the problems faced by adenoviruses. These viruses are found to integrate into chromosome 19 and thus are capable of being passed on from one generation to the next.

Disadvantage: These viruses are also not cell specific and thus certain techniques are performed to overcome this. The most common way in which this is being done is by engineering the envelope gene to have receptors of the target cells so that it can recognize and attach to target cells and enter them.
Example of viral vectors: HSV, common cold virus, HIV.

NON-VIRAL VECTOR SYSTEMS

These are usually physical or chemical methods that can be used in gene therapy to assist in transport of the gene of interest. Some common non-viral vector systems in use are:

Pure DNA construct: In this method the desired gene of interest (the DNA construct) is introduced into the host cells by physical methods such as the use of a biolistic gun, magic bullet, etc. however it has a low efficiency as it does not integrate with the genome and the protein degrades rapidly thus addressing the need for recurrent therapy.

Liposome/Lipoflexes mediated transport: Lipid DNA complexes are used in this case. They are non-toxic and non-immunogenic but have low efficiency and are prone to lysosomal degradation.

Liposome
Synthetically prepared veside composed of lipid bilayer. It is used as a vehicle to deliver nutrients and pharmaceutical drugs.

DNA molecular conjugate: This has been used to overcome the aspect of lysosomal degradation. With this method it is possible to deliver large DNA constructs (>10 kb). The molecule that DNA is conjugated to is usually a polymer like poly-L-lysine which has ligands specific for the target cell. The DNA enters the cell by receptor mediated endocytosis. There are also minimal chances of lysosomal degradation and an increase in efficiency.

HAC: Human Artificial Chromosome. This has a large amount of DNA carrying capacity and also has regulatory sequences for the gene. However since this is a relatively new discover, deliver methods have not yet been identified.

SPECIAL GENE THERAPY STRATEGIES

There are two ways in which this can be done:

TIL: Tumor Infiltrating Lymphocytes. These can be engineered to kill cancer cells. Genes for the TNFa are engineered into TIL and this aids in killing cancer cells.

TNF and neomycin are usually seen together, but neomycin is just used as a selection marker to check for transformation efficiency.

Suicide gene therapy: Thymidine kinase gene is used in this case. It is also called suicide gene. This gene encodes for the TK enzyme that phosphorylates nucleotides and aids in DNA replication. Gancyclovir is a prodrug that is a structural analog to thymidine and gets incorporated into the cell and so TK phosphorylates this and this is not recognized by the DNA pol and thus DNA replication is inhibited.

Antisense gene therapy: This is used in diseases where there is over-expression of proteins. cDNA is converted to cRNA and this cRNA is put into the cells and this has a complementary structure to that of the RNA and binds to it and thus inhibits translation. Or an antisense RNA strand can directly be prepared and used.

Gene therapy may also be classified as follows:

Germline gene therapy
An approach that delivers genes to sperm or egg.

Germline gene therapy: In germline gene therapy, germ cells, i.e., sperms or eggs are the targets. They are modified by inserting functional genes into their genomes. Therefore, the change due to therapy would be heritable and the effect will be passed on to the next generation, thus eliminating the diseased gene from the family. However, germline gene therapy in humans has raised a lot of ethical and legal issues and hence has not progressed towards application.

Somatic gene therapy
Alteration of the genetic makeup of the somatic/ body cells.

Somatic cell gene therapy: In somatic cell gene therapy, the gene is introduced only in somatic cells. Integration of the functional gene into the genome, relieves the patient to a large extent from the disorder however, this change is not heritable as it does not involve the germline. At present, somatic cell therapy is the only feasible option, and clinical trials are in progress.

IMPACT OF GENETIC CONDITION ON FAMILIES

Clinical genetics is concerned with the diagnosis and management of the medical, social, and psychological aspects of hereditary disease. As in all other areas of medicine, it is essential to make a correct diagnosis and to provide appropriate treatment, which must include helping the affected person and family members understand and come to terms with the nature and consequences of the disorder. When a disorder is diagnosed as heritable, there is an added dimension: the need to inform the members of the family about the disorder, emphasize on their risk and means available to modify these risks. The unique feature of genetic disease is its tendency to recur within families and hence counselling has to be focused not only on the original patient but also on members of the family, both present and future. Genetic counselling is therefore concerned not only with informing the patient and family but also with providing psychologically oriented counselling to help individuals adapt and adjust to the impact and implications of the disorder in the family.

The chapter on genetic counselling describes in detail the indications and processes of genetic counselling, while emphasizing on risk assessment and psychological support.

GENETIC COUNSELLING

Genetic counselling is a *communication process* that deals with the human problems associated with the occurrence or risk of occurrence of a genetic disorder in a family. The process aims at helping the individual or the family to:

1. **Understand** the diagnosis, prognosis and available management, the genetic basis and chance of recurrence, and the options available (including genetic testing).

2. **Choose** the course of action appropriate to their personal and family situations.

3. **Adjust** to the psychosocial impact of the genetic condition in the family. (*Adapted from American Society of Human Genetics, 1975*)

Genetic counselling is a new field that provides information to patients and others who are concerned about hereditary conditions. It is also an educational process that helps patients and family members deal with many aspects of a genetic condition. An individual who seeks genetic counseling is known as a **consultand**.

Genetic counselling includes the following:

1. Interpreting a diagnosis of the condition.

2. Providing information about clinical features/symptoms.

3. Diagnostic, carrier, predictive, and presymptomatic testing wherever appropriate.

4. Treatment/management and prognosis.

5. Explaining to the patient and family the mode of inheritance of the genetic condition.

6. Calculating probabilities/risks that family members might transmit/inherit the condition to future generations.

7. Provides information about the reproductive options that are available to those at risk for the disease.

8. Helping the patient and family cope with the psychological anxiety and physical stress that may be associated with their disorder.

Genetic counselling is done by a team of health professionals that includes counsellors, physicians, medical geneticists, therapists, dietician, laboratory personnel, and social workers.

Table 5.1 lists some common indications for genetic counselling, while Table 5.2 depicts the steps involved in genetic counselling.

Table 5.1 Indications for genetic counselling

1. Clinical history of genetic disease in individual/members in the family.
2. History of previous child with a genetic disease, birth defect, or chromosomal abnormality.
3. Previous child with mental retardation or a close relative suffers from mental retardation.
4. Advanced maternal age in women (>30–35 years).
5. Consanguinity (husband and wife are closely related).
6. When a foetal abnormality is detected during pregnancy.
7. Clinical history of spontaneous abortion/infertility.
8. Exposure to potential teratogen (drugs, chemicals, radiation, or other environmental agents that can cause birth defects).
9. Both parents are carriers for a recessive genetic disease.

Genetic counselling usually begins with a diagnosis of the condition. On the bases of a physical examination, biochemical tests, chromosome analysis, family history, and other information, a physician determines the cause of the condition. An accurate diagnosis is critical, because treatment and the probability of passing on the condition may vary, depending on the diagnosis.

For example, there are a number of different types of neurological disorders, which may be caused by chromosome abnormalities, single-gene mutations, hormonal imbalances, or environmental factors. People who have neurological disorders resulting from an autosomal dominant gene (as in Huntington's Chorea) have a 50% chance of passing the condition to their children, whereas people with neurological disorders caused by a rare recessive gene have a low likelihood of passing the trait to their children.

When the nature of the condition is known, a genetic counsellor takes time with the patient and other family members and explains the diagnosis. A family pedigree is constructed, and the probability of transmitting the condition to future generations can be calculated for different family members. The counsellor helps the family interpret the genetic risks and explains various reproductive options that are available, including prenatal diagnosis, artificial insemination, and in vitro fertilization. A family's decision about future pregnancies frequently depends on the magnitude of the genetic risk, the severity and effects of the condition, the importance of having children, and religious and cultural views. The genetic counsellor helps the family sort through these factors and facilitates their decision making.

Throughout the process, a good genetic counsellor uses *non-directed* counselling, which means that he or she provides information and facilitates discussions but does not bring his or her own opinion and values into the discussion. The goal of non-directed counseling is for the family to reach its own decision on the basis of the best available information. Genetic conditions are often perceived differently from other diseases and medical problems, because genetic conditions are intrinsic to the individual person and can be passed on to children.

Table 5.2 Steps involved in genetic counselling

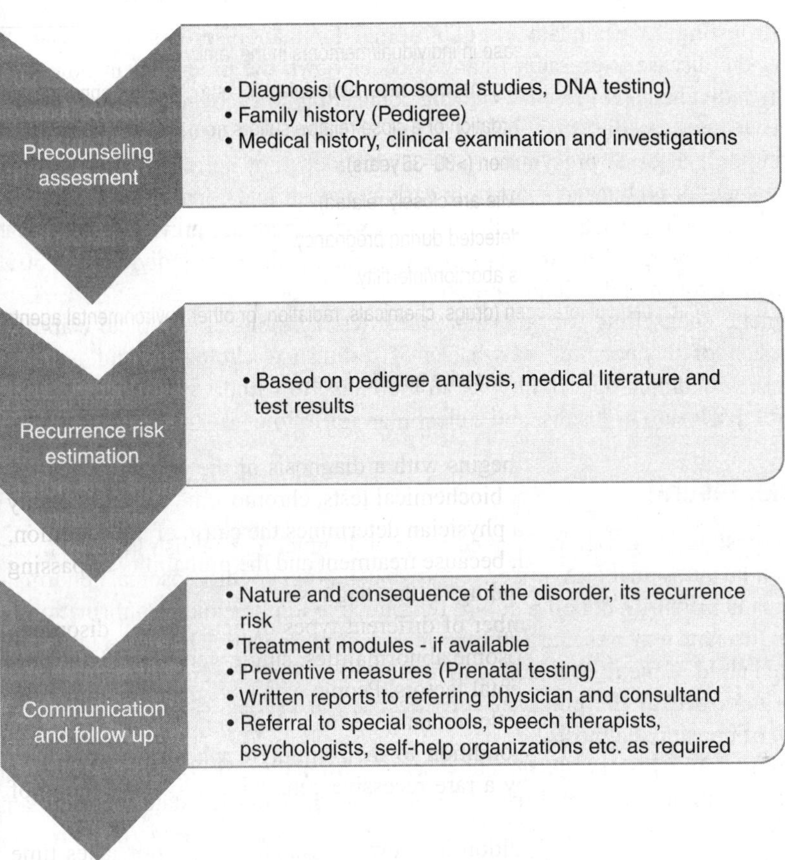

Such perceptions may produce feelings of guilt about past reproductive choices and intense personal dilemmas about future choices. Genetic counsellors are trained to help patients and family members recognize and cope with these feelings.

Genetic services (Counselling and genetic diagnostic testing)

Genetic counselling is an integral part of genetic diagnostic services. It is important as a follow-up service after a diagnostic test result to counsel the individual and the family about the genetic disease expression, mode of inheritance, recurrence risk, and management strategies. Also, genetic counselling is offered to individuals before a genetic test to guide the individual and the family about the undergoing genetic testing process (diagnostic, carrier, or prenatal testing), ensuring informed consent, and addressing issues related to the same.

Presymptomatic testing

Genetic testing in certain late onset autosomal dominant disorders is important to predict the disease expression (many decades down the time line) in otherwise healthy individuals (at present). Genetic counselling to such individuals is important as it helps predict their health status in advance. For conditions, such as Huntington's disease, presymptomatic testing does not currently alter medical management or prognosis (apart from early diagnosis and counselling measures), whereas for others, such as familial breast cancer, there are preventative options available. Presymptomatic testing is most commonly done for individuals at 50% risk of an autosomal dominant condition.

Genetic counselling for presymptomatic testing includes complete elaborate discussion of the potential drawbacks of testing (psychological and financial impact), with ample opportunity for an individual to withdraw from testing right up until disclosure of results, and a clear plan for follow up.

Carrier testing

Carrier testing is advised/performed on an individual to establish his/her carrier state for an autosomal or X-linked recessive condition or chromosomal abnormality. This is primarily done for future reproductive implications. Confirmation of the carrier state may indicate a substantial risk of reproductive loss or of having an affected child. Genetic counselling before carrier testing ensures that the individual is informed of the potential consequences of carrier testing including the option of prenatal diagnosis.

Strong family history of a genetic disease is often directive of carrier testing in individuals (young and mid teens) to establish their carrier status. For certain autosomal recessive diseases, it is best done along with the partner, as reproductive consequences are observed only if both the partners are carriers.

Prenatal testing

Prenatal diagnostic testing has come as a blessing to many couples with high genetic risk to continue their precious pregnancies that would have otherwise been terminated. However, prenatal testing, and the associated option of medical termination of pregnancy (in case of an abnormality detected), most often have an important psychological impact on pregnant women and their partners.

Genetic counselling is ideally offered to couples with a known family history in early pregnancy to give the couple ample time to make a considered choice. In couples without a previous family history but with a positive biochemical screening test result (as in Down syndrome), counselling is provided with benefits/risks associated with invasive prenatal diagnostic tests (like amniocentesis). Condition must be explained, its recurrence risk must be calculated, the details of the test procedure, its associated risks, the accuracy of the test, and the potential consequences of testing including the option of termination of pregnancy must be presented to the couples. This helps them take an informed choice of decision.

Couples at high genetic risk often require ongoing counselling and support during pregnancy. If the consequence of testing leads to termination of a precious pregnancy, follow-up support should be offered. Even if the results are favourable, couples may still have some anxiety until the baby is born and clinical examination in the neonatal period gives reassurance about normality. Constant and continuous psychological support to the couple and family is extremely important in prenatal genetic counselling service, and the reassurance provided by the counsellor and clinician would help an entire family combat stress and anxiety.

LEGAL AND ETHICAL ISSUES

The success of medical and clinical genetics have been accompanied by a parallel growth in the level of concern and anxiety that our knowledge be used judiciously for the benefit and not to the detriment of individuals, their families and society as a whole. With the initiation of the Human Genome Project in the United States, the US congress recognized the ethical dilemmas and the potential for serious societal harm from the misuse of this vastly expanded knowledge of human genetics. The congress responded by mandating that a portion of the US Human Genome Project budget be used to support research and education in the Ethical, Legal, and Social Implications (ELSI) of the project. Similar programs exist in other countries as well. The ELSI effort is designed to study the effect of the knowledge gained by the HGP in many areas, including the practice of medicine and other health care professions, the formulation and administration of public policy, the law and education.

Table 5.3 lists some critical ethical issues in medical genetics.

Table 5.3 Critical ethical issues in medical genetics

Genetic Testing
Prenatal testing for nondisease traits or sex
Testing for genes that predispose to late onset disease
Testing children for a carrier state

Privacy of Genetic Information
Access to an individual's genetic information

Misuse of Genetic Information
Discrimination in employment based on an employee's genotype
Discrimination in Life insurance underwriting
Discrimination in Health insurance underwriting

Genetic Screening
Stigmatization and Privacy

In any discussion of ethical issues in medicine, three cardinal principles are cited: **beneficence** (doing good for the patient), respect for individual **autonomy**

Autonomy (Medical Ethics)
The quality of being independent, free and self-directing.

(safeguarding an individual's rights) and **justice** (ensuring all individuals are treated equally and fairly). Complex ethical issues arise when these cardinal principles are perceived in conflict with one another. The role of ethicists working in interface between society and medical genetics is to weigh and balance conflicting demands. Table 5.4 provides details on the ethical principles in medicine.

Table 5.4 Ethical principles in medicine

Respect for the Autonomy of Persons
Respecting self determination of patients and protecting persons with diminished autonomy;

Beneficence
Highest priority to the welfare of patients and maximizing benefits to their health; also applies to concern for the health of populations;

Non-maleficence
Avoiding harm to patients or, at least, minimizing harm;

Justice
To give persons their due and distribute benefits of medicine fairly in society, according to need.

Non-maleficence (Medical Ethics)
Avoiding the causation of harm.

ETHICAL ISSUES IN PRENATAL DIAGNOSIS (ADAPTED FROM WHO GUIDELINES ON ETHICAL ISSUES IN MEDICAL GENETICS)

Proposed ethical guidelines for the provision of prenatal diagnosis are as follows

1. Equitable distribution of genetics services, including prenatal diagnosis, is owed first to those with the greatest medical need, regardless of ability to pay, or any other considerations (justice).
2. If prenatal diagnosis is medically indicated, it should be available regardless of a couple's stated views on abortion. Prenatal diagnosis may, in some cases, be used to prepare for the birth of a child with a disorder (autonomy).
3. Prenatal diagnosis is done only to give parents and physicians information about the health of the fetus. The use of prenatal diagnosis for paternity testing, except in cases of rape or incest or for gender selection, apart from sex-linked disorders, is not acceptable (non-maleficence).
4. Prenatal diagnosis should be voluntary in nature. The prospective parents should decide whether a particular genetic disorder warrants prenatal diagnosis or termination of a pregnancy with an affected fetus, rather than the doctor or the government (autonomy).
5. Prenatal diagnosis solely for relief of maternal anxiety, in the absence of medical indications, should have lower priority in allocation of resources than prenatal diagnosis with medical indications (justice).

6. Counseling should precede prenatal diagnosis (non-maleficence).

7. Physicians should disclose all clinically relevant findings to the pregnant woman or couple (autonomy).

8. The woman and/or couple's choices in an affected pregnancy should be respected and protected, within the framework of the law and culture of the nation. The couple, not the professional or the government, should make the choice (autonomy).

ETHICAL ISSUES IN GENETIC TESTING OF CHILDREN

Additional ethical problems arise when genetic testing involves children. As with adults, testing children for carrier status or presymptomatic testing could be beneficial when interventions that decrease morbidity and increase longevity are available. Testing in children however carries the risks of serious psychological damage, stigmatization, insurance and employment discrimination. Considering the principle of autonomy, their decision about their genetic constitution must be balanced with discussion with parents to help them to be prepared for a future possibility of the child developing the disease.

The preponderance of opinion among bioethicists is that unless there is a clear benefit to the child, testing for a late onset disease or for the carrier state should be done only when the child is old and mature enough to decide whether to seek such a testing.

PRIVACY OF GENETIC INFORMATION AND ITS MISUSE

The third main principle is justice i.e. everyone must be able to benefit equally from the progress in medical genetics. Employers and Insurance companies will definitely discriminate individuals based on their genetic composition. Premiums will be calculated in such a way that, those of them who have an abnormal genetic constitution will stand no gain on comparison with a normal person. Employers may show differences in hiring individuals with known genetic information which may help them choose healthy individuals and in turn low absenteeism and better performance and more profit. However these function much against the principle of justice. Medical genetics has a profound effect beyond the narrow impact those confines to medical practice. Integrating this knowledge into public policy will require coordinated efforts of the government, business and the public.

ROLE OF A NURSE

Nurses have a unique potential to contribute to the effective delivery of genetic services:

1. First, they are the single largest group of healthcare providers.
2. Second, they are employed in settings throughout the healthcare system.
3. Third, nurses are accustomed to providing and promoting a broad range of health and related services for individuals and the families they serve.

"Nursing, as an applied science, cannot afford to lag behind current scientific knowledge when that knowledge can enhance and enrich the care of patients and their families. Inclusion in the nursing curriculum of genetic theory and principles is but one small advance in expanding the dimensions of nursing practice through increased knowledge and understanding."—Brantl and Esslinger (1962).

Nursing educators took efforts to integrate genetics as a part of their curriculum to help nursing students acquire necessary knowledge. The undergraduate curriculum for nurses includes formal course work in the biological, physical, and social sciences. Concepts learned in basic sciences are expected to be carried into the clinical situation, where they are further reinforced by additional didactic content and practical experience. During the clinical sequence, nurses must develop skills in eliciting and interpreting information, providing support, counselling, and teaching, in addition to acquiring technical skills.

REVIEW QUESTIONS

Essay Question

1. Explain in brief the importance of understanding genetics in nursing and the role of a nurse in this perspective.
2. Explain in detail with diagrams the difference between prokaryotic and eukaryotic cell.
3. Explain the recent advances in gene therapy as a treatment option for genetic disorders. Classify gene therapy based on the mode of therapy. Explain with examples.
4. Define genetic counselling. Explain the indications of genetic counselling in detail.
5. Describe the different steps involved in genetic counselling.
6. Explain the importance of genetic counselling as a genetic service.
7. Explain the legal and ethical issues in medical genetics in detail.

Short Notes

1. Write short notes on the following:
   (a) Ex vivo therapy
   (b) In vivo therapy
   (c) Vectors used in gene therapy
   (d) Gene therapy in cancer
   (e) Somatic and germline gene therapy
   (f) Gene augmentation and gene inhibition

2. Write short notes on the following:
   (a) Ethical principles in medicine
   (b) Ethical issues in medical genetics
   (c) Ethics in prenatal diagnosis

Annexure 1

CULTURE OF HUMAN AMNIOCYTES FOR CYTOGENETIC ANALYSIS

Aim: To set up an **amniotic fluid culture by long term method**. This process is applicable for clinical services and to help in genetic counseling.

Principle: Amniotic fluid represents a heterogeneous population of fetal cells and the chromosomal analysis of the cultured cells can be used to rule out any structural and/or numerical chromosomal anomalies.

Sample Type:

- Collect approximately 20 ml of amniotic fluid in sterile sample containers.
- Process all samples on the same day if possible. If processing is done at a later date, samples can be stored at room temperature for 24 hrs.
- Do not use contaminated samples or samples received in wrong containers.

Equipment and Reagents

Equipments

- Laminar Hood
- Incubator (CO_2, water jacketed incubator)
- Centrifuge.

Reagents

- Amniomax Complete medium
- Colcemid
- Trypsin-EDTA
- Hypotonic solution (0.075 M potassium chloride: 1% Sodium citrate in the ratio of 6:4).

- Carnoy's fixative (Methanol and glacial acetic acid prepared in the ratio of 3:1).
- 25 cm^2 tissue culture radiation sterilized flasks
- Centrifuge tubes.
- Disposable pipettes / Micropipettes
- Disposable syringes / micro tips

Procedure

(i) Culture set up

- In a sterile hood, dispense amniotic fluid equally into pre-labeled centrifuge tubes.
- Centrifuge at 800–1000 rpm for 10 minutes.
- While the tube(s) are spinning, prepare the 25cm^2 tissue culture flask. Label.
- After centrifugation, remove the supernatant aseptically and re-suspend the cells in 10 ml Amniomax.
- Transfer 5 ml cell suspension into the pre-labeled flasks.
- Leave the flasks undisturbed in a CO_2 incubator for 5–7 days. Incubators are set for 37°C and 5% CO_2.
- After 5–7 days, examine the cultures under the inverted microscope. If small colonies have developed, remove the medium and feed with 4 ml Amniomax.
- If there are only single cell attachments seen under the microscope, then wait for 1–2 days before feeding.
- Feed the flasks once in 2–3 days until ready for harvest.
- Primary cultures are usually harvested after 10–12 days.

(ii) Prior to Harvesting

- Add 50–100 µl of colcemid and incubate at 37°C for 60 minutes.
- Pre-warm the hypotonic solution at 37°C.
- Pre-chill freshly prepared Carnoys fixative and store at 4°C.
- Pre-warm the trypsin-EDTA 1X at 37°C.

(iii) Harvesting

- Remove the medium from the flask and place it in the centrifuge tube.
- Rinse the flask with 1 ml of the pre-warmed trypsin-EDTA 1X solution and add wash to the corresponding centrifuge tube.
- Add another 4 ml of trypsin-EDTA 1X solution and leave the flask in the incubator for 5–7 minutes.

- At the end of 5 minutes, remove the flask and tap the bottom gently. Leave the flask in the incubator till the completion of the 7 minutes.
- Check to see if the cells have lifted. If the cells are still attached, leave in the incubator a little longer.
- When the cells have detached, aspirate gently and add suspension to the centrifuge tube and gently break the cell pellet by tapping the tube with fingers.
- Centrifuge at 800–1000 rpm for 10 minutes.
- Add 10 ml of pre-warmed hypotonic solution. Mix well and gently with a clean pasteur pipette.
- Incubate at 37°C for 20 minutes.
- Add 2 ml of pre-chilled fixative and mix gently by inverting the tube.
- Centrifuge at 800–1000 rpm for 10 minutes
- After centrifuging, decant the supernatant and re-suspend cells by gently tapping the tube.
- Add 5 ml of pre-chilled fixative drop by drop while vortexing.
- Keep at room temperature for 20 minutes.
- Centrifuge at 800–1000 rpm for 10 minutes
- Decant supernatant. Add 5 ml of fresh fixative. Refrigerate at 4°C overnight.

(iv) Slide preparation and GTG banding

- Prepare slides by dropping an appropriately concentrated suspension from an appropriate height onto clean, pre-chilled slides using a pasteur pipette.
- Place it on a hot plate, maintained at a temp of 45–50°C, till it dries.
- Remove the slide and view under a phase contrast microscope
- Age slides overnight at 60°C and perform GTG
- 25 metaphases analysed for numerical and/or structural anomalies.

CULTURE OF HUMAN CHORIONIC VILLI FOR CYTOGENETIC ANALYSIS

Aim: Chorionic villus sampling is usually performed to detect fetal chromosomal abnormalities between 11 and 13 weeks of pregnancy. This process is applicable to patients in order to help them with genetic counseling.

Principle: Chorionic villus sampling (CVS) is a prenatal test that involves taking a tiny tissue sample from outside the sac where the fetus develops. The tissue is tested to diagnose or rule out certain birth defects. The test generally is performed between 10 to 13 weeks after a woman's last menstrual period. CVS may be offered when there is an increased risk of chromosomal or genetic birth defects.

Required Equipment and Reagents

Equipments

- Laminar Hood
- Incubator (CO_2 water jacketed incubator)
- Centrifuge

Required reagents and consumables

- 25 cm^2 radiation sterilized tissue culture flasks
- 15 ml Centrifuge tubes
- Sterile pipettes
- Amniomax complete medium
- Colcemid
- Trypsin-EDTA
- Hypotonic solution (0.075 M potassium chloride: 1% Sodium citrate in the ratio of 6:4)
- Carnoy's fixative (Methanol and glacial acetic acid prepared in the ratio of 3:1).

Procedure

(i) Culture set up

- Clean the CVS sample in a sterile hood and tease in buffer.
- Label two 25 cm^2 tissue culture flasks
- Wash the sample well with medium
- Transfer a few villi to a sterile petridish.
- Using a sterile surgical blade, chop the villi till sufficiently dissociated.
- Add 8 ml amniomax to the petriplate. Mix well and gently.
- Transfer 4 ml of the cell suspension aseptically to two pre-labeled flasks.
- Leave the flask undisturbed in a CO_2 incubator for 5–7 days. Incubators are set for 37°C and 5% CO_2.
- After 5–7 days, examine the cultures under the inverted microscope. If small colonies have developed, remove the medium and feed with 4 ml of amniomax.
- If there are only single cell attachments seen under the microscope, then wait for 1–2 days before feeding.
- Feed the flasks once in 2–3 days until it is ready for harvest.
- Primary cultures are usually harvested after 10–12 days.

(ii) Prior to Harvesting

- Add 50–100 µl of colcemid and incubate at 37°C for 60 min.
- Pre-warm the hypotonic solution at 37°C and pre-chill freshly prepared Carnoy's fixative at 4°C.
- Pre-warm trypsin-EDTA 1X at 37°C

(iii) Harvesting

- Remove the medium from the flask and place it in the centrifuge tube.
- Rinse the flask with 1 ml of the pre-warmed trypsin-EDTA 1X solution and add wash to the corresponding centrifuge tube
- Add another 4 ml of trypsin-EDTA 1X solution and leave the flask in the incubator for 5–7 minutes
- At the end of 6 minutes, remove the flask and tap the bottom gently. Leave the flask in the incubator till completion of the 7 minutes.
- Check to see if the cells have lifted. If the cells are still attached, leave in the incubator a little longer.
- When the cells have detached, aspirate gently and add suspension to the centrifuge tube. Gently break the cell pellet by tapping against the tube with fingers
- Centrifuge at 800–1000 RPM for 10 min.
- Add 10 ml of pre-warmed hypotonic solution and mix well.
- Incubate at 37°C for 20 minutes.
- Add 2 ml of pre-chilled fixative and mix gently by inverting the tube.
- Centrifuge at 800–1000 rpm for 10 min
- After centrifugation, decant the supernatant and re-suspend cells by gently tapping the tube.
- Add 5 ml of pre-chilled fixative drop by drop while vortexing.
- Keep at room temperature for 20 min.
- Centrifuge at 800–1000 rpm for 10 min
- Decant supernatant and add 5 ml fresh fixative. Refrigerate at 4°C overnight.

(iv) Slide preparation and GTG banding

- Before slide preparation the fixative wash is repeated.
- Prepare slides by dropping an appropriately concentrated suspension from an appropriate height onto clean, pre-chilled slides using a pasteur pipette.
- Place it on a hot plate, maintained at a temp of 45–50°C, till dry.
- Remove the slide and view under a phase contrast microscope.
- Age slides overnight at 60°C and perform GTG banding
- 25 metaphases analysed for numerical and/or structural anomalies.

CULTURE OF HUMAN CORD BLOOD FOR CYTOGENETIC ANALYSIS

Aim: To set up a 72 hr cord blood culture. This process is applicable for clinical services and to help in genetic counseling.

Principle: Cord blood is collected for the study of constitutional chromosome abnormalities. The sample is collected in heparinized vacutainer. The lymphocytes are stimulated to enter cell cycle using phytohemagglutinin (PHA) for 72 hours and arrested at metaphase using colchicine. The metaphase chromosomes are banded and analysed to identify the constitutional chromosome abnormalities.

Equipment and Reagents

Equipments

- Laminar Hood
- Incubator (CO_2 water jacketed incubator)
- Centrifuge

Reagents

- RPMI – 1640
- Foetal Bovine Serum (FBS
- Phytohaemagglutinin (PHA)
- Ethidium bromide (EtBr) stock concentration 1 mg/ml
- Colchicine Himedia stock concentration 1 mg/ml
- Hypotonic solution Potassium chloride 0.075 M
- Carnoy's fixative (Methanol: Glacial acetic acid in the ratio of 3:1).
- Micropipettes / Disposable pipettes
- Microtips / disposable syringe
- T_{25} Tissue culture flasks
- Centrifuge tubes (15 ml)

Procedure

(i) Culture set up

- Label the culture flasks date and time of culture initiation i.e. time of PHA addition.
- Add 8 ml RPMI medium, 2 ml FBS and 400 µl PHA to the pre-labeled culture flask followed by 1 ml blood sample and mix well.
- Incubate at 37°C for 66½ in 5% CO_2 incubator.

(ii) Prior to Harvesting

- Add 100 µl of Etbr at the 66½ and incubate at 37°C for 30 minutes.
- Add 100 µl of colchicine and incubate at 37°C for 60 minutes.
- Pre-warm the potassium chloride solution at 37°C and pre-chill freshly prepared Carnoys fixative at 4°C.

(iii) Harvesting

- Transfer the contents of the culture flask to a clean 15 ml centrifuge tube and label appropriately.
- Centrifuge at 800–1000 rpm for 10 minutes.
- Add 10 ml of pre-warmed hypotonic solution and incubate at 37°C for 20 minutes.
- Add 2 ml of pre-chilled fixative to the cell suspension and mix well.
- Centrifuge at 800–1000 rpm for 10 minutes. Remove supernatant.
- Add 8 ml of pre-chilled fixative to the cell pellet while vortexing.
- Incubate at room temperature for 20 minutes.
- Centrifuge at 800–1000 rpm for 10 minutes. Remove supernatant
- Add 10 ml of fixative and keep at 4°C for 2 hours or until slide preparation.

(iv) Slide preparation and GTG banding

- Prepare slides by dropping an appropriately concentrated suspension from an appropriate height onto clean, pre-chilled slides using a pasteur pipette.
- Place it on a hot plate, maintained at a temperature of 45–50°C, till it dries.
- Remove the slide and view under a phase contrast microscope
- Slides aged overnight at 60°Care banded by GTG banding

Calculating results

25 metaphases are scored for numerical and/or structural anomalies, at least 10 from each of two cultures. The analysis is increased to 50 metaphases in case of abnormality or mosaicism.

CULTURE OF HUMAN PERIPHERAL BLOOD FOR CYTOGENETIC ANALYSIS

Aim: To set up a peripheral blood lymphocyte (PBL) culture by 72-hour culture. This process is applicable for clinical services, for the patients and to help them in genetic counseling.

Principle: Peripheral blood is collected for the study of constitutional chromosome abnormalities. The sample is collected in a heparinized container. The lymphocytes are stimulated to enter the cell cycle using phytohemagglutinin (PHA) for 72 hours and arrested at metaphase using colchicine. The metaphase chromosomes are banded and analysed to identify constitutional chromosome abnormalities.

Required equipment and reagents

Equipments

- Laminar Hood
- Incubator (CO_2 water jacketed incubator)
- Centrifuge

Reagents and consumables

- Disposable pipettes / Micropipettes
- Disposable syringes / micro tips
- 25 cm^2 radiation sterilized culture flasks
- RPMI-1640
- Foetal Bovine Serum (FBS)
- Phytohaemagglutinin (PHA)
- Ethidium bromide (EtBr) stock concentration 1 mg/ml
- Colchicine Himedia stock concentration 1 mg/ml
- Hypotonic solution - Potassium chloride - 0.075 M
- Carnoy's fixative (Methanol and glacial acetic acid prepared in the ratio of 3:1).

Procedure steps

(i) Culture set up

- Label the culture flasks date and time of culture initiation i.e. time of PHA addition.
- Add 8 ml RPMI medium, 2 ml FBS and 500 µl PHA to the pre-labeled culture flask followed by 1 ml blood sample and mix well.
- Incubate at 37°C for 66½ in 5% CO_2 incubator.

(ii) Prior to Harvesting

- Add 100 µl of Etbr at the 66½ and incubate at 37°C for 30 minutes.
- Add 100 µl of colchicine and incubate at 37°C for 60 minutes.
- Pre-warm the potassium chloride solution at 37°C and pre-chill freshly prepared Carnoy's fixative at 4°C.

(iii) Harvesting

- Transfer the contents of the culture flask to a clean 15 ml centrifuge tube and label appropriately.
- Centrifuge at 800–1000 rpm for 10 minutes.
- Add 10 ml of pre-warmed hypotonic solution and incubate at 37°C for 20 minutes.
- Centrifuge at 800–1000 rpm for 10 minutes. Remove supernatant.
- Add 8 ml of pre-chilled fixative to the cell pellet while vortexing.
- Incubate at room temperature for 20 minutes.
- Centrifuge at 800–1000 rpm for 10 minutes. Remove supernatant
- Add 10 ml of fixative and keep at 4°C for 2 hours or until slide preparation.

(iv) Slide preparation and GTG banding

- Prepare slides by dropping an appropriately concentrated suspension from an appropriate height onto clean, pre-chilled slides using a pasteur pipette.
- Place it on a hot plate, maintained at a temperature of 45–50°C, till it dries.
- Remove the slide and view under a phase contrast microscope
- Slides aged overnight at 60°Care banded by GTG banding.

Karyotyping: 25 metaphases analysed for numerical and/or structural anomalies. 25 metaphases are scored for numerical and/or structural anomalies. The analysis is increased to 50 metaphases in case of abnormality or mosaicism.

GIEMSA STAINING

Aim: To stain metaphase chromosomes with Giemsa stain and trypsin to elicit a banding pattern throughout the chromosome arms designated as G-Banding. It is used for studying cytogenetic abnormalities.

Principle: Giemsa banding (G-Banding) is the most commonly used technique for the routine staining of mammalian chromosomes. The structural and functional composition of chromosomes leads to the differential banding patterns. The slides are treated with a protease (Trypsin) enzyme and stained with Giemsa. Dark bands contain A-T rich DNA, replicate their DNA late in S-phase and appear to contain relatively few active genes. They may also differ from light bands in terms of protein composition. Differential extraction of protein during fixation and banding pre-treatments from different regions of the chromosome may be important in the mechanism by which G-bands are obtained.

Equipments

Equipments

- Microscope with 100× oil immersion magnification.
- Coplin jars
- Stop watch
- Measuring cylinders

Reagents and consumables

- Giemsa stain stock
- Giemsa working solution (50 ml): 5 ml of Giemsa stock dissolved in 45 ml of distilled water.
- Trypsin from bovine: 5 mg of trypsin dissolved in 50 ml of pre-warmed phosphate buffer saline.
- Phosphate buffer saline (PBS) 1× solution prepared using commercially available 10× PBS stock. Distilled water.

Procedure Steps

- Prepare aged slides for the respective cultured sample.
- Prepare the solutions in coplin jars separately and keep at 37°C (jar 1: trypsin solution, jars 2 and 3: PBS, jar 4: Giemsa working solution, jars 5 and 6– distilled water).
- Treat the slides for 10–20 seconds by slowly agitating in trypsin solution kept at 37°C.
- Rinse the slides in two series of PBS.
- Stain the slides in Giemsa working solution for 3–5 minutes.
- Rinse the slides in two series of distilled water and air-dry.
- Mount the slides and use for analysis.

Note: If the chromosomes appear fuzzy, insufficient aging of slides is the most likely explanation. Over-trypsinized chromosomes appear fat and pale while under trypsinized chromosomes are dark with poor distinction between light and dark bands. If the chromosomes appear pale and blue in colour, check the pH. Chromosomes, which appear to be stained too darkly, can often be improved simply by rinsing the slide in distilled water.

The time and concentration of trypsin treatment is very critical as it determine the morphology and banding pattern of the chromosomes. If the temperature of trypsin and pH of the stain is changed the test will not produce the desired results.

REFERENCES

The AGT Cytogenetics Laboratory Manual Third Edition. M. J. Barch, T. Knutsen, J. L. Spurbeck (eds). pp 217–218. Lippincott-Raven Publishers.

Human Chromosomes – Principles and Techniques. Second Edition (1995), Verma, R. S and Arvind Babu (eds), pp – 16–72. McGraw-Hill, Inc.

ISCN (2013): An International System for Human Cytogenetic Nomenclature. L.G. Shaffer, Jean McGowan-Jordan, M. Schmid (eds); S. Karger publishing. (2013)

Annexure 2: Rare Genetic Disorders

XERODERMA PIGMENTOSUM

Xeroderma pigmentosum (XP), more commonly referred as dry pigmented skin condition, is a rare hereditary disorder inherited in an autosomal recessive pattern that predominantly sensitizes the affected individual to develop skin related infections on exposure to sunlight, along with higher susceptibility to developing skin cancer. Mostly in around 60% of total cases, XP affected individuals have an exaggerated response to developing sunburns with blisters, persistent erythema, and sunlight-induced ocular abnormalities depending upon the period of exposure to sunlight. In the remaining 40% of cases, patients experience varying degrees of neurological dysfunction (acquired microcephaly, progressive sensorineural hearing loss, cognitive impairment and ataxia) with no sunburn reaction. However, this minor category of patients will have increased number of lentigines – freckle like pigmentations on sun-exposed regions predominantly on their nose, zygoma and forehead of the face as well as on sides of the neck.

The prevalence of XP varies across different regions of the world wherein, in Japan the prevalence of XP is estimated at 1:22,000 and around 1:1,000,000 in the US. In communities where consanguineous marriages and endogamy are quite common, the prevalence of XP is as high as 1:10,000, particularly in countries of the Middle East, North Africa. The genetic basis for developing XP arises from mutations in products of eight genes corresponding to eight XP complementation groups that are involved in DNA repair pathways. Components XP (A to G) are involved in repair of UV-induced DNA damage, whereas XPV (DNA polymerase η) is involved in replication of DNA containing unrepaired damage.

Diagnosis of XP has its own challenges and limitations since there are certain other genetic disorders that have common features as that of this skin disease. As a first line of choice, clinical findings of the patient such as acute sun sensitivity, sunlight induced eye damages, and development of skin neoplasms such as basal cell carcinoma, melanoma, squamous cell carcinoma potentially signify criteria for XP diagnosis. Genetic diagnostic test are performed after establishing clinical findings and gathering family history. Generally, molecular genetic testing involves combination of multigene panel i.e. gene-targeted testing and comprehensive genomic testing – exome sequencing and genome sequencing.

Identifying biallelic pathogenic variants in one of the following genes namely *DDB2, POLH, XPA, XPC, ERCC1, ERCC2, ERCC3, ERCC4, ERCC5*, marks the confirmatory molecular diagnosis of XP. Apart from molecular genetic testing, the most commonly used test includes the measurement of unscheduled DNA synthesis (UDS) in cultured skin fibroblasts. This test is performed by taking tissue biopsy from unexposed areas of the skin (e.g. inner arms). The fibroblasts present in the skin biopsy sample are then UV-irradiated in a petri dish, and the level of UDS is measured with the help of either autoradiography, liquid scintillation counting or by fluorescent assays. Reduced levels of UDS confirm the diagnosis of XP disease. For individuals who have XP-V disease condition, the above mechanism of culturing protocol may not be suitable, because nucleotide excision repair pathway (NER) is not affected. Rather, cultured fibroblasts of XP-V cells are first exposed to UV then they are incubated in caffeine for few days. Later, these cells viability are then compared to normal cells. Specific sensitivity towards UV irradiation in the caffeine component's presence along with normal UDS, thus confirms XP-V diagnosis. For antenatal diagnosis, DNA mutation analysis can be performed either in amniocytes or chorionic villus (CVS) cells.

Treatment strategies for XP patients include management of skin lesions and removal of cancerous lesions depending upon the type of skin ailment caused. Premalignant skin lesions like actinic keratosis can be treated by freezing them with liquid nitrogen; much larger areas of the affected skin can be treated with topical applications of 5-fluorouracil or imiquimod products. Skin cancer lesions that are more recurrent or those that are present in locations that have high recurrence can be treated with Mohs micrographic surgery. Oral isotretinoin or acitretin can be used to prevent formation of new skin neoplasms but can cause other side effects. Eye abnormalities can be treated surgically, whereas corneal injury coupled with eyelid abnormality can be ameliorated with usage of eye drops or soft contact lenses. Hearing loss may be managed with hearing aids.

THROMBOPHILIA

Thrombophilia is a type of blood disorder that can either be acquired or inherited during the course of one's life, where, the affected individuals develop a hypercoagulable condition. The disorder renders the patient's blood to develop severe clots (thrombosis) more readily in both of the major blood vessels – arteries and veins. There was a remarkable discovery made by the scientist Rudolf Virchow in the year 1856, where he proposed and postulated a hypothesis by explaining the etiology of pulmonary embolism (PE) which further lead to deciphering the three primal causes of arterial and venous thrombosis – stasis, injury to the blood vessel wall and abnormalities in circulating blood. The predisposition to form inappropriate blood clots within the blood vessels can arise from several factors such as genetic, acquired alterations in blood coagulation mechanism and also by the extensive interactions between genetic and acquired factors. Thrombotic events are identified to be an inevitable source of morbidity and mortality in patients. It is therefore crucial to accurately diagnose, analyse and employ appropriate therapeutic interventions at the earliest, to prevent the affected individuals from facing such end stage crisis.

Thrombophilia is broadly categorised as acquired and hereditary forms of disease based on the causative mechanisms of disease pathogenesis. Acquired thrombophilia is generally caused because of acquired disorders of the homeostasis system. These acquired forms of thrombotic disorders can promote prothrombotic states in patients through elevation of procoagulant factors, decreased anticoagulants, pro-inflammatory/autoimmune mechanisms, and multiple alterations in the blood coagulation homeostasis mechanisms. Some of the disorders that are associated with acquired forms of thrombophilia include antiphospholipid antibody syndrome, transiently/permanently enhanced levels of procoagulant factors, hyperomocisteinaemia and decreased levels of natural anticoagulants. On the other hand, inherited (hereditary) forms of thrombophilia have genetic predisposition behind the disease pathogenesis. Inherited forms of thrombophilia have the propensity to induce more fatal life-threating conditions such as the development of venous thromboembolism (VTE). Of all causes, the factor V Leiden and mutations in the prothrombin gene G20210A, accounts for nearly 50–70% majority of inherited thrombophilia disorders. The remaining less frequent however those that have more severe defects include defects in the antithrombin (AT), protein S (PS), and protein C (PC). In the recent times, several other novel genetic defects for this disease development have been identified namely pseudo-homozygosity for activated protein C (APC) resistance, resistance to AT and the hyperfunctional factor IX Padua. Lastly, the ABO blood grouping is the most common genetic risk factor for developing VTE in thrombophilia patients. Individuals who have inherited thrombophilia are particularly more prone to develop acute PE, especially amongst younger population. Another intriguing component of this blood disorder condition is that, thrombophilic disorders are further categorized based on its coagulation abnormality with loss-of-function and the other with gain-of-function.

Clinical evaluation of thrombophilic disorder involves a series of screening and confirmed diagnostic tests and that has to be implemented with appropriate measures. Global thrombophilia diagnosis is recommended in all patients who have indication of thromboembolism whereas the disease-specific laboratory diagnostic testing is recommended only in certain specific cases. Inherited thrombophilia screening is advised for neonates and adolescents who have VTE. This condition is more likely in children who develop sepsis, dehydration, has any underlying congenital heart diseases, and congenital anomalies in the inferior vena cava of the heart. Thrombophilia screening is highly recommended for neonates who have purpura fulminans, skin necrosis or idiopathic VTE, and also in adolescents who have idiopathic VTE. In adults, thrombophilia screening is essential if the patients are presented with VTE. Basic laboratory tests that are required for initial examination of thromboembolism includes coagulation profile involving the estimation of Prothrombin time (PT), activated partial thromboplastin time (aPTT), D-Dimer, and fibrinogen functional assays. In addition to this, evaluation of factor VIII level, lupus anticoagulants, anti-cardiolipin, anti-β2 glycoprotein I antibodies are also necessary. Genetic screening and diagnosis is recommended when any of the following conditions are observed in the patients such as patients who have VTE before 40 years of age, VTE at a younger age (ideally less than 50) with weaker risk factor, presence of VTE in unusual sites and positive family history of having VTE in two generations. Commonly, genetic testing for thrombophilia includes testing factor V Leiden (FVL), genetic mutations in the prothrombin gene (*PGM*) and mutation analysis in the methylenetetrahydrofolate reductase (*MTHFR*) gene by using PCR-based methods.

Treatment strategy for management of thrombophilia relies on the usage of anticoagulant therapy as it aids in prevention of thrombosis rather than clearing the thrombotic clots that are already formed within the patient's vasculature. The standard care of therapy for patients with acute VTE comprises of unfractionated or low-molecular-weight heparin and anticoagulation therapy with either warfarin or other vitamin K antagonists. Warfarin is required and can be started the first 24 hours and then low-molecular-weight heparin (LMWH) is started and the dosage can be maintained for 5 days till the desirable levels of PT is achieved within the range of 2.0–3.0 in International Normalized Ratio (INR). Special and cautious precautionary managements are required for patients who have antithrombin deficiency or inherited protein C deficiency.

RETT SYNDROME

Rett syndrome (RTT) is a rare progressive neurodegenerative disorder that predominantly affects 1 in 10,000 of the female population, and a much less fraction of males. This syndrome belongs to MECP2-related phenotypes where it is further categorized as classic and variant Rett syndrome. Girls who are affected by classic form of Rett syndrome tend to have normal psychomotor development during the first 6 to 18 months of age, beyond which the child will undergo developmental stagnation along with rapid decline in language and motor skills function. The developing child is characterized with repetitive stereotypic hand movements particularly during the rapid phase of regression. Additionally, symptoms such as autistic features, fits of screaming and uncontrolled crying, bruxism, gait ataxia, apraxia, tremors, seizures, acquired microcephaly are relatively common. In affected males, the most common identifiable characteristic is severe neonatal-onset encephalopathy which is followed by progression of involuntary moments, abnormal tone, breathing difficulties and seizures. Most of the Rett syndrome affected male children do not survive beyond 2 years of age.

Nearly 95% of the classic RTT disease is caused because of mutations in the *MECP2* gene and are *de novo* in nature that mostly occurs in paternal germline. Loss-of-function mutations in the *MECP2* gene results in inappropriate expression of genes that are involved in the brain development. The severity of this disease condition varies in each of the affected female because of the effects of random X inactivation. In mildly affected females, a large proportion of the X chromosome that bears the mutated gene has been found to be randomly inactivated. RTT syndrome follows X-linked dominant pattern of inheritance.

The diagnosis of RTT is achieved through molecular genetic testing in a female proband who has suggestive clinical findings and a heterozygous *MECP2* pathogenic variant. In a male proband, the diagnosis is established by evaluation of clinical suggestive findings, and a hemizygous pathogenic variant in the MECP2 gene. There is no cure for this disease; however the patient's symptoms can be well managed by using appropriate medications for relieving various signs and symptoms along with special emphasis on providing psychosocial support including the family members. Risperidone might be of usage in ameliorating agitation and melatonin is used to mitigate sleep disturbances.

RETINOBLASTOMA

Retinoblastoma is a condition that results in formation of malignant tumors along the retinal region of the eye during its developmental stage in children below five years of age. The disease is caused in nearly 1 in 20,000 children worldwide. The tumor formation usually begins 12 weeks after conception and at 4 years wherein the retinal cells are actively dividing and proliferating. Approximately 60% of the cases are caused because of somatic mutations in the *RB1* gene that are not heritable in nature. Non-hereditary forms of this disease affect both the alleles of the gene. The remaining 40% of the cases are caused because of germline hereditary mutations in one of the allele of the *RB1* gene and thus it is identified to be inherited in autosomal dominant pattern. An intriguing feature in the hereditary forms of the disease is that around 30% of its total cases are caused because of *de novo* mutations which are mostly transmitted to the progeny through paternal lineage. The other 10% of hereditary cases are transmitted to the progeny from either of the parent who tends to carry the retinoblastoma mutation in all of his/her cells. Apart from these, there are nearly 10% of inherited cases wherein the proband doesn't develop the disease although they carry the disease causing mutation. This condition is because of reduced penetrance.

The development of the disease is either unifocal or multifocal. For instance, around 60% of the affected individuals have unilateral retinoblastoma (mean age of diagnosis – 24 months) and 40% of cases are diagnosed as bilateral retinoblastoma (mean age of diagnosis – 15 months). Diagnosis of retinoblastoma can be inferred first with visual examination of the eye's fundus region using indirect ophthalmoscopy. Hereditary forms of this disease can be diagnosed by clinical examination followed by family history evaluation and inspection of heterozygous germline pathogenic variant in the *RB1* gene.

With regard to treatment strategies, care to the patients can be best provided by multidisciplinary team combined of ophthalmology, radiation oncology, pediatric oncology and pathology. Treatment can be availed depending upon the number of tumor foci, tumor stage, size and locality of the tumor in the eyes, extent of extraocular extension. If diagnosis has been established earlier, the eye tumor can be treated with cryotherapy (freezing method) or laser photocoagulation. In more severe cases of retinoblastoma disease, chemotherapy, radiation therapy or removal (enucleation) of the eye may be required and necessary. Moreover, careful monitoring of consequent tumor formations and avoiding agents that could induce second mutations are also inevitable for management of patients with retinoblastoma.

PRADER-WILLI SYNDROME

Prader-Willi Syndrome (PWS) is a classic example of an uncommon genetic phenomenon called as genomic imprinting. PWS is caused because of deletion of about 4 Mb segment of the long arm of chromosome 15. Children affected with PWS tends to have short stature, small hands and feet, mild to moderate intellectual disability, obesity and hypogonadism. Most importantly, the affected child has poor muscle tone (hypotonia) and in general the motor functions and language development are delayed. Other features of a child affected with PWS include characteristic facial features, scoliosis and strabismus.

Being a genetic disorder, this inheritance pattern of this particular deletion on chromosome 15 poses a striking and an intriguing observation. If the progeny inherits the deletion on chromosome 15 from the father, the developing child gets affected with PWS. On the other hand, if the progeny inherits the same deletion on chromosome 15 from the mother, the child is presented with Angelman syndrome (AS). In addition to genomic imprinting, PWS is also caused because of uniparental disomy (UPD)– a condition in which the progeny inherits both copies of a particular chromosome from the same parent. (No copies of that specific chromosome from another parent). For instance, if two copies of the maternal chromosome 15 are inherited, the child will be affected with PWS since there are no active paternal genes present in the critical region. Lastly, PWS can also be manifested in the child if there are defects in the imprinting control center on the chromosome 15.

Diagnosis of PWS is established by accurate analysis of DNA methylation patterns in the Prader-Willi critical region (PWCR) on chromosome 15 at 15q11.2–q13. The molecular causative mechanism and diagnosis in a proband could be identified by performing simultaneous oligo-SNP combination array (OSA) and DNA methylation analysis. The difference and significance between the aforementioned dual tests is that DNA methylation analysis can identify the maternal-only imprinting within the PWCR on chromosome 15. On the other hand, the cause for identification of 15q11.2–q13 deletion, uniparental isodisomy, segmental isodisomy and imprinting center deletion, the OSA technique could be utilized. In the case of maternal-only genomic imprinting (identified through DNA methylation analysis) and normal OSA, DNA polymorphism analysis can be employed for distinguishing UPD from an imprinting defect caused by epimutation.

Therapeutic management of PWS affected children includes careful monitoring and guidance throughout their life stages. During childhood period, strict precautions should be followed for maintain proper body mass index (BMI) - BMI z score <2. Growth hormone therapy can be commenced for improving and normalizing body height, increase lean body mass along with mobility, and decrease the fat mass. Since the children with PWS develop hypogonadism that results in genital dysplasia and causes eventual infertility issues, sex hormone therapy should be implemented at the time of puberty for both males and females. During the adulthood stage, a residential facility for individuals affected with PWS that aids in regulating behavior and weight management could potentially contribute enormous benefits in helping them to maintain a healthy lifestyle. This is particularly necessary since these patients could become obese easily and have increased risk of mortality. In addition, growth hormone supplementation may help in maintenance of muscle mass.

LYNCH SYNDROME

Lynch syndrome predisposes the affected individual to having higher risk of developing colorectal cancer (CRC) and cancers of the ovary, endometrium, stomach, small bowel, brain (in the form of glioblastoma), skin, prostate and pancreas. The risk of developing cancer and the age of onset varies based on the underlying genetic susceptibility and defects. Lynch syndrome is typically caused because of germline mutations in genes that are involved in DNA mismatch repair namely *MLH1*, *MSH2*, *MSH6*, *PMS2*, and *EPCAM*. The syndrome follows autosomal dominant pattern of inheritance by posing 50% risk of inheriting the disease in each of the offspring that are born to a couple wherein even if one of the parent is affected with this given syndrome. More commonly, Lynch syndrome is also known as hereditary nonpolyposis colorectal cancer (HNPCC).

Lynch syndrome contributes for nearly 3% of all endometrial and colorectal cancers. Diagnosis of this syndrome comprises of series of multiple procedures that includes recognition of typical features, and appropriate genetic testing. Importantly, it is not easy to distinguish Lynch sundrome-associated CRC and endometrial cancers from the sporadic forms of colon and endometrial cancer. Moreover, lack of availability of family history details could make the diagnosis quite difficult. Thus, it is imperative to follow up with the affected (suspected) individual and also to gather family history details about at-risk individuals. To counteract these limitations, universal screening has been put forward for enabling differential diagnosis of this syndrome.

Universal screening of Lynch syndrome is performed by identification of a germline heterozygous pathogenic variant in the *MLH1*, *MSH2*, *MSH6*, or *PMS2* or deletion in *EPCAM* for individuals who have cancers of the colon and/or endometrium. This is to inspect for genetic defects in the DNA repair pathway – Mismatch repair pathway (MMR). Immunohistochemistry (IHC) and microsatellite instability (MSI) are two such screening methods that can be used for diagnosis of Lynch syndrome in the suspected individuals. MSI is an indication of proper functioning of the MMR system in the cells. Loss of function of the MMR system which is either caused because of Lynch syndrome or by the epigenetic silencing of the *MLH1* gene, results in the MSI. This MSI can be detected by PCR on colon tumor specimen of the suspected individual. If MSI is detected through PCR, then further confirmatory tests are needed in order to rule out the possibilities of Lynch syndrome pathogenesis. IHC, on the contrary, helps in identification of either the presence or absence of MMR proteins in the tumor. If IHC testing reveals any absence of a protein(s), then there is a possibility of mutation in the corresponding gene.

Apart from these there are certain guidelines that have been imposed by two groups namely the Amsterdam criteria and the Bethesda guidelines for identification of individuals who are susceptible to Lynch syndrome. All the following criteria commonly referred as the 3–2–1 rule must be present for aiding in diagnosis of Lynch syndrome such as

(i) Minimum three relatives should be histologically confirmed to have CRC, where one should be a first-degree relative to the other two
(ii) Spanning of at least two consecutive generations
(iii) One of the CRC confirmed patient should have their diagnosis established before 50 years of age.

Here, apart from the above a condition of familial adenomatous polyposis must be excluded.

Treatment strategies for Lynch syndrome comprises of management of the disease clinical symptoms and presentations. For management of adenomas of the colon, a complete endoscopic polypectomy surgery followed by a follow-up colonoscopy should be performed every 1–2 years gap period. In the case of colon cancer management, segmental or extended colonic resection should be implemented depending upon the current clinical conditions of the patient e.g. age, disease duration etc. Those who suffer with rectal adenocarcinoma, either proctectomy or total proctocolectomy surgical maneuver is recommended.

FRAGILE X SYNDROME

Fragile X syndrome (FXS) occurs in individuals who have full mutation or loss-of-function variant in the *FMR1* gene present on 'X' chromosome. The prevalence of this syndrome is higher in males (1/4000) than in the case of females (1/8000). The fragile X syndrome is readily characterized by the appearance of distinctive facial pattern that has long face with large ears, hypermobile joints, and macroorchidism (increased volume in the testicular region) in postpubertal males. An important attribute of this condition is the degree of intellectual disability which varies amongst males and females. The extent of intellectual disability is milder amongst females than in the males. Reduced penetrance and variable expressivity of the syndrome in females, is a reflection of the effects of variation in X chromosome inactivation. Nearly in 50%–70% of FXS affected patients, autism spectrum disorder (ASD) is more common. FXS follows Mendelian genetics and is inherited in X-linked dominant pattern of inheritance.

Being an X-linked hereditary disorder, the transmission and expression of the mutated gene varies per se. This is because those who are affected with FXS have trinucleotide repeat expansion i.e. CGG repeats. Individuals who have CGG repeats of 200–1000 or more are identified to have full mutation in the *FMR1* gene. Individuals who have CGG repeats in an intermediary range of around 50–200 copies do not manifest the disease; however they are termed as carriers. This phenomenon is called as premutation. Premutation is generally observed in normal transmitting males and their female progeny. An intriguing observation is here that when these above mentioned females transmit their genes to their offspring, the CGG repeat expansion would increase i.e. premutation of 50–200 repeats will increase to a full mutation of 200 or more repeats in number. This expansion of premutation to full mutation will not occur in male transmission. Moreover, as the generations expands, the probability of premutation to convert to a full mutation increases successively. This phenomenon is what has been explained by the Sherman paradox.

Diagnosis of FXS could be readily established by the use of specialized molecular testing (PCR) in detecting CGG repeat expansion in the 5' UTR of *FMR1* gene along with abnormal DNA methylation for most of the alleles with more than 200 repeats. Ideally, the diagnosis of FXS inevitably requires the presence of full length mutation – CGG repeats more than 200 in number. Multigene panel and comprehensive genomic testing are required in practice only when no CGG repeat expansion is detected through PCR, but the syndrome FXS is still suspected. With regard to therapeutic intervention, there is no definite cure for FXS. Supportive and symptom-based therapy consisting of psychopharmacologic treatment and therapeutic services such as speech and language therapy, behavioral intervention, occupational therapy and individualized educational support could pave the way for better management of FXS affected children and adult individuals.

GLUCOSE 6 PHOSPHATE DEHYDROGENASE DEFICIENCY

Glucose-6-phosphate dehydrogenase (G6PD) is an enzyme that is predominantly involved in prevention of oxidative damage caused to the cytoplasm of cells through reactive oxygen species (ROS). G6PD helps in providing substrates to the cells for eliminating oxidative stress damage. Erythrocytes (RBCs) are particularly more prone to developing ROS induced damage since they are involved in cellular transport of oxygen. Thus, deficiencies in G6PD enzyme commonly referred as G6PD deficiency results in acute hemolytic anemia in the affected individuals. G6PD is a hereditary disorder that exclusively follows X-linked dominant pattern of inheritance. Currently, nearly four-hundred million people across the globe are known to be affected with G6PD deficiency and the disease is relatively more prevalent to the people who belong to the African, Asian and the Mediterranean descent.

The severity of this disease level varies from individual to individual and is dependent on the residual enzyme activity and its substrate binding which gets altered because of a genetic mutation. The World Health Organization (WHO) has categorized the disease severity into following five classes:-

(i)   Class I – very severe G6PD deficiency - with less than 1% enzyme activity, commonly caused by the Mediterranean mutation.

(ii)   Class II – severe G6PD deficiency – enzyme activity between 1% and 10%

(iii)   Class III – moderate G6PD deficiency – enzyme activity between 10% and 60%

(iv)   Class IV – normal G6PD – enzyme activity is between 60% and 150%

(v)   Class V – G6PD enzyme activity is greater than 150%

Gd gene codes for the enzyme G6PD and this gene is located on the long arm of X chromosome. Its cytogenetic location is Xq28. This gene has a high rate of heterogeneity and around 300 variants have been found till date. Currently, 217 precise mutations in this gene have been identified so far. Major mutations that are observed along this gene are a point mutation that occurs at the coding DNA, introns, and 5' and 3' UTRs. The most prevalent variants found in G6PD-deficient patients are S188F (Mediterranean mutation) in the Arab population, C131G and G487A in Bangladesh, and A376G in North America, Yemen, Saudi Arabia and Africa. Apart from the stress and damage that is caused to RBCs because of inherited G6PD, exposure to specific foods that contains huge amount of oxidative substances and exposure to anti-malarial agents can induce hemolytic anemia in patients with this particular enzyme deficiency.

Screening and diagnosis of G6PD deficient patients could be performed through clinical examination, collection of family history details, risk assessment and laboratory testing. For neonates, newborn screening is highly recommended if signs and symptoms of severe jaundice that are resistant to phototherapy along with a family history or suggestive ethnicity for G6PD deficiency are observed. The most popular screening technique is a quick fluorescent spot test to find NADP production as NADPH. Additionally, quantitative spectrophotometric analysis can be used for screening. For adults, laboratory tests including complete blood count, bilirubin levels, reticulocyte count, serum aminotransferases, and lactate dehydrogenase can be performed for evaluation of G6PD deficiency. Hemolysis indicators like schistocytes may be visible on a peripheral blood smear.

Treatment for neonatal patients should be concentrated on controlling jaundice and aversion of kernicterus. This includes using phototherapy in accordance with accepted, published standards. An exchange transfusion can be required in extreme circumstances. Management of adult patients is mostly based on the overall clinical picture. Less severe manifestations can be treated with supportive care, and by avoiding exposure to harmful agents that can induce hemolytic anemia.

Case Studies

This book presents 10 interesting case studies in varied topics of genetics ranging from genetic disorders following different inheritance patterns, biochemical genetic disorders, and food allergy to prenatal diagnostic tools, identification, analysis, recurrence risk calculation and genetic counselling. This would enable the students to understand and relate to the clinical perspective of genetics in a hospital scenario. The case studies described are illustrative and the names mentioned are imaginary.

Case Study 1

Jacob, a 47-year-old man presented initially with declining memory and concentration. His intellectual function progressively deteriorated along with motor, cognitive and psychiatric abnormalities. He developed involuntary movements of his fingers and toes and facial grimacing and pouting. He also experienced weight loss, sleep disturbances, incontinence and mutism. He was previously healthy with no family history of such a disorder. His DNA analysis revealed 57 CAG repeats. Identify the disorder and comment on its etiology, inheritance, phenotype and management.

Solution: The disorder is identified as Huntington's disease (HD).

Background and etiology: HD was first described by the physician George Huntington in 1872. The neuropathology is dominated by degeneration of the striatum and the cortex. Patients express the disease in early forties and manifest a characteristic phenotype of motor abnormalities (chorea, dystonia), personality changes, a gradual loss of cognition and ultimately death.

Pathogenesis and inheritance: HD is an Autosomal Dominant progressive neurodegenerative disorder that is caused by mutations in HD gene. The HD gene product huntingtin is ubiquitously expressed and its function remains unknown.

The inheritance of HD is explained by the discovery of trinucleotide expansion. An expansion of a stretch of triplet repeats, CAG, the codon coding for the aminoacid glutamine, in the coding region of a gene for a protein of unknown function called huntingtin. Normal individuals carry between 9 and 35 CAG repeats in their HD gene, with an average of 18 to 19. Individuals affected with HD have 40 or more repeats with the average being 46.

Expansion of HD polyglutamine tract appears to confer delirious gain of function. In addition to the diffuse, severe atrophy of the neostriatum that is the hallmark of HD, expression of mutant huntingtin causes neuronal dysfunction, generalized brain atrophy, changes in neuroreceptor levels and accumulation of neuronal nuclear and cytoplasmic aggregates. Ultimately, expression of mutant huntingtin leads to neuronal death.

Risk of inheritance: Each child of a parent with HD has a 50% risk of inheriting a mutant allele. Except for those alleles with 36 to 41 CAG repeats, all children inheriting mutant HD allele will develop HD if they have a normal life span.

Phenotype: HD is characterized by progressive motor, cognitive and psychiatric abnormalities. The motor disturbances include voluntary and involuntary movement. Chorea which is present in 90% of patients is the non-repetitive, non-periodic jerks that cannot be suppressed voluntarily. Cognitive abnormalities include language and behavioral disturbances like sexual deviation, aggression, outbursts, increased appetite, etc., while psychiatric manifestations include personality changes, psychosis and schizophrenia. They also experience sleep disturbances, weight loss, incontinence and mutism.

Management: Currently, no curative treatments are available for HD. Therapy focuses on supportive care and management of behavioral and neurological problems.

Presymptomatic and prenatal testing are available through analysis of the number of CAG repeats within exon 1 of the HD gene.

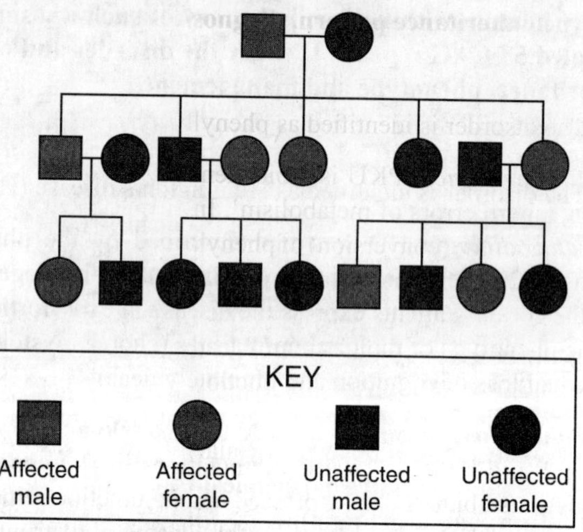

Autosomal inheritance of HD: Pedigree. (See page 252 for the colour image.)

Case Study 2

Joshua, a 5-year-old girl was referred to a genetic clinic with clinical symptoms of fair skin, blond hair and blue eyes. She developed skin eczema and suffered from epileptic seizures. She also suffered from severe mental retardation. She was asked to undergo urine and blood test to check for aminoacid levels and was also advised diet restriction. Identify the disorder; add a note on its phenotype, inheritance pattern, diagnosis and treatment module.

Solution: The disorder is identified as phenylketonuria (PKU).

Phenotype and inheritance: PKU is a biochemical/metabolic disorder which is grouped under 'inborn errors of metabolism'. In children with PKU, the enzyme necessary for metabolism (conversion) of phenylalanine to tyrosine, phenylalanine hydroxylase (PAH) is deficient. As a result of the enzyme defect, phenylalanine accumulates and is converted to phenylpyruvic acid and other metabolites which are excreted in the urine. The enzyme block leads to a deficiency of tyrosine with a consequent reduction in melanin production. Affected individuals therefore have fair skin, blond hair and blue eyes. The mental retardation observed in children with PKU is due to elevation of phenylalanine and its metabolites.

PKU is an **autosomal recessive** biochemical disorder with an incidence rate of 1 in 10,000 (Western European origin).

Diagnosis

New born screening: Urine and blood screening is routinely performed in newborns in most countries.

Urine test: To detect the presence of phenylpyruvic acid in urine with ferric chloride.

Guthrie blood test: Blood test done during the first week of birth to check the elevated levels of phenylalanine in blood.

Treatment and management

Diet restriction: Removal of phenylalanine from diet. This has proved to be an effective treatment module. If PKU is detected in early infancy, mental retardation can be prevented by giving diet containing restricted minimal amounts of phenylalanine. Phenylalanine is an essential aminoacid and cannot be entirely removed from the diet. By monitoring the level of phenylalainine in blood, it is possible to supply sufficient amounts to meet normal requirements and avoid levels which would result in mental retardation.

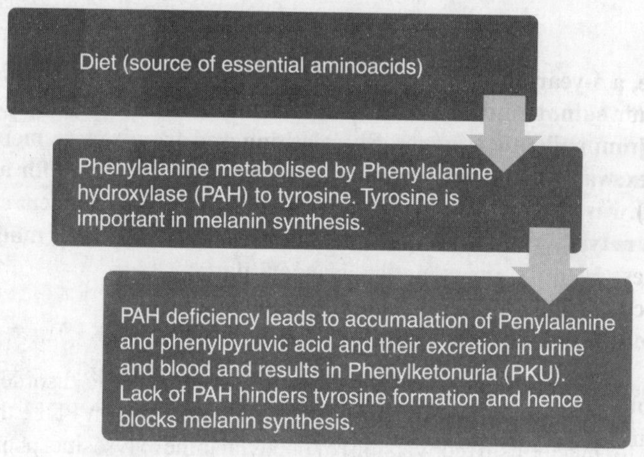

Figure 1 Biochemistry of phenylketonuria

Case Study 3

George, a 4-year-old boy was brought to a genetic clinic with a chief complaint that the boy showed difficulty with motor skills (walking, running, hopping, jumping) accompanied by breathing difficulty, fatigue and frequent falls. On examination he was found to have scoliosis (deformities of the chest and back). An electromyography (EMG) revealed pseudohypertrophy, loss of muscle mass (wasting), muscle contractures in the heels, legs and muscle deformities. Identify the genetic disorder, pathogenesis, clinical features, inheritance pattern, diagnosis and management.

Solution: The disorder is identified as Duchene Muscular Dystrophy (DMD). DMD is an **X-linked recessive** genetic disorder which results in progressive muscle degeneration and loss of motor skills and is most often fatal.

Genetics and inheritance pattern: Both males and females are affected. However since it is a X-linked recessive disorder, males are more frequently affected than females; females are more often carriers. Males have only a single X chromosome and if they receive the defective X, they are affected. However females have to receive two defective X chromosome to express the disease. When they carry one defective X, they are referred to as carriers and can transmit the disease condition to the following generations.

The sons of females who are carriers of the disease (women with a single defective X) each have a 50% chance of having the disease. The daughters each have a 50% chance of being carriers. Fathers cannot pass X-linked traits on to their sons, so the mutation is transmitted by the mother. The incidence rate of DMD is 1 out of every 3,600 male infants.

Pathogenesis: The disorder is caused by a mutation in the dystrophin gene, located in humans on the X chromosome (Xp21). The dystrophin gene codes for the protein dystrophin, an important structural component within muscle tissue. It connects the cytoskeleton of the muscle fiber to the extracellular matrix. The absence of dystrophin allows excess calcium to enter the sarcolemma. Changes in the signaling pathways alters mitochondrial function which results in increase of stress induced cytosolic calcium signals and amplification of reactive oxygen species (ROS) production. This increase in oxidative stress within the cell further damages the sarcolemma and results in cell death. Muscle fibers undergo necrosis and muscle cells are replaced by fat cells (adipose) and connective tissue and results in fibrosis.

Clinical features: The disease expresses in boys before the age of five. However symptoms may be observed in early infancy when the child fails to show proper motor skills. The clinical symptoms include wasting of muscles, enlargement of calf muscles (pseudohypertrophy), and progressive loss of motor skills (loss of ability to stand, walk or ascend stairs unaided). Muscle weakness of the legs, pelvis, arms and neck are significant. Most often children require braces to assist them to walk and are confined to wheel chair by the age of 12. Paralysis, scoliosis and mental retardation are also often observed. The average life expectancy varies from 14 years to mid-920s.

Gower's sign: This is classically seen in Duchenne muscular dystrophy but is also seen in other conditions associated with muscle degeneration like BMD (Becker muscular dystrophy and myotonic dystrophy. Gower's sign is a distinct clinical expression that indicates degeneration of the proximal muscles (most often of the lower limb) The patient uses his hands and arms to "climb" up on his own body from a sitting position because of their inability to lay strength on the hips or thighs due to muscle degeneration.

Diagnosis: Clinical examination reveals muscle degeneration, wasting, pseudo-hypertrophy, scoliosis, lack of motor skills, Gower's sign, fatigue, frequent falls, etc. The clinical features indicative of DMD are confirmed by various diagnostic tests. They include:

1. Molecular genetic testing: can detect errors/mutation in Xp21 gene. The dystrophin gene is composed of 79 exons and DNA PCR test reveals the specific mutation in the exon/exons. DNA testing is often the confirmatory test employed.

2. Muscle biopsy: Immunohistochemistry/Immunoblotting is done on the muscle tissue sample to detect the presence of dystrophin. This is often done when DNA testing does not yield confirmatory results.

3. Serum CPK levels: are tested in the blood. Creatine kinase (CPK) levels are extremely high in DMD.

4. Electromyography (EMG): is done to detect degree of muscle degeneration.

5. Prenatal testing: Genetic counseling is advised for people with a family history of the disorder. DMD can be detected prenatally with 90–95% accuracy. Mutations can be detected from samples obtained from amniocentesis, fetal blood sampling or chorionic villus sampling.

Treatment: Treatment modality is often not directed to cure as in most genetic conditions. Management options however are available which can improve the quality of life and life expectancy.

Corticosteroids are administered to improve muscle strength and increase energy levels.

Mild physical activity is recommended to improve muscle tone and activity. Physical therapy helps maintain muscle strength and function and prevents total loss of muscle flexibility. Physical therapists help patients by providing them with muscle exercises which minimize contractures and deformities. They also plan and execute breathing exercises to monitor respiratory function. Massage therapists are employed to relieve patients from pain due to muscular distress.

Independence in patients is promoted by aiding them with braces and wheel chairs, which improve their mobility and confidence.

Case Study 4

Joe is 15-months-old. At birth he was unable to tolerate cow's milk-based formulas. He showed severe diarrhea and vomiting after each feeding. The paediatrician recommended that her mother switch to a casein hydrolysate formula, which Joe tolerated well. Within two months he developed eczema that was treated with steroid creams. Cow's milk was introduced when Joe was 12 months of age. Skin symptoms increased remarkably. When eggs and peanut butter were later introduced he experienced immediate wheezing, watery swelling eyes, hives, increased skin itch and diarrhea. His paediatrician has sent him to a allergist and nutritionist.

1. How many food allergen suspects are there and what are they?
2. What nutrient substitutions must be considered?
3. What special care and instructions must be noted by parents and care takers?

Solution:

1. Four food allergen suspects—Cow's milk, casein hydrolysate, eggs and peanut butter.
2. Avoid cow's milk and products, eggs and peanut butter. Fruit juices, soy-based infant formula, soy milk and milk-free infant formulas can be used. Apple puree and bananas can substitute the nutrients derived from eggs and peanut butter.
3. Avoidance of food allergen must be remembered at all times. The parents must make Joe eating at home pleasurable and prepare substitutes to give him a variety and avoid dining out. Parents and care takers must remember to read the labels of products during grocery shopping to avoid foods containing milk products, eggs and peanut butter.

Case Study 5

Nancy had a routine 18-week Level II sonogram that revealed the foetus had isolated echogenic bowel. Nancy, age 27, and her spouse, Mike, age 30, were referred for genetic counseling to discuss the potential implication of this finding. The couple was understandably anxious, as this was their first pregnancy and no pregnancy complications had been noted previously.

Solution: As is standard in any genetic counseling session, a 3-generation family history is obtained. No relatives with mental retardation, birth defects, or genetic disorders were reported on either side of the family. The genetic counselor explained the ultrasound finding and informed the couple that the majority of foetuses with isolated echogenic bowel are born without associated problems. Given the finding, however, several possibilities were reviewed.

The first possibility was that of a maternal infection, such as toxoplasmosis or CMV. Since approximately 3–4 % of cases of echogenic bowel are related to such infections, the genetic counselor contacted the obstetrician and confirmed that Nancy did not have any known infection during her pregnancy. The couple inquired about other causes of echogenic bowel, and the genetic counselor explained that an underlying chromosomal abnormality, such as Down syndrome, can also cause echogenic bowel. Mike expressed confusion because he thought that only women over age 35 could have babies with Down syndrome. The genetic counselor proceeded to review the concepts behind chromosomes and non-disjunction, and informed the couple that while foetal chromosome problems are unlikely for most 27-year-old women, approximately 3 % of fetuses with iso-lated echogenic bowel have aneuploidy. Amniocentesis as a prenatal tool to detect such abnormalities was discussed and offered to the couple.

Finally, the genetic counselor discussed the association of echogenic bowel with obstruction, as seen in pregnancies with Cystic fibrosis (CF). Nancy stated that she already had CF testing and was indeed found to be a carrier. At that time, her husband was tested for CF and found to be negative. The genetic counselor obtained these reports from the obstetrician and confirmed that Nancy was tested for the standard panel of 31 mutations and was identified as a carrier of the delta

F508 mutation. Mike was also tested for this standard panel and was found to be negative. The genetic counselor notes, however, that Nancy was half Northern European and her husband was entirely Puerto Rican. The couple is informed that many different mutations can lead to CF, and the detection rate for Puerto Rican mutations using the standard CF panel is low. To err on the side of caution, an expanded panel of CF mutations was offered to the patient's husband and his blood was drawn for carrier screening.

The ability of amniocentesis to prenatally detect CF in addition to chromosome abnormalities was reviewed. Since Nancy was already 18 weeks pregnant, and prenatal diagnosis for CF can take up to four weeks, she opted to pursue the amniocentesis procedure immediately following the counseling session. This would allow time to consider the option of termination if the fetus was determined as affected with either a chromosome abnormality or CF. Two weeks later, the fetus was found to have normal chromosomes; however, Mike was found to be a carrier of a CF mutation that was not part of his original screening panel. The genetic counselor reviewed autosomal recessive inheritance with the couple and they learned that their risk was one quarter, or 25 %, to have a child with CF. The genetic counselor coordinated CF testing on the available cultured foetal cells. Approximately, 3 weeks later, it was determined that the fetus inherited 2 CF mutations and was therefore affected with CF. At 23 weeks of pregnancy, the couple was in the predicament of choosing between continuation or termination of pregnancy prior to the 24-week legal limit for termination. The genetic counselor helped the couple deal with the emotional reaction to this news and answered their questions regarding the clinical manifestations of CF. The supportive treatments available for CF were reviewed and the counselor informed the couple that while research is progressing, no cure existed for the disorder. The counselor facilitated a discussion between the couple about their options for the current pregnancy. Literature was provided to the couple and the genetic counselor remained open to phone calls and follow-up visits to help the couple make a decision that best suited their values. In the end, they elected to terminate the pregnancy, mainly because of the inability of genetic testing to determine the degree of severity of the CF.

The genetic counselor reviewed the information with Nancy's obstetrician, and it was discussed that while the standard panel of CF mutations picks up the majority of carriers, ethnic-based screening can be used to increase the detection rate and clinical utility of genetic testing. When Nancy was initially determined to be a CF carrier, a consultation with a genetic counselor would have helped the obstetrician determine which test to proceed with for her husband. If the couple had learned this information earlier in the pregnancy, prenatal testing and diagnosis could have been offered in the first trimester.

Case Study 6

A couple brought their 8-month-old daughter, Miriam, for the third time to the paediatrician for refusing to bear her weight on her feet. There was no history of fever, infection and all her previous medical history was otherwise normal except for low haemoglobin and enlarged spleen. She had palpable spleen tip and swollen feet. Her feet were very tender to palpation and she refused to bear weight. In view of this history and recurrent swelling her paediatrician tested Miriam for sickle cell disease by hemoglobin electrophoresis and the result documented sickle cell haemoglobin in Miriam.

Solution: Sickle cell anemia is an **autosomal recessive** disorder of haemoglobin in which the β subunit genes have a missense mutation causing the substitution of valine for glutamine at amino acid 6. The sickle cell mutation appears to have evolved because it confers some resistance to malaria and thus a survival advantage to individuals heterozygous for the mutation. The Val6Glu mutation in β globin decreases the solubility of deoxygenated hemoglobin and causes it from a gelatinous network of fibrous polymers that stiffen and distort the cell, sickle shaped cells. The rigid sickled erythrocytes occlude capillaries and cause infarctions. Repeated sickling and unsickling produce irreversibly sickled cells that are removed from the circulation. The removal of erythrocytes from the circulation exceeds the production capacity of the marrow and causes a haemolytic anemia.

Patients with sickle cell anemia generally present in the first 2 years of life with anemia, failure to thrive, splenomegaly, repeated infections, and dactylitis (painful swelling of the hands or feet from the occlusion of the capillaries in small bones). Vaso occlusive infarctions occur in many tissues causing strokes, renal papillary necrosis, leg ulcers, bone aseptic necrosis and visual loss. The functional asplenia, from infarction and other poorly understood factors, increases susceptibility to bacterial infections.

Current treatment options available are only supportive. No specific therapy that prevents or reverses the sickling process in vivo has been identified. Although gene therapy has the potential to ameliorate and cure this disease, effective gene transfer has not been achieved. Allogenic bone marrow transplantation is the only treatment currently available that can cure sickle cell disease.

Case Study 7

Joe and Felicia, an Ashkenazic Jewish couple were referred to a genetics clinic for evaluation of their risk of having a child with Tay Sachs disease. Felicia had a sister who died of Tay Sachs as a child. Joe had a uncle who suffered from some psychiatric disorder but did not know what disease his uncle suffered from. Enzymatic carrier testing showed both Joe and Felicia had extremely reduced hexosaminidase *A* activity. Subsequent molecular analysis for *HEXA* mutations confirmed that Joe carried a disease causing mutation, whereas Felicia had a pseudo deficiency allele but no disease causing mutation.

Solution: Tay Sachs disease, infantile G_{M2} gangliosidosis, is a **autosomal recessive** disorder of ganglioside catabolism that is caused by a deficiency of hexosaminidase A. The incidence of Tay Sachs disease ranges from 1 in 3600 Ashkenazic Jewish births to 1 in 360,000 non-Ashkenazic Jewish births.

Gangliosides, a type of sphingoglycolipid, are a group of ceramide oligosaccharides that have at least one sialic acid residue. Gangliosides reside in all cell surface membranes but are more abundant in the brain. They function as receptors for various glycoprotein hormones and bacterial toxins and are involved in cell differentiation and cell cell interaction.

Hexosaminidase A is a lysosomal enzyme that is composed of two subunits. The α subunit is encoded by the *HEXA* gene on chromosome 15 and β subunit by the *HEXB* gene on chromosome 5. Mutations of the α subunit or the activator protein causes accumulation of G_{M2} in the lysosome and thereby Tay Sachs disease.

Infantile onset G_{M2} gangliosidosis is characterized by neurological deterioration beginning ages 3 and 6 months and progressing to death by 2 to 4 years. Regression of motor development, visual loss along with "cherry red" spot on funduscopic examination and seizures are characteristic features observed.

Tay Sachs disease is currently an incurable disorder, therefore treatment focuses on management of symptoms and palliative care. Nearly all patients require pharmacological management of their seizures.

Case Study 8

Fiona, a 15-year-old girl, was referred to an endocrinology clinic for evaluation of absent secondary sexual characteristics (menses and breast development). Although born small for gestational age, she was in good health and normal intellect through her childhood. The findings on her examination were short stature, broad chest and widely spaced breasts. Her physician requested as follicle stimulating hormone (FSH) level, growth hormone (GH), bone analysis and chromosome analysis. These tests showed normal GH level, an elevated FSH level and abnormal karyotype (45, X). The physician explained that Fiona had Turner syndrome.

Solution: Turner syndrome (TS) is caused by complete or partial absence of second X chromosome in females.50% of TS is associated with 45, X karyotype, 25% with a structural abnormality of the second X chromosome and 25% with 45,X mosaicism.

Monosomy of X chromosome can arise either by failure to include a sex chromosome in one of the gametes or by loss of a sex chromosome from the zygote or early embryo. The mechanism by which X chromosome monosomy causes TS is poorly understood. The X chromosome contains several loci necessary for ovarian maintenance and female fertility. Although oocytes development requires only a single x chromosome, maintenance of those oocytes requires two X chromosomes. In the absence of the second X chromosome, therefore, oocytes in fetuses and neonates with TS degenerate, their ovaries atrophy into streaks of fibrous tissue.

All patients with TS have short stature, and more than 90% ovarian dysgenesis. Many individuals also have webbed neck, low nuchal hairline, broad chest, cardiac and renal anomalies, edema of hands and feet and dysplastic nails. Women with TS have increased risk for osteoporosis, diabetes mellitus and cardiovascular disease.

TS patients are treated with growth hormone supplements. Estrogen therapy promotes development of secondary sexual characteristics, and progesterone therapy is added to induce menses. In addition medical management includes echocardiography for evaluation of heart disease, ultrasound for evaluation of renal anomalies and glucose tolerance test for detection of diabetes.

Case Study 9

Diana, a 17-year-old high school girl, was referred to a genetics clinic for evaluation of Marfan syndrome. She was a thin tall girl. On physical examination, Diana has an asthenic habitus with high arched palate, mild pectus carinatum, archnodactyly, diastolic murmur and stretch marks on her shoulders and thighs. Her echocardiography showed dilatation of the ascending aorta with aortic regurgitation. An ophthalmologic examination showed bilateral iridodonesis and slight displacement of lens. Based on physical examination and test results geneticist explained to Diana that she had Marfan syndrome.

Solution: Marfan syndrome is an **autosomal dominant** condition. It is characterized by three major systems: ocular, skeletal and cardiovascular. The ocular defects include myopia and ectopia lentis (displaced lens). The skeletal defects include dolichostenomelia (unusually long and slender limbs), pectus excavatum (hollow chest), pectus carinatum (pigeon chest), scoliosis and arachnodactyly (spider fingers). Marfan patients also exhibit joint hypermobility. Most patients with Marfan syndrome develop prolapse of the mitral valve (this can result in mitral regurgitation), ascending aorta, cardiomyopathy and congestive heart failure.

All these defects involve excessively stretchy connective tissue. The role of connective tissue is apparent for defects such a aortic dilatation and detached lens. Patients with Marfan syndrome have mutations of the chromosome 15 gene that encodes fibrillin, a connective tissue protein which is found in aorta, suspensory ligament of the lens and periosteum. The location of the gene product and its role as a component of the connective tissue explains the pleiotropic effects that causes disturbances in they eye, the skeleton and the cardiovascular system.

Treatment for Marfan syndrome includes regular opthalmological examinations, avoidance of heavy exercises and administration of β adrenergic blockers to decrease abruptness of heart contractions.

Case Study 10

Jenny, a 3-year-old girl, was referred to a paediatric clinic to evaluate poor growth. She suffered from diarrhea, colic and, malodorous stools during infancy. During her second year, she developed chronic cough and frequent upper respiratory tract infections. The paediatrician suggested many routine tests along with sweat chloride test. The sweat chloride level was 75 mol/L, a level consistent with CF (normal values 40 mol/L). The parents and Jenny were referred to a genetic clinic for further counseling and treatment.

Solution: Cystic Fibrosis (CF) is one of the most common single gene disorders. Pancreas develop fibrotic lesions; one of the principal organs affected in this disease. 85% of CF patients have pancreatic insufficiency. The intestinal tract is also affected and 10–20% of newborns with CF have meconium ileus (a thick plug that blocks the colon). Sweat glands of CF patients are abnormal, resulting in high levels of chloride in sweat. More than 95% of males with CF are sterile due to the absence or obstruction of vas deferens. The most serious problem faced by CF patients is obstruction of lungs by heavy thick mucus. Because this mucus cannot be cleared effectively, the lungs are highly susceptible to infection by bacteria like *Staphylococcus aureus* and *Pseudomonas aeruginosa*. Chronic obstruction and infection lead to destruction of the lung tissue, resulting eventually in death from pulmonary disease.

The gene responsible for CF was mapped to chromosome 7q. It is a large gene, spanning 250 kb and including 27 exons. This gene encodes a protein product labelled "cystic fibrosis transmembrane regulator" (CFTR). CFTR forms cyclic AMP regulated chloride ion channels that span the membranes of specialized epithelial cells, such as those that line the bowel and lung. In addition, CFTR is involved in regulating the transport of sodium ions across epithelial cell membranes. Defective ion transport results in salt imbalances, depleting the airway of water and producing the thick, obstructive secretions seen in the lungs. The pancreas is also affected by thick secretions leading to fibrosis and pancreatic insufficiency. The chloride ion transport defect explains the abnormally high concentration of chloride in the sweat secretions of CF patients: chloride is secreted instead of being absorbed by the sweat gland.

CFTR mutations can be identified by DNA analysis along with sweat chloride test to confirm diagnosis of CF in patients. Improved antibiotics, aggressive chest physical therapy and pancreatic enzyme replacement therapy have improved the survival rate of CF patients over the last three decades.

Index

Illustrations

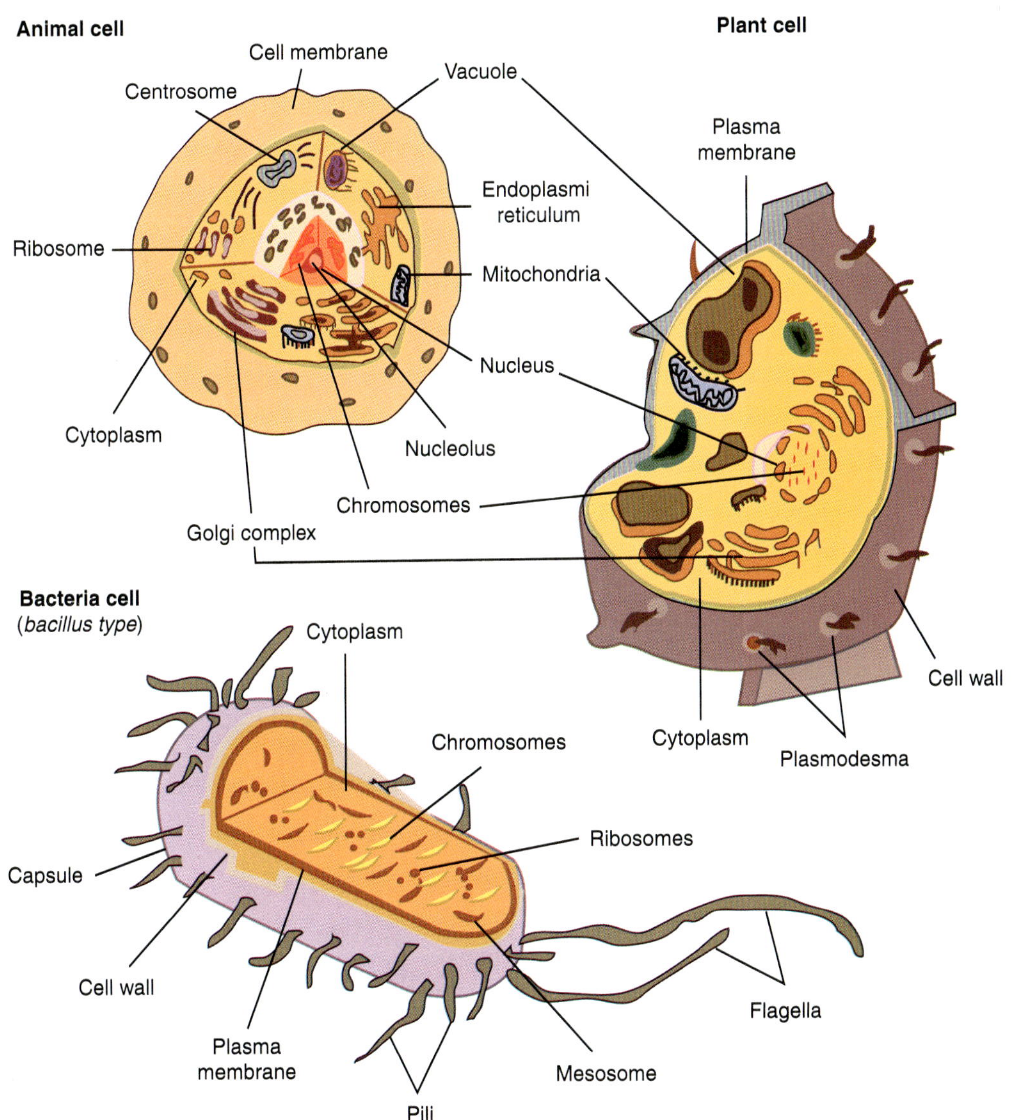

Figure 1.1 Prokaryotic and eukaryotic cells. (See also figure 1.1 on page 3.)

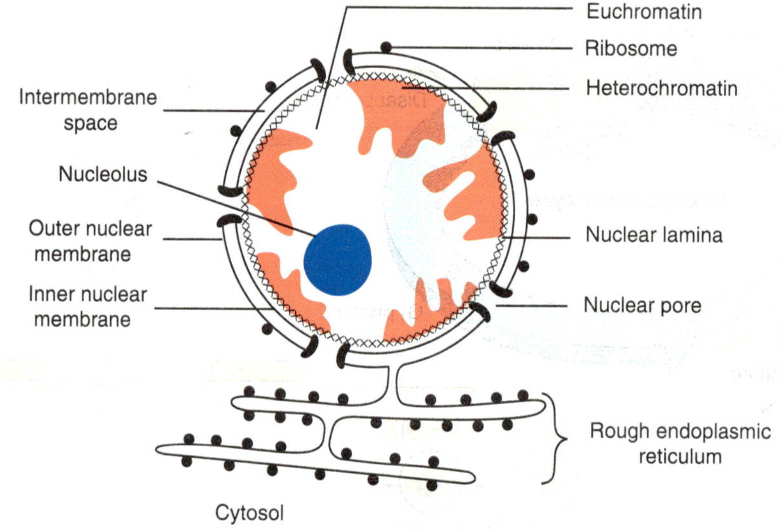

Figure 1.2 Nucleus. (See also figure 1.2 on page 6.)

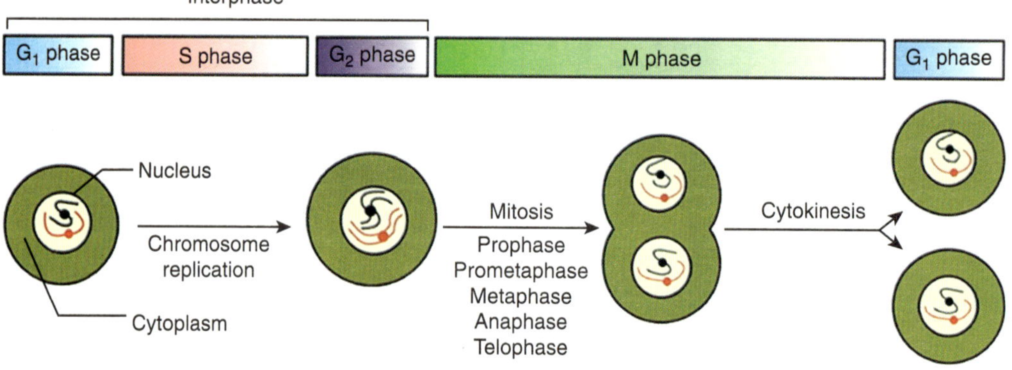

Figure 1.3 The cell division cycle. (See also figure 1.3 on page 7.)

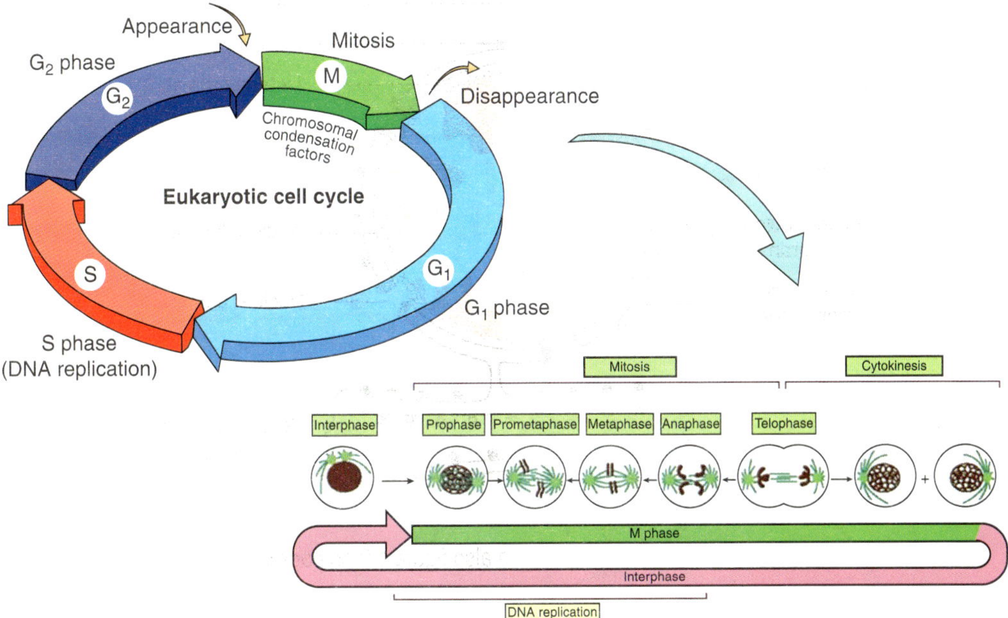

Figure 1.4 The eukaryotic cell cycle. (See also figure 1.4 on page 8.)

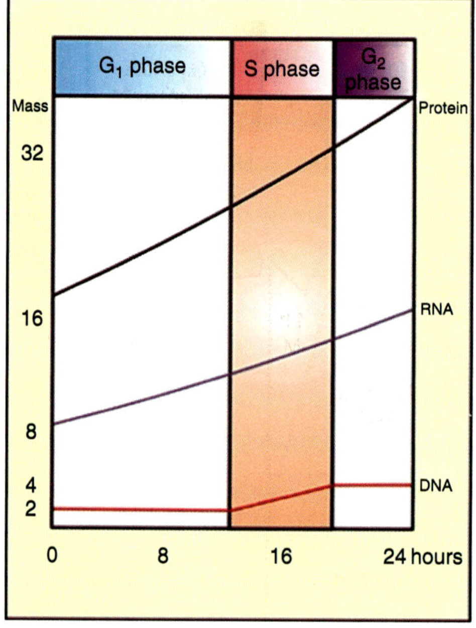

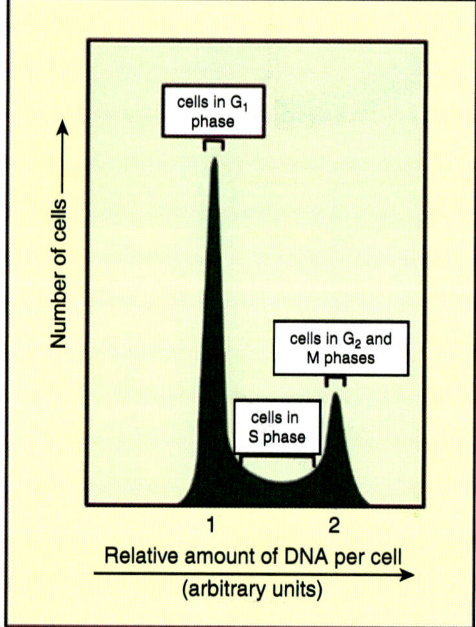

Synthesis of RNA and proteins occurs continuously, but DNA synthesis occurs only in the discrete period of S phase.

Figure 1.5 Changes in cellular components during cell cycle. (See also figure 1.5 on page 9.)

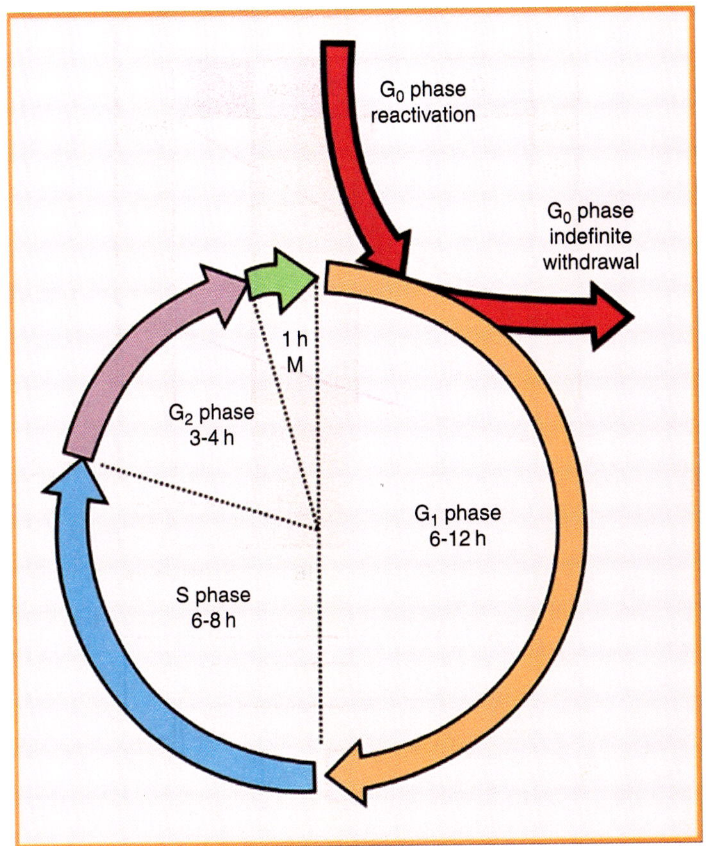

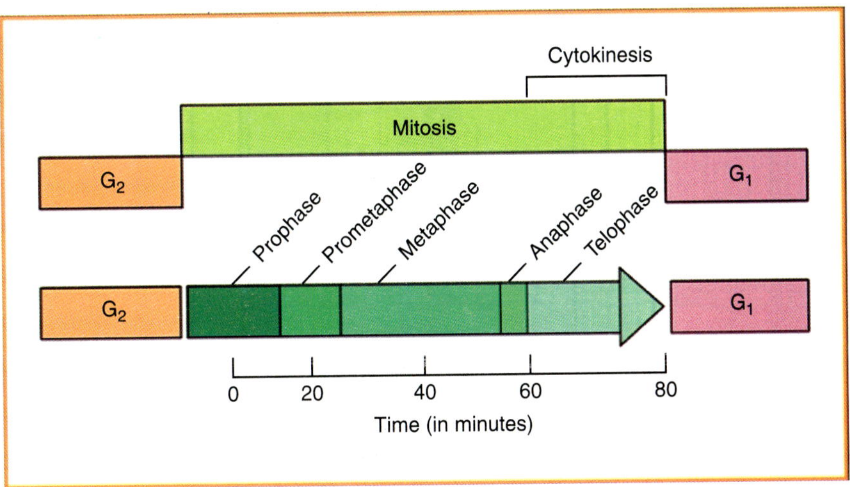

Figure 1.6 Duration of the cell cycle. (See also figure 1.6 on page 11.)

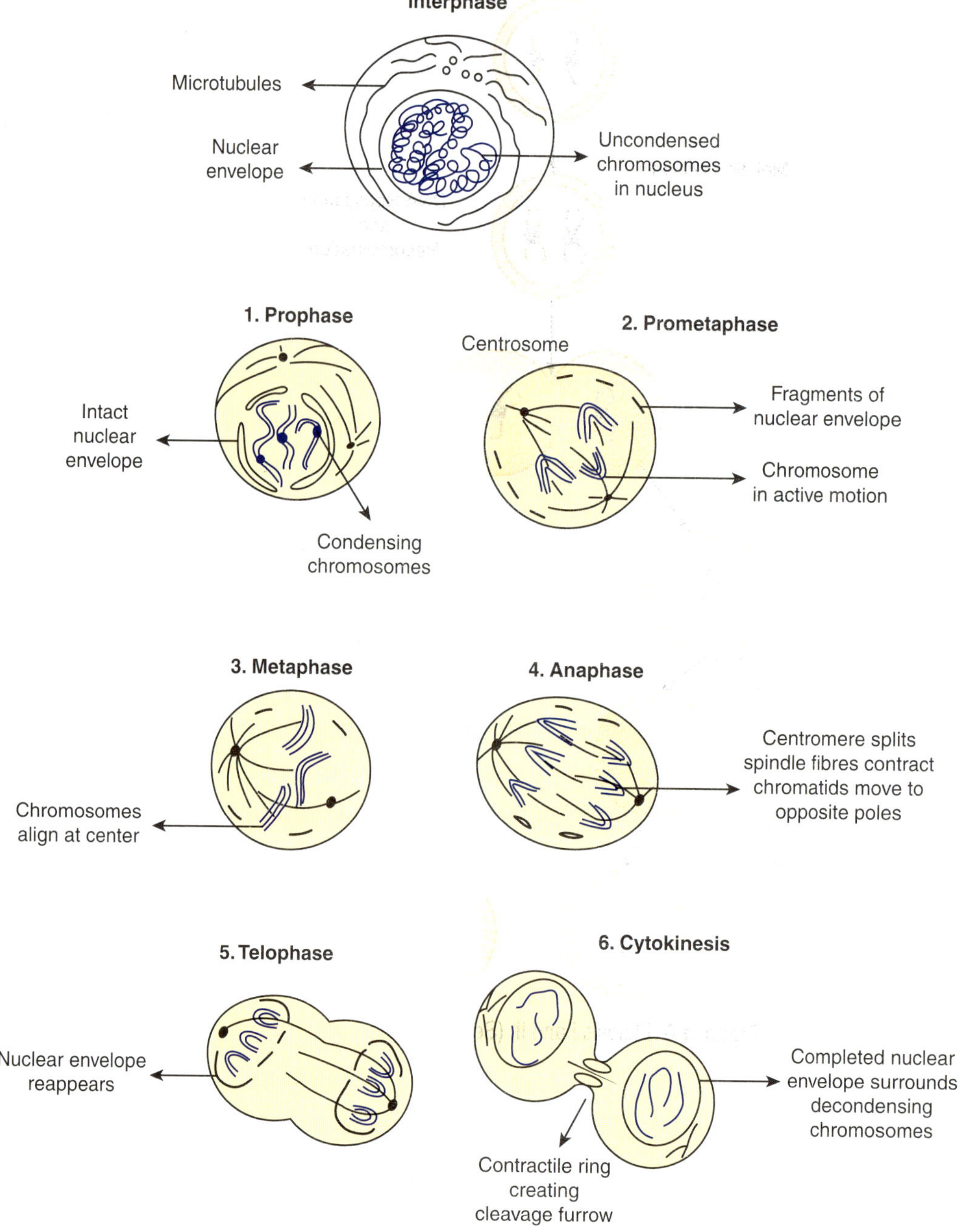

Figure 1.7 The phases of mitosis. (See also figure 1.7 on page 14.)

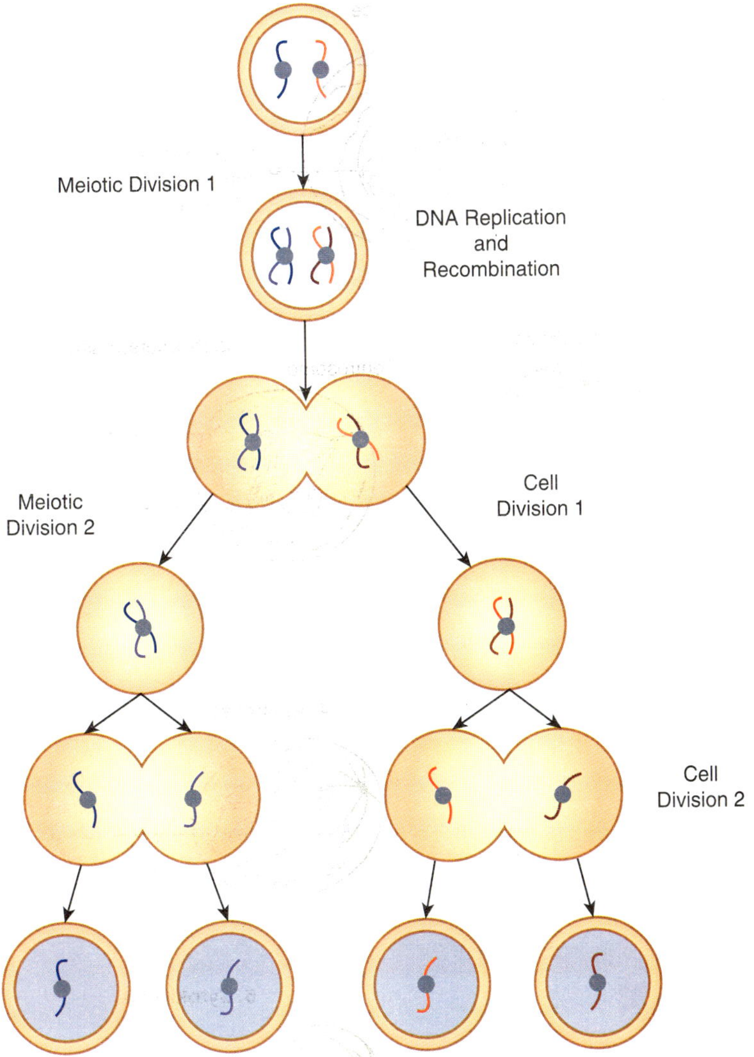

Figure 1.8 Meiosis I and II. (See also figure 1.8 on page 18.)

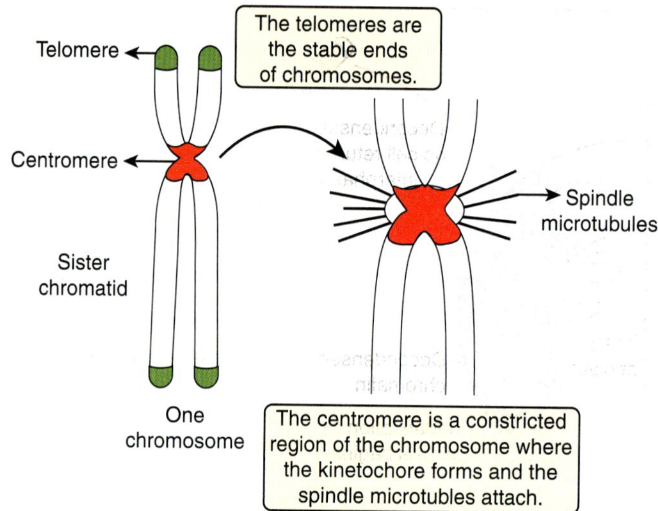

Figure 1.9 Structure of a eukaryotic chromosome. (See also figure 1.9 on page 22.)

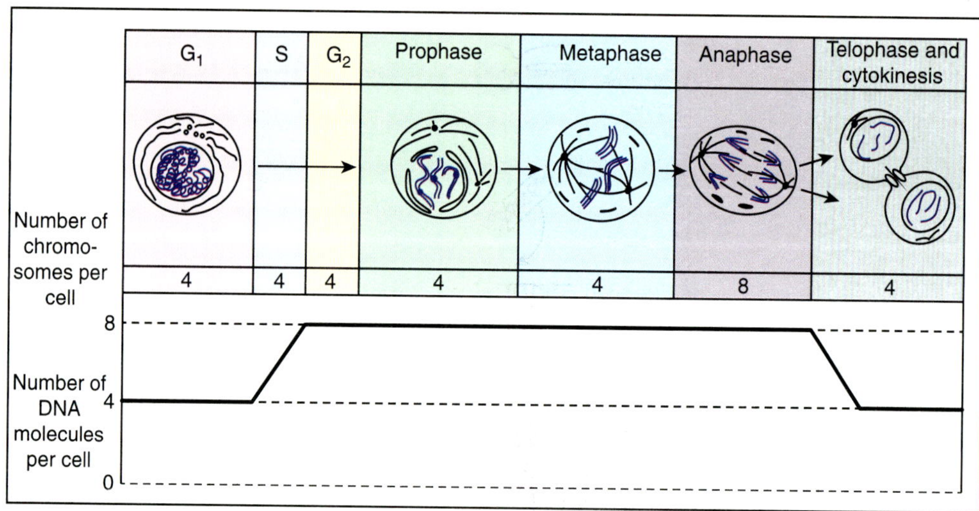

Figure 1.10 The number of chromosomes and DNA molecules changes in the course of the cell cycle. (See also figure 1.10 on page 22.)

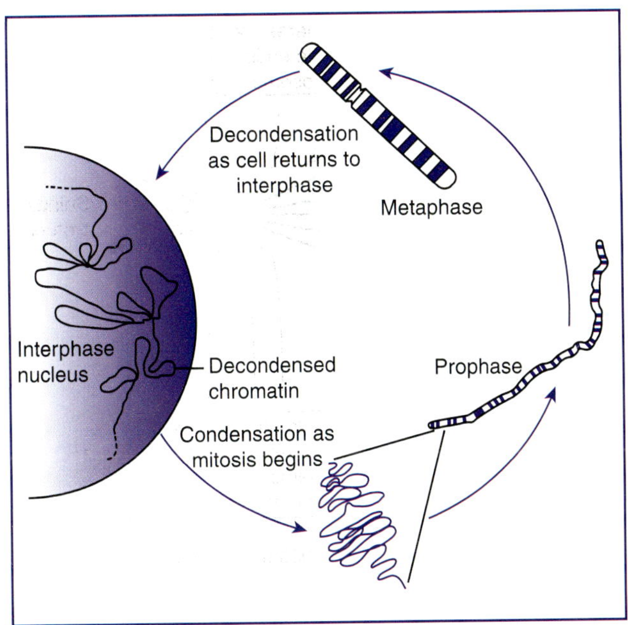

Figure 1.11 Cycle of condensation and decondensation and levels of chromatin packing. (See also figure 1.11 on page 23.)

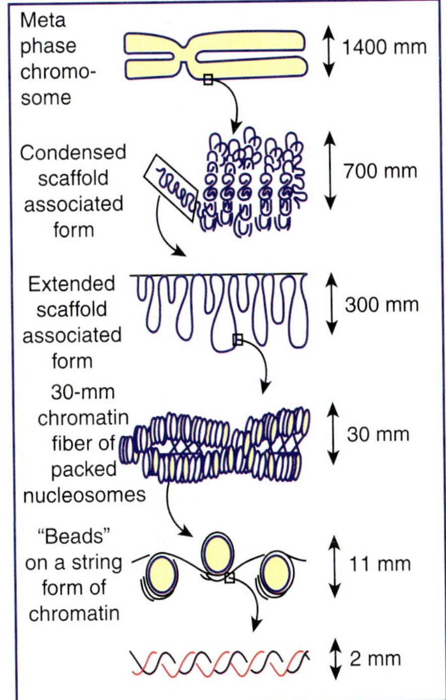

Figure 1.12 Organization of DNA into chromosomes. (See also figure 1.12 on page 24.)

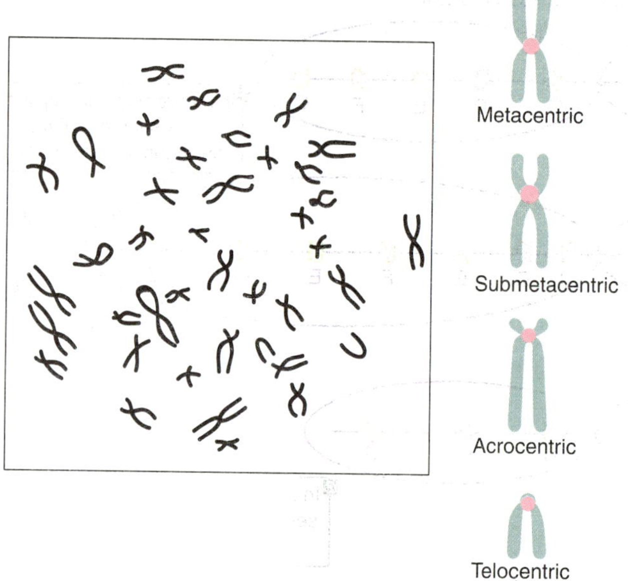

Figure 1.13 Forms of chromosomes. (See also figure 1.13 on page 25.)

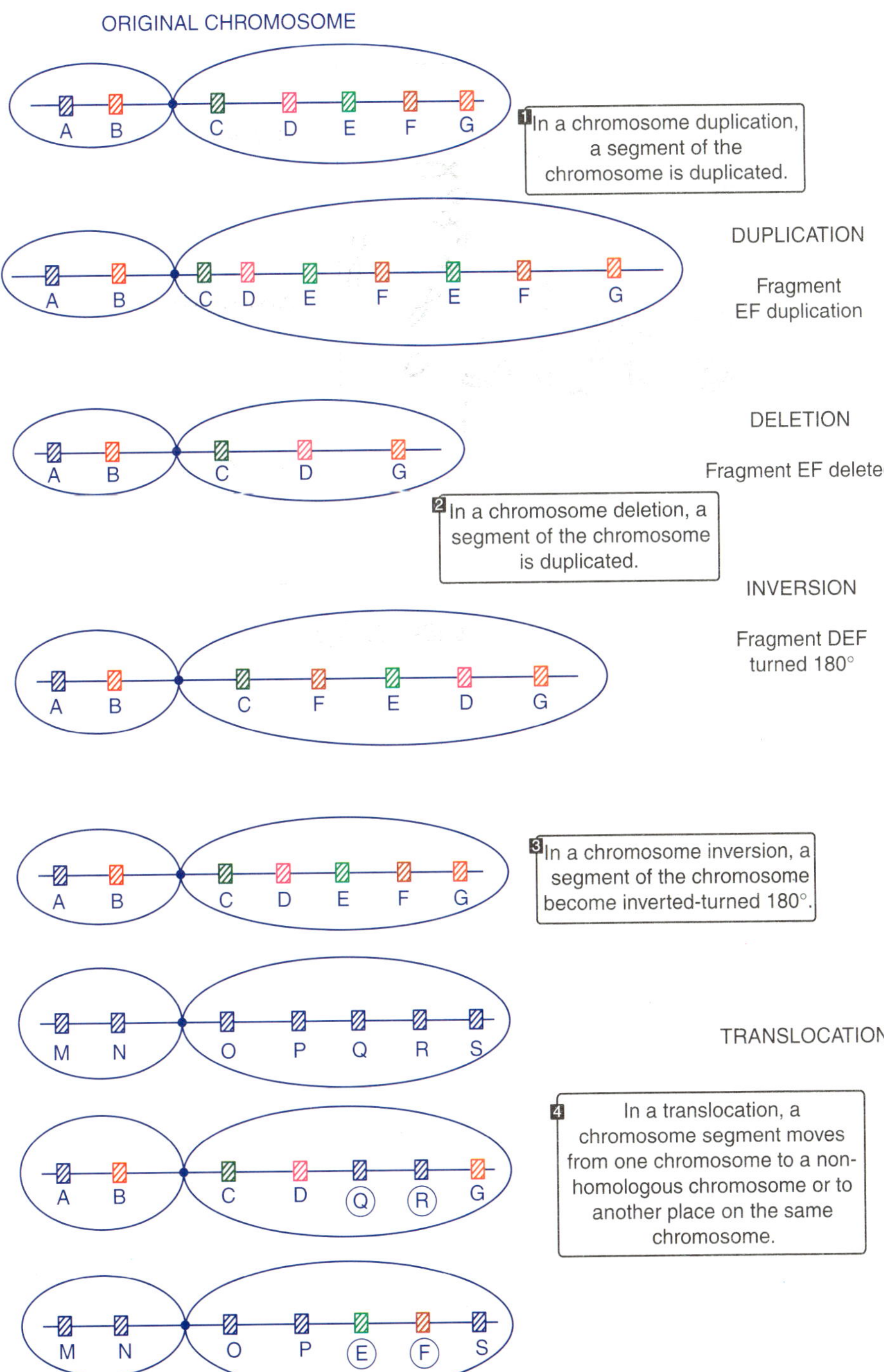

Figure 1.15 Structural chromosomal abnormalities. (See also figure 1.15 on page 29.)

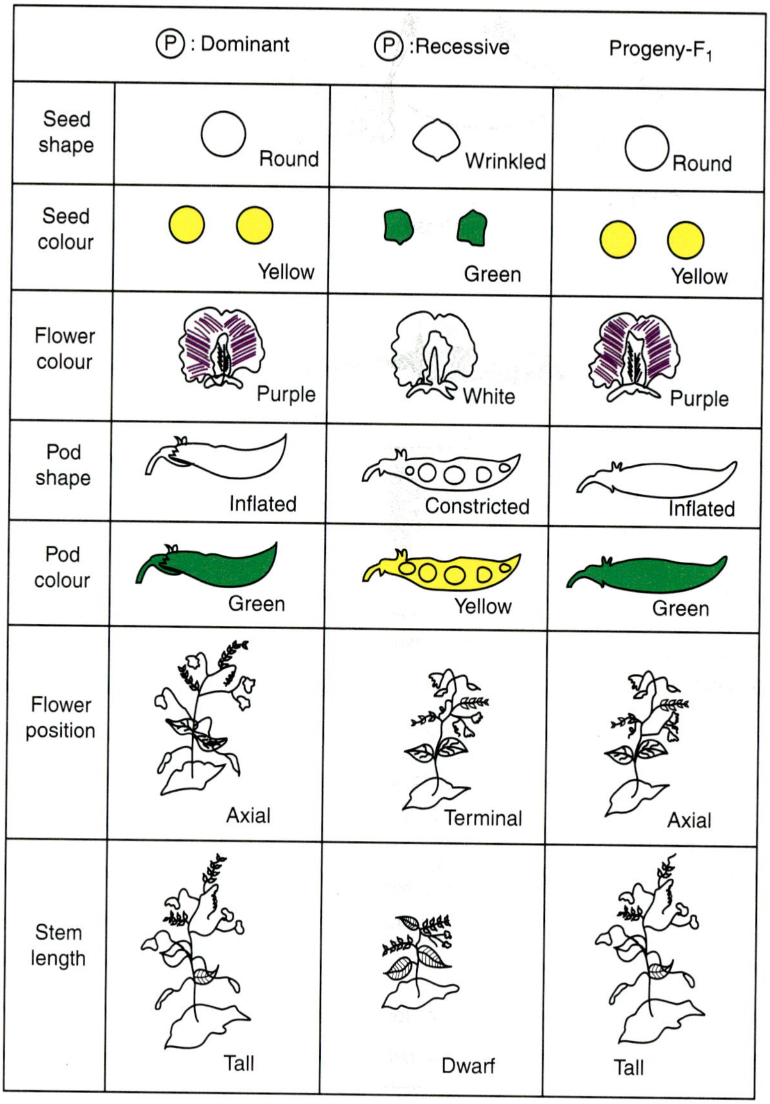

	(P) : Dominant	(P) :Recessive	Progeny-F$_1$
Seed shape	Round	Wrinkled	Round
Seed colour	Yellow	Green	Yellow
Flower colour	Purple	White	Purple
Pod shape	Inflated	Constricted	Inflated
Pod colour	Green	Yellow	Green
Flower position	Axial	Terminal	Axial
Stem length	Tall	Dwarf	Tall

Figure 1.16 Seven contrasting characters of Mendel's experimental organism. (See also figure 1.16 on page 38.)

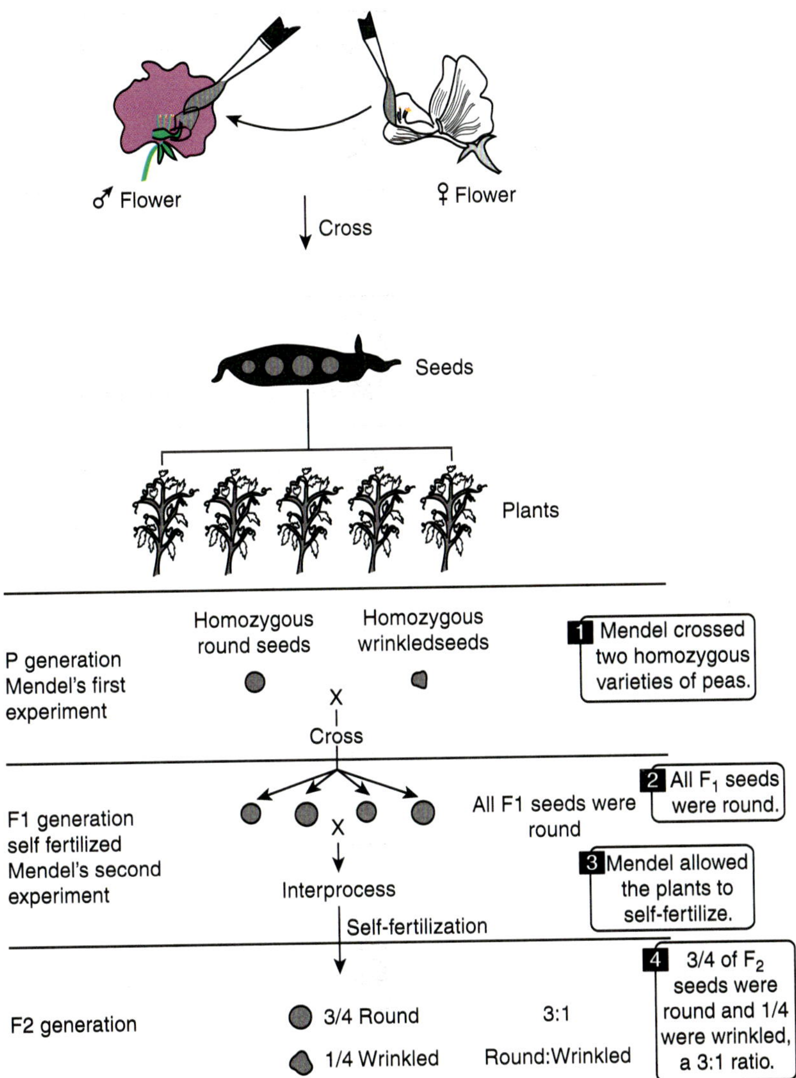

Figure 1.17 Monohybrid cross. (See also figure 1.17 on page 39.)

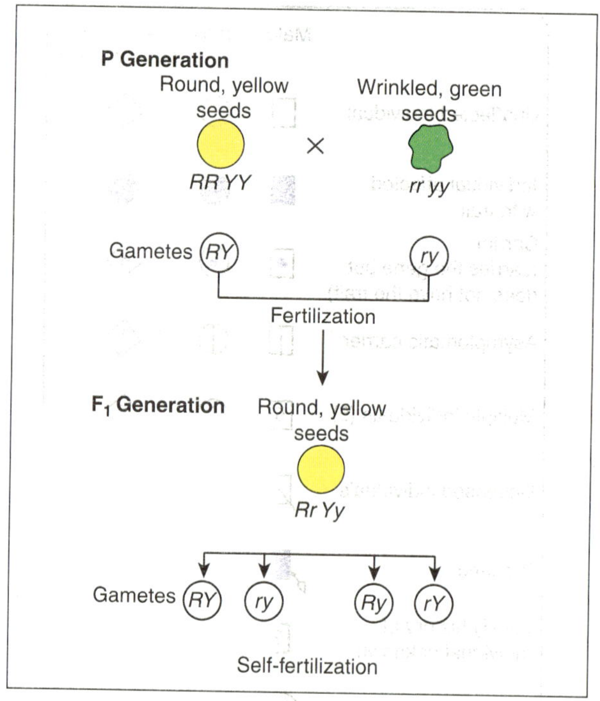

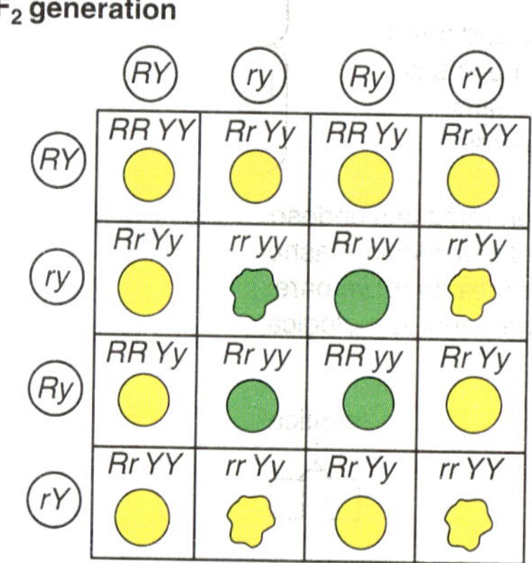

9 Round, yellow
3 Round, green
3 Wrinkled yellow
1 Wrinkled, green

Figure 1.18 Dihybrid cross. (See also figure 1.18 on page 41.)

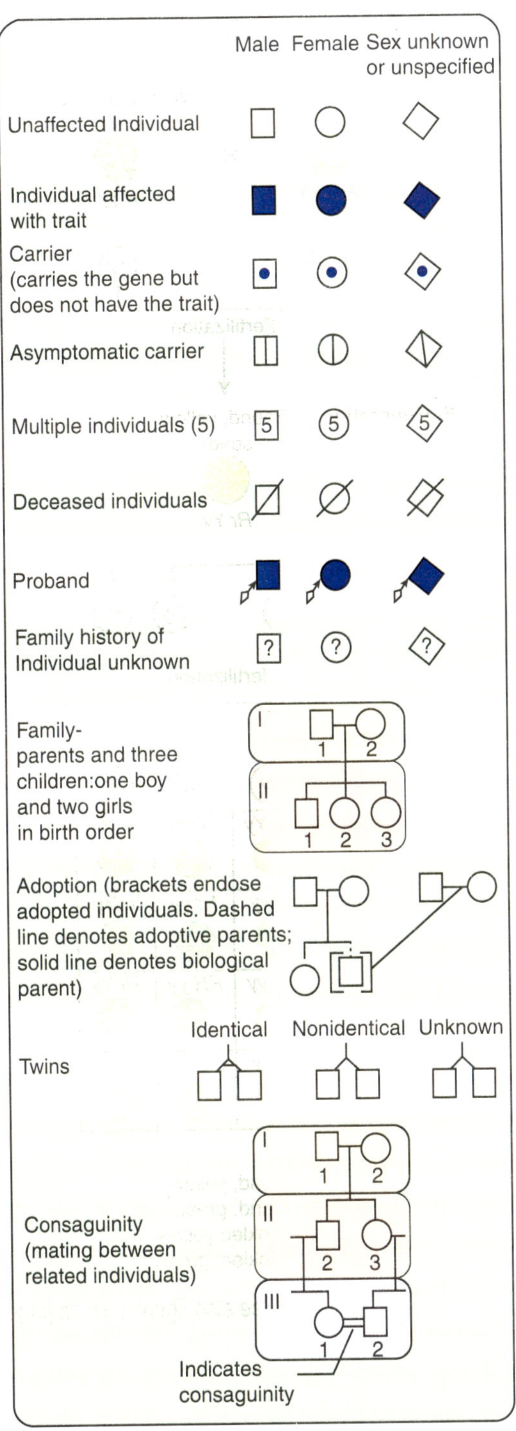

Figure 1.19 Pedigree notations. (See also figure 1.19 on page 43.)

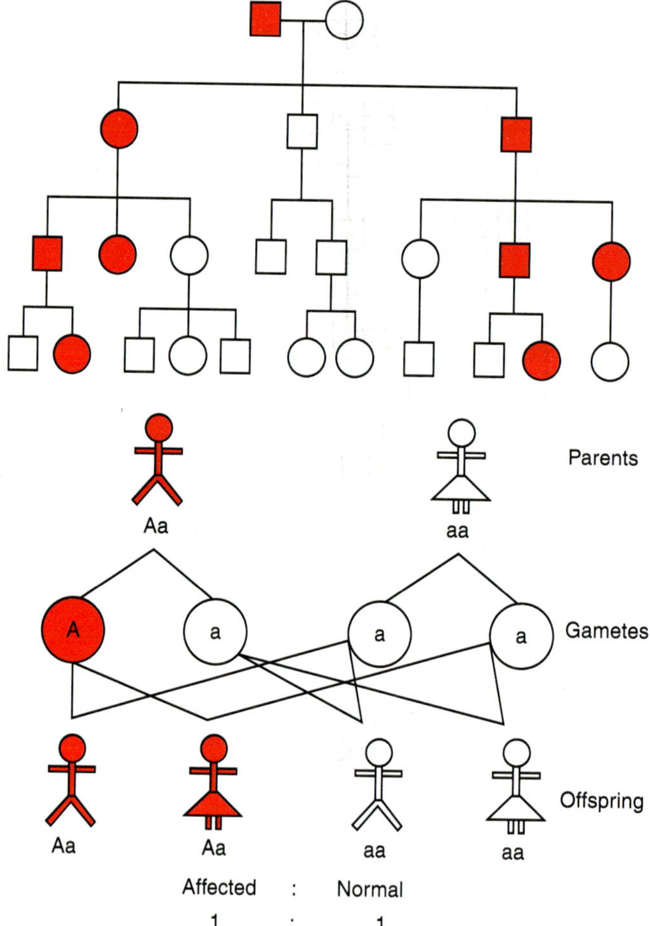

Figure 1.20 Autosomal dominant inheritance. (See also figure 1.20 on page 45.)

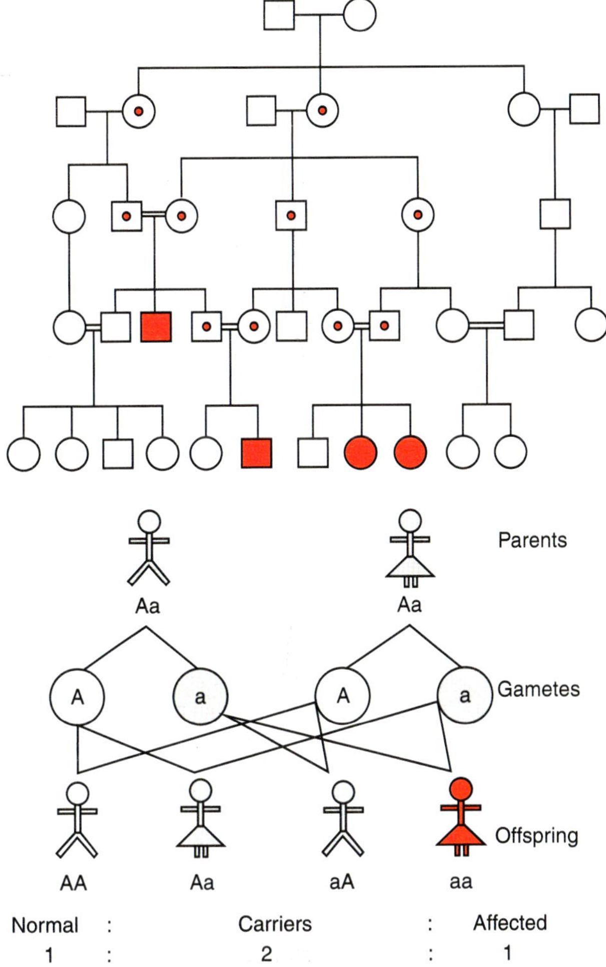

Figure 1.21 Autosomal recessive inheritance. (See also figure 1.21 on page 46.)

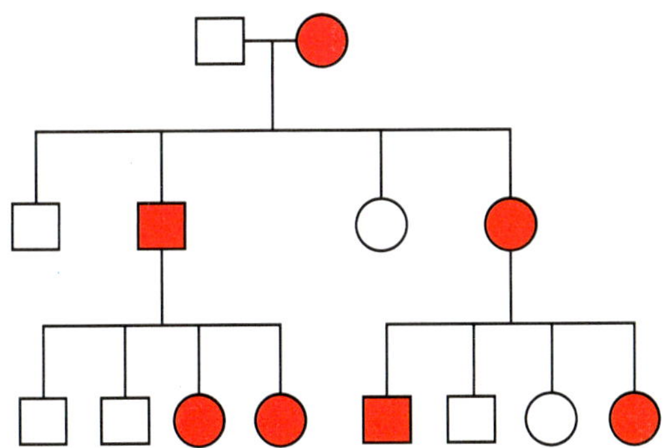

Figure 1.22 X-linked dominant inheritance. (See also figure 1.22 on page 47.)

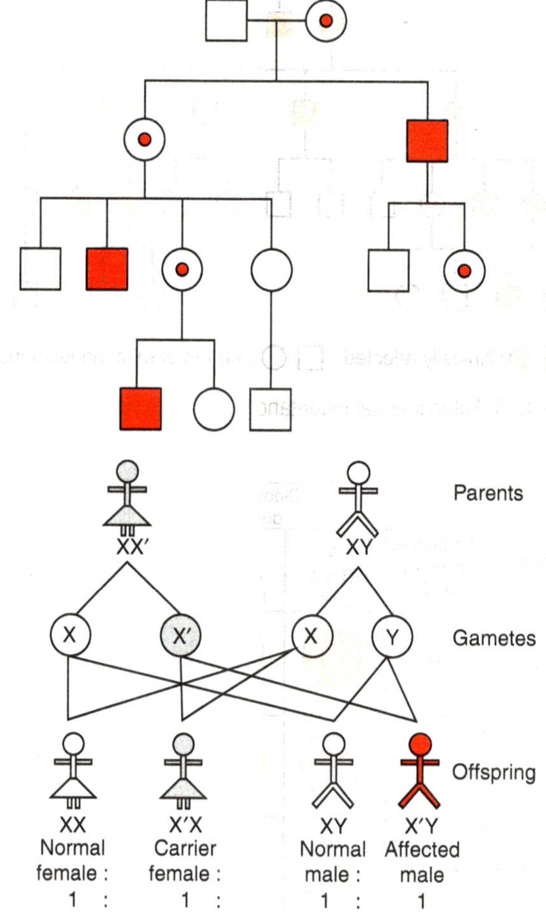

Figure 1.23 X-linked recessive inheritance. (See also figure 1.23 on page 47.)

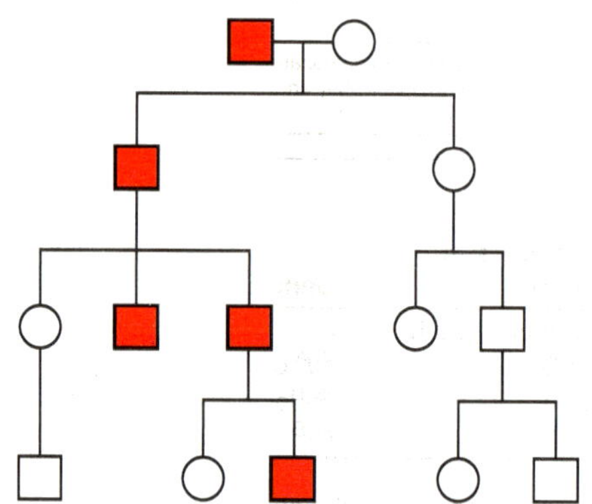

Figure 1.24 Y-linked inheritance. (See also figure 1.24 on page 48.)

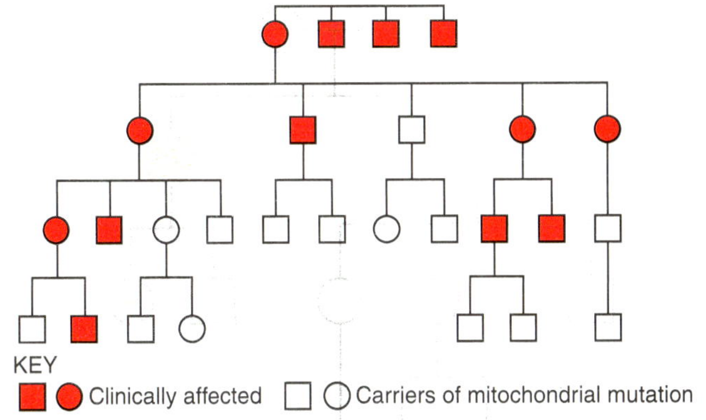

Figure 1.25 Mitochondrial inheritance. (See also figure 1.25 on page 48.)

Pheno type	Geno type	Antigen type	Antibodies made by body	Blood-recipient reactions to donor-blood antibodies			
				A (B anti bodies)	B (A anti bodies)	AB (no anti bodies)	O (A and B antibodies)
A	I^AI^A or I^Ai	A	B	●	⦿	●	⦿
B	I^BI^B or I^Bi	B	A	⦿	●	●	⦿
AB	I^AI^B	A and B	None	⦿	⦿	●	⦿
O	ii	None	A and B	●	●	●	●

Red blood cells that do not react with the recipient antibody remain evently disposed. Donor blood and recipient blood are compatiable.

Blood cells that react with the recipient antibody clump together. Donor blood and recipient blood are not compatible.

Type O donors can donate to any recipient: they are universal donors.

Type AB recipients can accept blood from any donor: they are universal recipients

Blood Type Corresponding to Antigens on Red Blood Cells	Antibodies in Serum	Genotype	Reaction of Red Cells to Anti-A Antibodies	Reaction of Red Cells to Anti-B Antibodies
O	Anti-A and anti-B	ii	−	−
A	Anti-B	I^AI^A or I^Ai	+	−
B	Anti-A	I^BI^B or I^Bi	−	+
AB	None	I^AI^B	+	+

Figure 1.26 ABO blood group system—Genotypes and phenotypes. (See also figure 1.26 on page 50.)

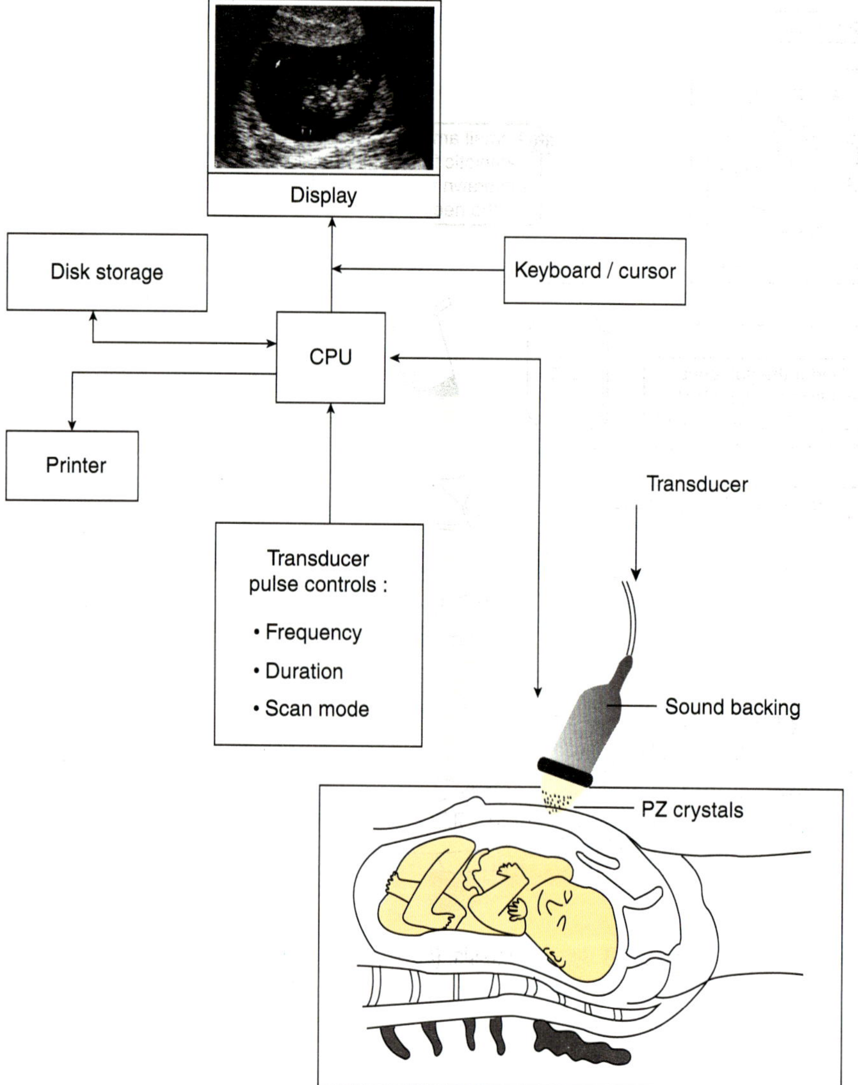

Figure 2.5 Ultrasound. (See also figure 2.5 on page 75.)

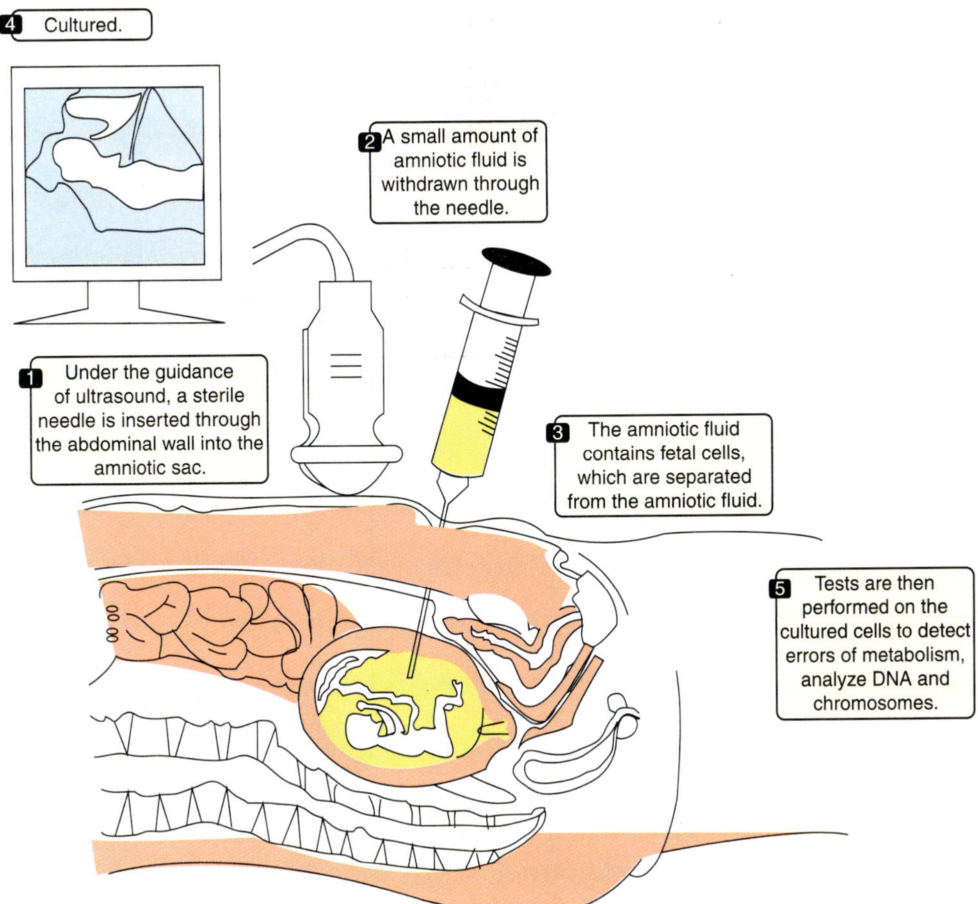

Figure 2.6 Amniocentesis. (See also figure 2.6 on page 78.)

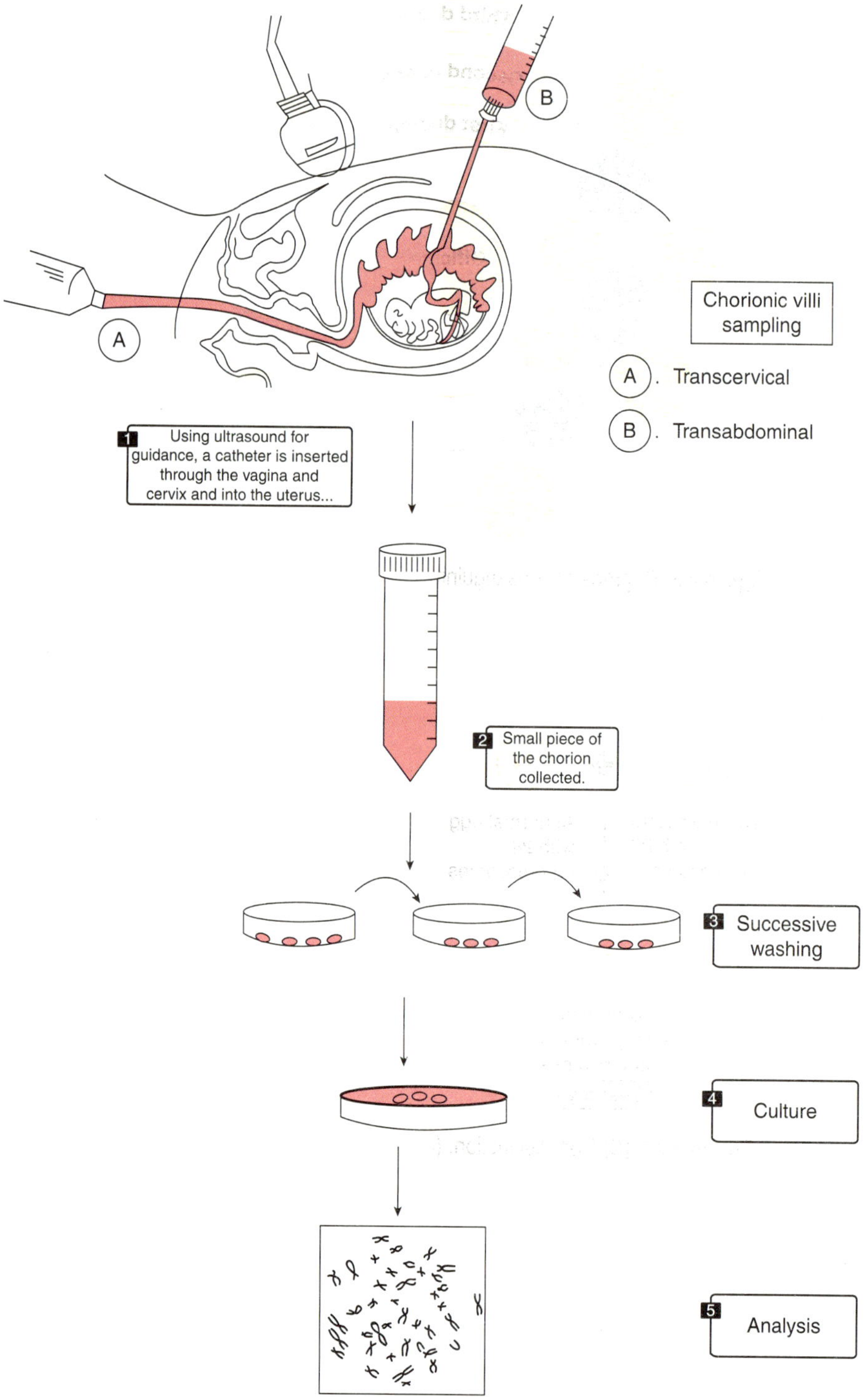

Figure 2.7 Chorionic villus sampling. (See also figure 2.7 on page 80.)

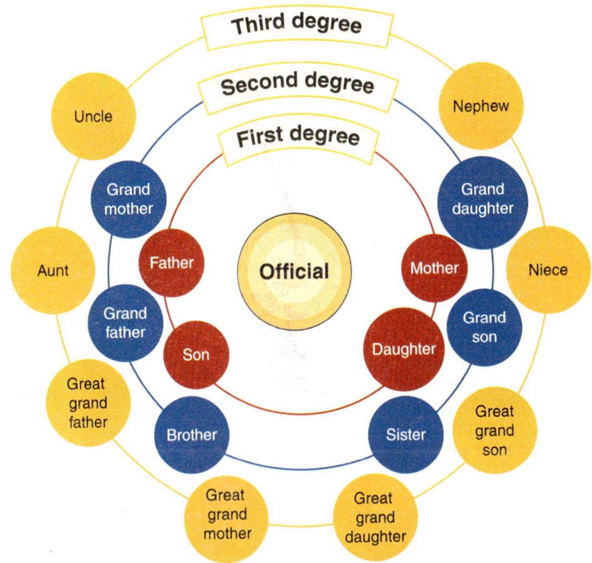

Figure 2.2 Degrees of consanguinity. (See also figure 2.2 on page 60.)

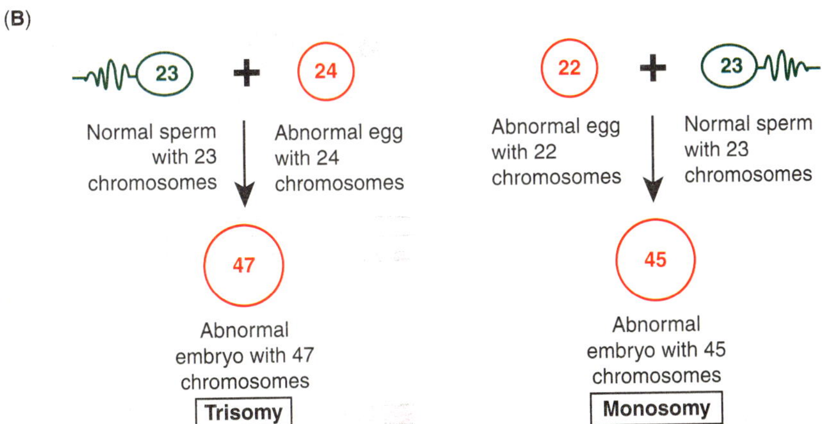

Figure 2.23 (B) Non-disjunction. (See also figure 14.1 on page 116.)

(C)

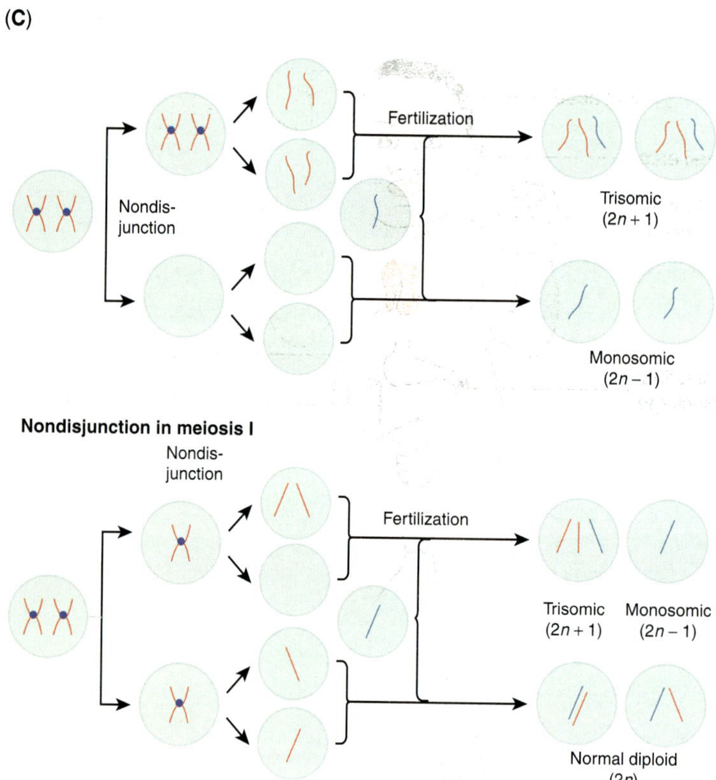

Figure 2.23 **(C)** Mechanism of Non-disjunction. (See also figure 2.23 on page 116.)

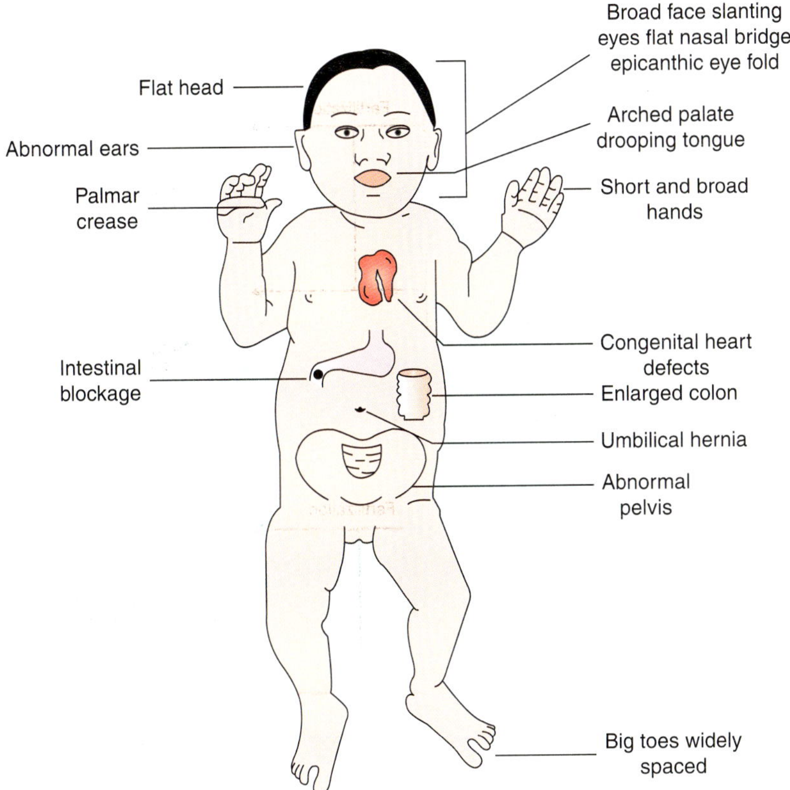

Figure 2.24 Clinical features of Down syndrome. (See also figure 2.24 on page 119.)

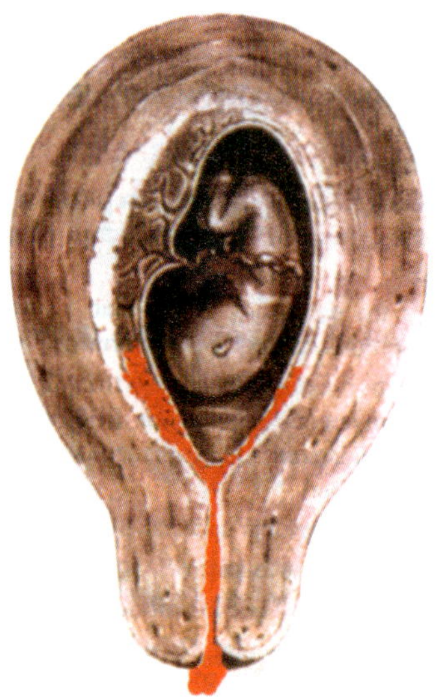

Figure 2.12 Threatened abortion—slight bleeding, membranes intact, and cervical os closed. (See also figure 2.12 on page 101.)

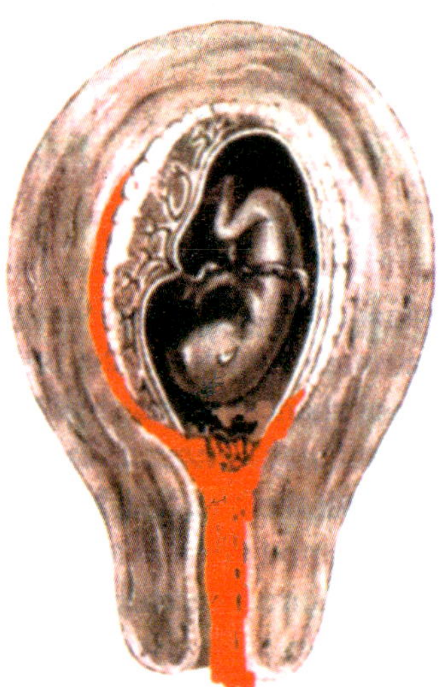

Figure 2.13 Inevitable abortion—moderate bleeding with pain, and cervical os dilated. (See also figure 2.13 on page 101.)

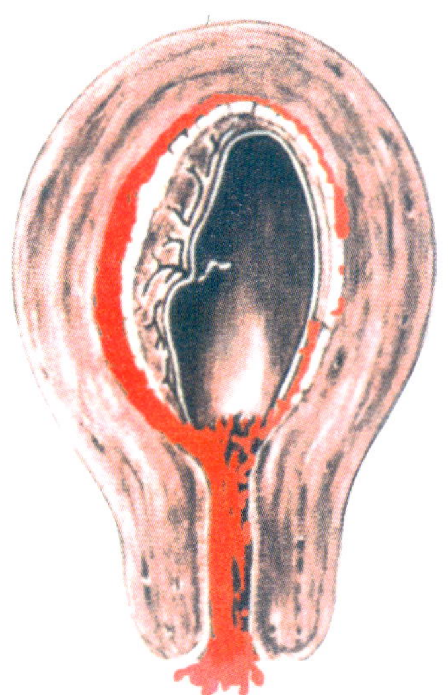

Figure 2.14 Incomplete abortion—free bleeding, foetus expelled, and cervical os dilated. (See also figure 2.14 on page 102.)

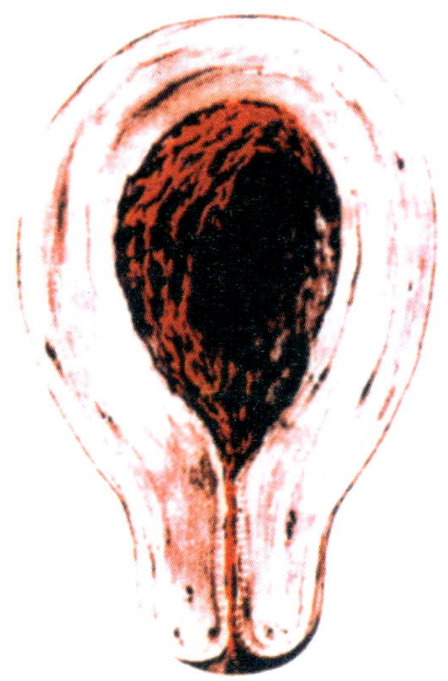

Figure 2.15 Complete abortion—foetus and placenta expelled, bleeding scanty, and cervical os closed. (See also figure 2.15 on page 102.)

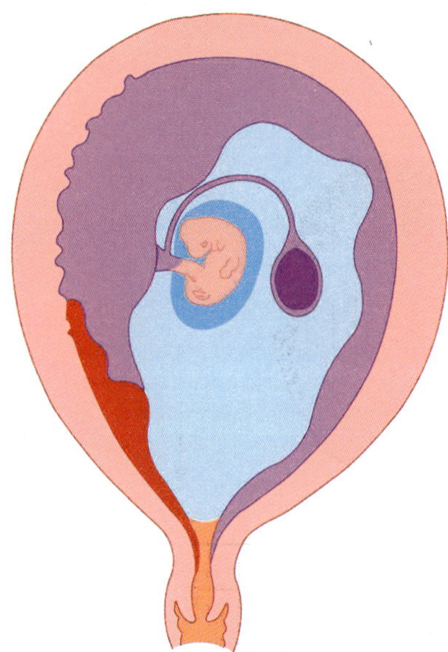

Figure 2.16 Missed abortion—intrauterine death of the foetus. (See also figure 2.16 on page 103.)

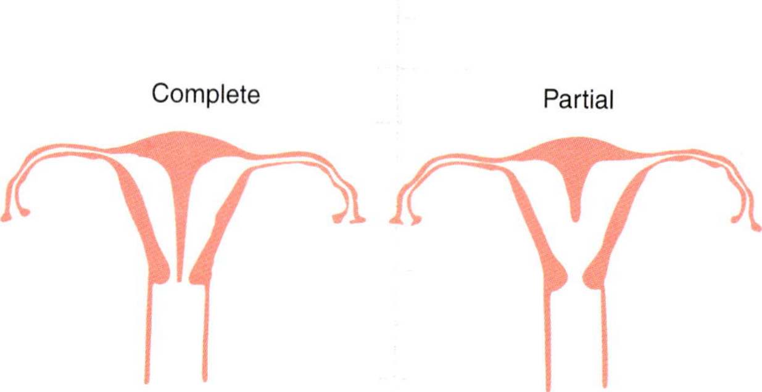

Figure 2.18 Uterine septate. (See also figure 2.18 on page 108.)

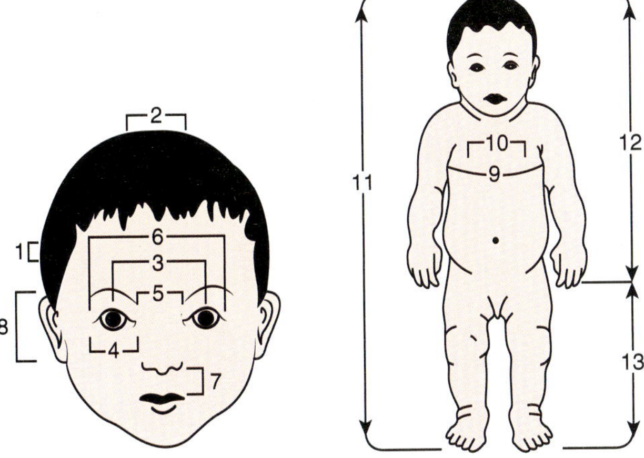

Measurement	Range (cm)	
	Term **(38–40 wk)**	**Preterm** **(38–40 wk)**
1 Head circumference	32–37	27–32
2 Anterior tontanelle $\left(\dfrac{L-W}{2}\right)$	0.7–3.7	...
3 Interpupillary distance	3.3–4.5	3.1–3.9
4 Palpebral fissure	1.5–2.1	1.3–1.6
5 Inner canthal distance	1.5–2.5	1.4–2.1
6 Outer canthal distance	5.3–7.3	3.9–5.1
7 Philtrum	0.6–1.2	0.5–0.9
8 Ear length	3–4.3	2.4–3.5
9 Chest circumference	28–38	23–29
10 Internipple distance*	6.5–10	5–6.5
11 Height	47–55	39–47
12 Hand (palm to middle finger)	5.3–7.8	4.1–5.5
13 Ratio of middle finger to hand	0.38–0.48	0.38–0.5
14 penis (pubic bone to tip of glans)	2.7–4.3	1.8–3.2

* Internipple distance should not exceed 25 % of chest circumference.

Figure 3.2 Physical evaluation of dysmorphic infant. (See also figure 3.2 on page 130.)

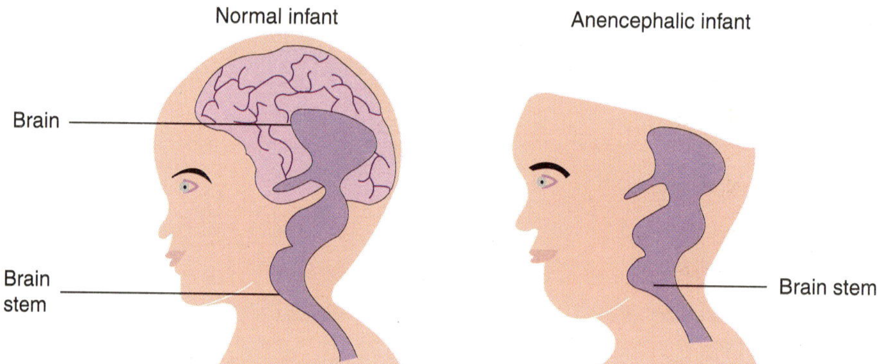

Figure 2.21 Anencephaly. (See also figure 2.21 on page 112.)

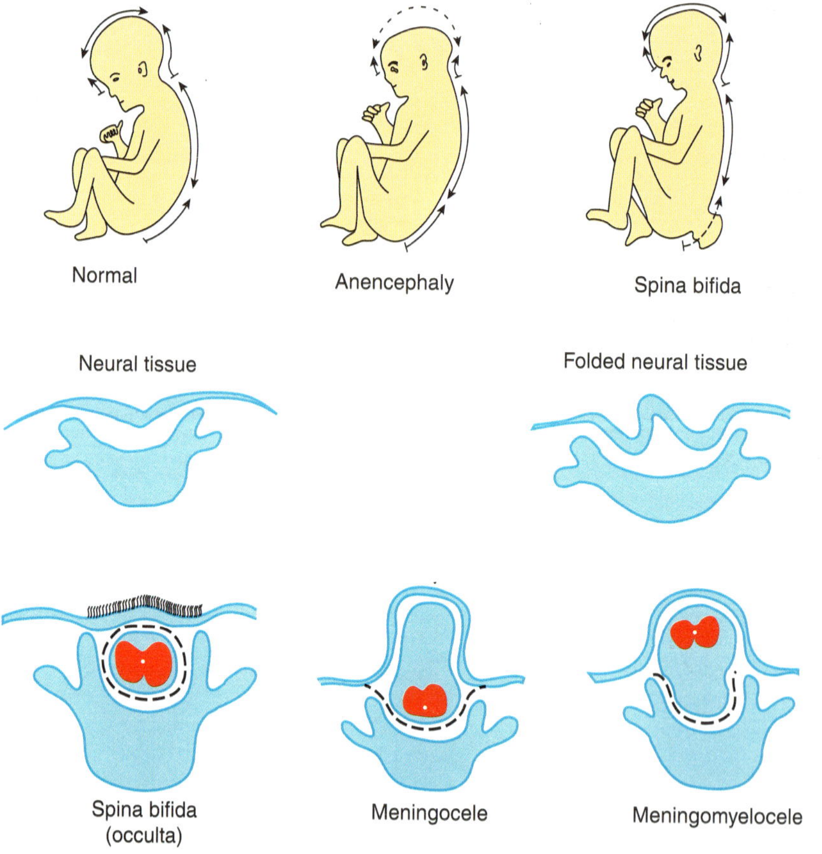

Figure 2.22 Spina bifida, meningocele, and meningomyocele. (See also figure 2.22 on page 113.)

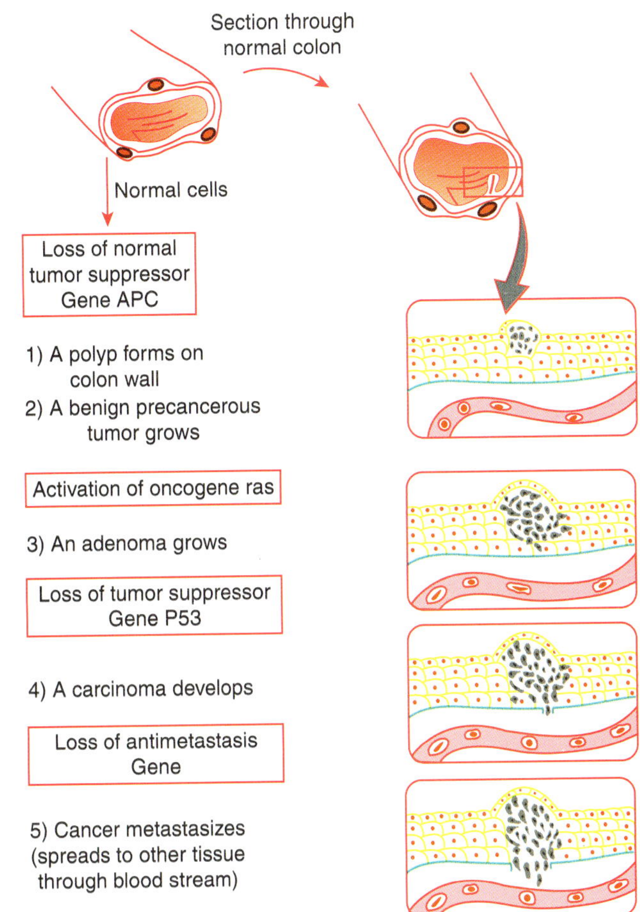

Figure 4.5 Mutations in multiple genes contribute to progression of colorectal cancer (See also figure 4.5 on page 147.)

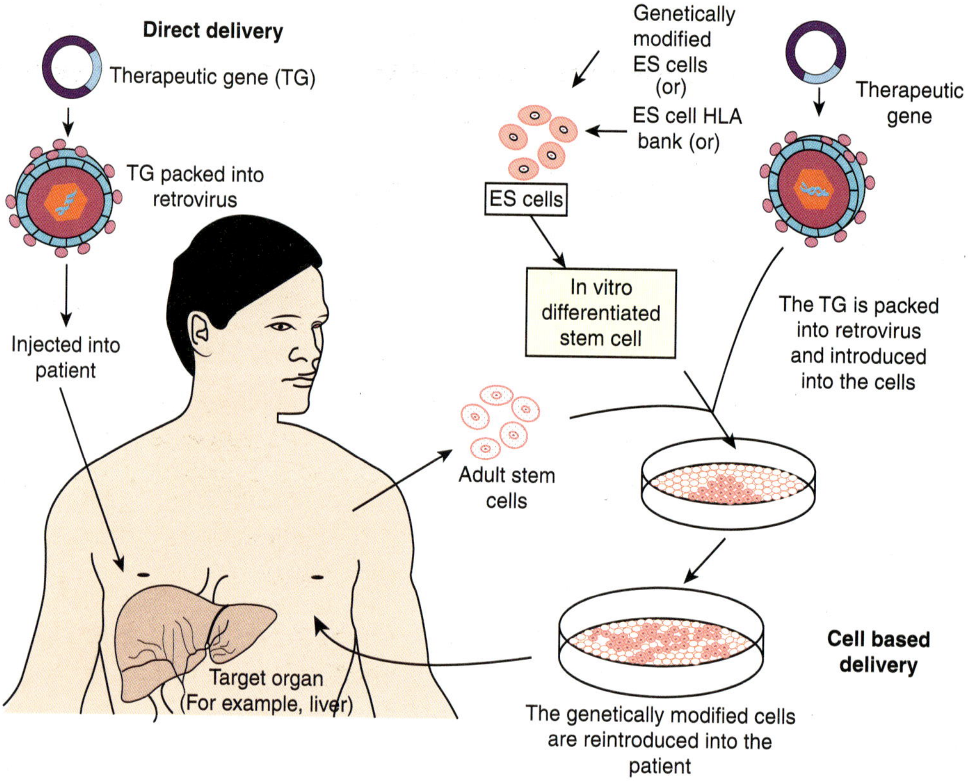

Figure 5.1 Modes of gene therapy. (See also figure 5.1 on page 169.)

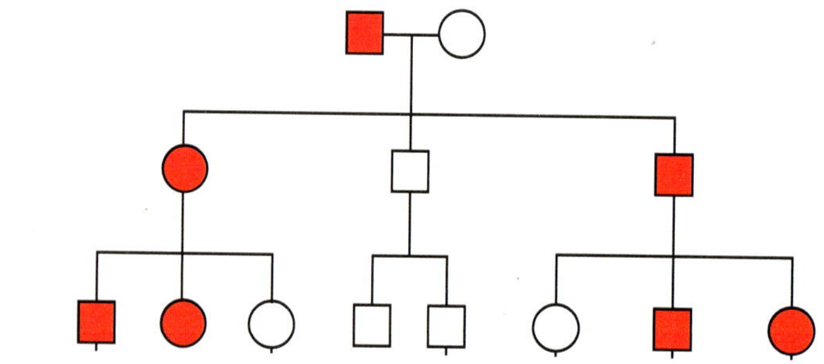

Autosomal inheritance of HD: Pedigree. (See also figure on page 206.)